CONTESTED EPIDEMICS

Policy Responses in Brazil and the US
and What the BRICS Can Learn

CONTESTED
EPIDEMICS

Policy Responses in Brazil and the US
and What the BRICS Can Learn

Eduardo J Gómez

King's College London, UK

Imperial College Press

Published by

Imperial College Press
57 Shelton Street
Covent Garden
London WC2H 9HE

Distributed by

World Scientific Publishing Co. Pte. Ltd.
5 Toh Tuck Link, Singapore 596224
USA office: 27 Warren Street, Suite 401-402, Hackensack, NJ 07601
UK office: 57 Shelton Street, Covent Garden, London WC2H 9HE

Library of Congress Cataloging-in-Publication Data
Gómez, Eduardo J., 1973– author.
  Contested epidemics : policy responses in Brazil and the US, and what the BRICS can learn /
Eduardo J. Gómez.
    p. ; cm.
  Includes bibliographical references and index.
  ISBN 978-1-78326-514-5 (hardcover : alk. paper)
  I. Title.
  [DNLM: 1. Epidemics--Brazil. 2. Epidemics--United States. 3. Acquired Immunodeficiency
Syndrome--epidemiology--Brazil. 4. Acquired Immunodeficiency Syndrome--epidemiology--United
States. 5. Health Policy--Brazil. 6. Health Policy--United States. 7. Obesity--epidemiology--Brazil.
8. Obesity--epidemiology--United States. 9. Tuberculosis--epidemiology--Brazil. 10. Tuberculosis--
epidemiology--United States. WA 105]
  RA463
  614.4'981--dc23

                                                                        2014019377

British Library Cataloguing-in-Publication Data
A catalogue record for this book is available from the British Library.

Typeset by Stallion Press
Email: enquiries@stallionpress.com

Printed in Singapore

To my father, Guillermo L. Gómez, and my grandparents,
Januario and Lucila Gómez

Acknowledgements

This book was long in the making. It was the product of not only my hard work, but also the support and encouragement of many others. In graduate school, my doctoral thesis advisor, Professor James Morone in the Department of Political Science at Brown University, was invaluable in mentoring me throughout the process of research and writing. I'll never forget our long chats over coffee and scones; my bickering and frustrations over incessant emails that drove him nuts; and the amazing wisdom he imparted on the dos and don'ts of publishing. Professors Marion Orr in the Department of Political Science at Brown, James Mahoney, then in the Department of Sociology at Brown (now at Northwestern University), and James Green in the Department of History at Brown also provided wonderful encouragement and guidance during the beginning stages of this project. Finally, I give much thanks to the late Professor Alan Zuckerman in the Department of Political Science at Brown. Alan pushed me to work hard and to understand the meaning of comparative politics.

In Brazil, several colleagues were also very helpful when conducting research for this book. Professors Gilberto Hochman of the Fundação Oswaldo Cruz and Marta Arretche in the Department of Political Science at the University of São Paulo helped tremendously when conducting archival work on the history of public health in Brazil. Over the years, several other Brazilian colleagues provided excellent comments and suggestions, namely Draurio Barreira, Ezio T. Santos-Filho, Fernando Cardoso, Pedro Chequer, Paulo Teixeira, Carlos Basilia, Mauro Sanchez, and Lorena Barberia. And in the US, Tom Bossert, Varun Gauri, Jon Oberlander, Michael Sparer, Helen Gale,

Kurt Weyland, Yanzhong Huang, Laurie Garrett, Elena Hoffnagle, and Jen Kates were wonderful in providing suggestions and guidance.

Finally, I wish to thank my wonderful father, Guillermo L. Gómez, for encouraging me and being there for me throughout the writing of this book, especially during my difficult times. At home, throughout the long nights in which I poured out my ideas over my iMac, my two lovely cats, 'Pitos and 'Mitas, provided much warmth and comfort. Finally, I wish to thank my grandparents, Januario and Lucila Gómez. I'll never forget their support throughout my difficult years in graduate school. Januario and Lucila's sacrifice and courage in emigrating from Colombia to the US during the 1950s made my opportunity and success possible.

Contents

Chapter 1

Introduction

No one responds to health epidemics the same way. When news of a health threat emerges, some are quick to point the finger, blame others, and attribute it as accountable to their faults and their sins. Others believe that it is not the individual, but changes in the broader socio-economic and biological context that is to blame. People are simply unpredictable in how they view and react to disease. Governments are no different. Regardless of politicians happily proclaiming their commitment to healthcare needs, and regardless of how stable their democratic institutions are, health epidemics often prompt conflicting perceptions, interests, and contradictory policy views among political leaders, bureaucrats, and civil society. This vexing problem often leads to political contestation, policy inaction, and ongoing death.

In part because of these daunting political challenges, better understanding of the politics of government response to health epidemics has emerged as a new area of scholarly research. As transitions to democracy, the wealth of nations, and healthcare inequalities increase over time, political scientists have become increasingly concerned and puzzled by the large degree of variability in the timing and depth of government response to epidemics as well as citizens' broader healthcare needs. In the past two decades, especially with the arrival of the HIV/AIDS epidemic amidst these political and economic transitions, political scientists have begun to provide theoretical and empirical answers for why some governments fair better in their policy response.

For example, some scholars claim that advanced industrialized nations exhibiting enduring and effective democratic institutions provide, although to varying degrees, the best bureaucratic and policy responses (Baldwin, 2007; Barnett and Whiteside, 2006; Ruger, 2005; Sen 1999; Whiteside, 1999). In these systems, the presence of a long history of national and local elections as well as accountability to civil society, often facilitated through the presence of a free press, generates political incentives to aggressively respond, in turn helping stunt the growth of HIV/AIDS and other diseases (Bor, 2007; Ruger, 2005; Sen, 1999). In this context politicians seeking reelection have also strategically used epidemics to garner electoral support through their advocacy of human rights, anti-discrimination, and help for the sickly and poor while adhering to international norms of equality in access to medicines (Ruger, 2005; Sen, 1999). To varying degrees, countries such as the US, the UK, France, Germany, and the Nordic states (Denmark, Finland, Iceland, Norway, and Sweden) have provided the best examples of this process (Baldwin, 2007; Nathanson, 1996; Vallgarda, 2007). Alternatively, nondemocracies as well as nations recently transitioning to democracy, such as China, Brazil, India, Uganda, Russia, and South Africa, were not as timely and successful in their initial response to HIV/AIDS and other diseases (Huang, 2006; Lieberman, 2009; Parker, 2003; Putzel, 2004). In these nations, the presence of political dictatorships and/or unaccountable electoral institutions engendered few political incentives to respond, while upholding international norms of equality in access to healthcare was never seen as a priority.

Alternatively, others claim that governments that have had sound and enduring commitments to listening to and meeting the needs of civil society have been the best responders to epidemics. This is often exhibited by the creation of national or sub-national institutions, such as committees or commissions, that formally invite and permanently represent the policy interests of civil society. With the information obtained through these institutions, moreover, government officials have the knowledge needed to effectively meet citizen needs, to help civil society avoid infection, and the ability to create policies that promote non-discrimination, awareness, and social acceptance (Barnett and Whiteside, 2006; Immergut, 1992; Whiteside, 1999). Yet again, scholars claim that it is the advanced industrialized democracies, such as the US, the UK, France, Germany, and the Nordic states, that have established these civic representational institutions and, consequently, engendered early policy responses to HIV/AIDS and other diseases (Aggleton, 2001; Altman, 1986; Baldwin, 2007; Rosenbrock and Wright, 2000; Vallgarda, 2007). Conversely, nondemocracies, as well as recently transitioned democracies, have not had a long history of working closely with civil society in response to epidemics; this, in turn, has not led to the creation of formal institutions representing the needs of civil society and better informed policy. South Africa, China, India, and a myriad of African nations have exhibited these shortcomings (Huang, 2006; Lieberman, 2009; Patterson, 2005).

Finally, others claim that nations with wealthier healthcare systems, technical expertise, and greater financial resources have tended to be more effective policy responders to epidemics. Once again, the well-established, wealthier democracies, such as the US, the UK, France, Germany, and the Nordic states provide good examples (Nathanson, 1996; Price-Smith, 2002; Price-Smith *et al.*, 2004). By possessing hospitals with the latest healthcare technologies, sufficient infrastructure, such as beds and surgical equipment, and highly trained doctors and nurses, these democracies have been more capable of responding to HIV/AIDS and other health threats when compared to lesser-developed nations that do not have this state capacity (Nathanson, 1996; Price-Smith, 2002; Price-Smith *et al.*, 2004).

This research seems to suggest, therefore, that well-established democracies exhibiting wealthier and advanced healthcare systems are better positioned to respond to health epidemics; nevertheless, this position has recently been challenged by scholars claiming that the effectiveness of government response is never preconditioned by political regime type and the overall level of healthcare resources (Gauri and Khaleghian, 2002; Gauri and Lieberman, 2006). That is to say, at times nondemocracies as well as lesser-developed, nascent democracies with comparatively weaker healthcare systems, limited funding and infrastructure seem to be equally as capable of aggressively responding to epidemics (Gauri and Khaleghian, 2002; Gauri and Lieberman, 2006; McGuire, 2010). Cuba, for instance, was praised for its ability to quickly identify and prevent the spread of HIV/AIDS throughout the 1980s, sustaining an effective policy response over the years (Anderson, 2009), while Vietnam and China have repeatedly exhibited a strong ability to immunize children from disease (Gauri and Khaleghian, 2002).

If the type of political system present, healthcare systems, and wealth of nations do not determine a government's ability to respond to epidemics, then what factors do? Answering this question effectively requires a more in-depth comparative historical analysis of how wealthier, more established democracies respond to epidemics in comparison with poorer, nascent democracies. To that end, in this book I examine how the US and Brazil reacted to different types of epidemics that were questioned and indeed heavily debated between politicians and bureaucrats with respect to their overall threat to society — or what I call *contested epidemics*. In-depth case study evidence seems to suggest that Brazil may have done better than the US when it came to responding to contested epidemics, and that Brazil's response had nothing to do with the overall quality and durability of its democratic system, financial and infrastructural wealth, as well as the presence of representative civil society institutions.

But what exactly are contested epidemics? I argue that these epidemics emerge when new health threats arise and politicians and health officials immediately debate their overall threat to society. Good examples include syphilis, polio, tuberculosis (TB), and malnourishment historically, and HIV/AIDS, TB, and obesity today. While their mode of transmission, contagiousness, mortality rate, type of medical treatment, and technological and infrastructural needs are different from each other — thus potentially requiring a different type of policy response — they are nevertheless viewed as similar for several reasons. First, contested epidemics are not considered "flash epidemics," such as the Spanish Flu of 1918, because they do not kill thousands of individuals in a short period of time; second, they are often relegated to marginalized minority groups and the poor; and third, these epidemics carry with them a form of social stigma. Slothfulness, sexual promiscuity, and drug addiction are often viewed as the reasons why individuals succumb to these diseases. In this context, stigma and discrimination, often the byproduct of moral belief, instigates contestation between those politicians and health officials transfixed by these moral values versus those that are mainly motivated by scientific evidence and progressive social welfare.

However, why have I compared the US to Brazil? Why not any other group of nations which, like the US and Brazil, have been exposed to several types of contested epidemics? I compared the US and Brazil because of their uniquely similar type of demographic, geographic, and socioeconomic characteristics. Furthermore, I compared these nations because to my knowledge, it is the first attempt to compare the US and Brazil's historic institutional and policy response to health epidemics. Because of their similar types of economic development and political stability, the US is often compared to western European nations (especially the UK and Germany) when comparing health politics and policy (Hacker, 2004; Marmor *et al.*, 2005; Sparer *et al.*, 2011), while the study of Brazil on this topic is often relegated to case studies of Brazil and/or comparisons of Brazil to other Latin American nations (Weyland, 1995, 2007).

With respect to the US and Brazil's similarities, in terms of population and geographic size, both nations were also selected because they are the biggest governments in the western hemisphere. In terms of total population size, the US has approximately 313.9 million people compared to 198.7 million in Brazil (United States Census Bureau, 2013; World Bank, 2013); the next largest populations in the western hemisphere are Mexico at 112.3 million, Colombia at 47.7 million, and Argentina at 41.09 million (United States Census Bureau, 2013; World Bank, 2013). US geographic territory spans 9,629,091 square kilometers (km^2); Brazil is 8,514,877 km^2, the two largest — next to Canada's 9,984,670 km^2 — in the western hemisphere (United Nations, 2008). The US and Brazil were also compared because they are the largest federal systems in the region, with a great deal of financial, administrative, and social welfare policies decentralized to local governments (Allard, 2009; Arretche, 2003). Both nations also have very diverse ethnic and racial populations, and a long history of slavery (Bendix, 1964). Finally, there is a large degree of income inequality in both countries. In 2007, the US, for example, had a Gini coefficient (which measures income distribution, with a score of 0 being completely equal versus 100 being completely unequal) of 45.1 compared to 51.9 in Brazil in 2012 (CIA, 2013). (In fact, both nations rank in the top 50 most unequal societies in the world (CIA, 2013).) Finally, these nations were compared because of their similar geographic bias in access to healthcare: that is, the presence of better quality healthcare services and infrastructure in the wealthier urban versus poorer rural areas (Kepp, 2008; The National Advisory Committee, 2000).

Despite these similarities, it is also important to point out that the US and Brazil have exhibited several differences. First, the US has been a stable electoral democracy for several decades, with a nationally elected president and elected House of Representatives since 1788 (with senators elected for the first time in 1913), an independent judiciary since 1789, and state elections since 1776. In contrast, Brazil has gone through several phases of democracy and dictatorship: during the 19th and early 20th century, it was a democracy with a nationally elected president and Congress (House and Senate); from 1930 to 1945 it returned to a presidential dictatorship (when all state elections and governments were demolished and the central government retained complete political and economic authority); from 1945 to 1964 it returned to a limited form of presidential democracy; it moved back to a fully fledged military dictatorship between 1964 to 1986; and finally returned to a presidential democracy in 1986 while establishing a democratic constitution in 1988 (Skidmore, 2007).

In addition, the US has a long history of developing a vast military structure while being engaged in — and often leading — foreign military campaigns (Clemens, 2000). Brazil, on the other hand, has no such history and has always pursued peaceful multilateral cooperation (Cervo, 2011; Garcia, 2012). US foreign policy has always been focused on helping lead and influence global policy, on essentially every policy issue of importance to the international community (Clemens, 2000). Conversely, Brazil has never had these types of foreign policy interests, preferring instead to engage in peaceful multilateralism and cooperation (Cervo, 2011; Garcia, 2012). Nevertheless, in recent years, as Brazil's economy has grown and its global importance increased, especially in the area of development, it appears that the government has become more interested in establishing itself as an important, influential nation (Dauvergne and Farias, 2012).

Finally, a major difference between the US and Brazil stems from the fact that Brazil has a fully fledged universal healthcare system, whereas the US does not. In 1988, the Brazilian government introduced a universal healthcare system known as SUS (*Sistema Único de Saúde*) (Weyland, 1995). This system is decentralized, and is managed by state and municipal governments, from tax revenues obtained from national, state, and municipal governments. In Brazil, moreover, universal healthcare access is written into the 1988 democratic constitution as a "human right," which, in turn, has led to the distribution of free medications and treatment for all. In contrast, no universal healthcare system exists in the US. Instead, the US has a mixed public–private healthcare system, where government healthcare policies are provided for the poor and elderly (Medicaid and Medicare, respectively), the military, and children, while most of the rest of the population is either enrolled in private healthcare insurance or has no health insurance (Blumenthal and Morone, 2009). Because of this, and as we will see in Chapters 3 and 5 of this book, there is often a shortage of medication and access to quality healthcare.

Despite these differences in healthcare systems, if one considers the acute differences in financial and technical capacity between both nations, one would expect the US to do better than Brazil in its response to contested epidemics. Just because Brazil has a generous universal healthcare system by no means guarantees that it will have the same financial and technical capacity as the US in its ability to effectively respond to epidemics. What is more, the US has also been the world leader in providing financial and technical assistance to combat epidemics (Bliss, 2012), thus suggesting that the government has been unwaveringly committed to saving and protecting lives. In 2010, for example, 54.2% of total global funding for AIDS was provided by the US, 13% by the UK, 5.8% by France, 5.1% the Netherlands, 4.5% Germany, and 2.5% Denmark (Kaiser Family Foundation, 2011). Therefore, if it is indeed the case that Brazil did eventually outpace the US in its response to contested epidemics, then precisely *how* did Brazil achieve this?

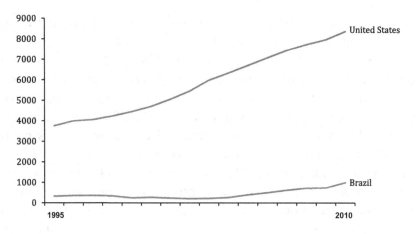

Figure 1.1   Per capita total expenditure on health at average exchange rate (US dollars) in the US and Brazil
Source: World Health Organization, 2012

This notion is even more puzzling when one considers the vast difference in per capita spending for healthcare between both nations, with the US far outpacing Brazil between 1995 and 2010 (see Figure 1.1). In terms of human resources and infrastructure, Brazil also pales into insignificance in comparison. In 2000, the World Health Organization (WHO) reported that in the US, there were a total of 730,801 physicians compared to 198,153 in Brazil; 2,669,603 registered nurses in the US compared to 659,111 in Brazil; 611,993 lab technicians in the US compared to 44,095 in Brazil; and finally, 7,056,080 healthcare management support workers in the US compared to 839, 376 in Brazil. Given these stark differences, should not the US's wealth in health have led to a more aggressive response to AIDS and obesity? Why, then, has this not occurred?

Solving this puzzle requires a historical analysis of how and why government leaders in the US and Brazil eventually differed in their response to shifting international and domestic contexts. While governments in both nations did not immediately respond to their respective contested epidemics, eventually I argue that Brazil outpaced the US because of how its political leaders responded to and worked with the international community as well as civil society. With the emergence of international criticisms and pressures for a more aggressive government response by the late 1980s, in contrast to the US, Brazil's presidents saw these pressures as an opportunity to increase the government's international reputation through the implementation of new bureaucratic and policy reforms while working with international financiers to facilitate this process. In order to ensure that these reforms continued, moreover, Brazil's health officials strategically used their partnership with social health movements and non-governmental organizations (NGOs) in order to increase their legitimacy and influence when seeking ongoing support for their policy efforts; conversely, politicians and health officials in the US never pursued these types of international and domestic strategies, thus failing to respond in a centralized, effective manner.

And therein lies the main outcome of interest in this book: overcoming what Remy Prud'homme (1995) once referred to as the "dangers of decentralization" through an *ongoing* centralized bureaucratic and policy response to contested epidemics. By *ongoing*, I refer to continuous federal spending and policy innovations in response to epidemics. Here, I define a "centralized bureaucratic and policy response" as the creation and ongoing expansion of national public health agencies focused on particular epidemics, on one hand, and the creation of federal policies that provide state and municipal governments with fiscal and technical resources while holding them accountable to national policy mandates, on the other. The latter often entails the creation of new partnerships between public health officials and civil society, such as NGOs, with the goal of monitoring local governments and holding them accountable to national policy mandates.

My argument essentially builds on the emerging consensus within international health agencies, policymakers, and scholars that bureaucratic and policy centralization is needed in order to respond effectively to epidemics (Lieberman, 2009; Nathanson, 1996; Pritchett and Woolcock, 2004; UNAIDS, 1999; World Health Organization, 1992). This consensus has emerged mainly because healthcare decentralization processes, especially in developing nations, are often poorly implemented and are typically a consequence of poor timing and planning, sub-national fiscal imbalances, weak administration, and corruption (Prud'homme, 1995; Rodden, 2006).[1]

But it is important to note that a centralized response may not always be the best policy solution. Governments may at times exhibit an inability to achieve this outcome. This may be due to factors such as the lack of a preexisting political cultures favoring a centralized response to health challenges as well as simply not having the appropriate technical skills and funding needed to engender a skilled public health bureaucracy (Nathanson, 1996). Others have instead emphasized the *principal–agent* problems that reside within the bureaucracy and how this hampers a centralized bureaucratic response (Pritchett and Woolcock, 2004). Here, the *principals*, such as agency directors, Congress, or federal courts may have a difficult time creating incentives for bureaucratic officials, i.e. the *agents*, to effectively implement policy (Pritchett and Woolcock, 2004; Kerwin, 2003). These principal–agent coordination problems may also be due to either a lack of communication between these principals and agents or because the latter are often disobedient to central government commands, striving to get away with their own policy preferences due to their distant location from the center, personal interests and incentives (Kerwin, 2003).

Despite these challenges, when the appropriate historical, bureaucratic, and political context is in place, as seen in Brazil, I agree with the aforementioned scholars that a centralized bureaucratic and policy response is the appropriate course of action to take. In fact, even those critics of a centralized response to social welfare policies claim that when it comes to public health emergencies, such as providing vaccines for polio and other diseases, a centralized response is more appropriate and necessary (Gauri and Khaleghian, 2002; Pritchett and Woolcock, 2004). This is because, ultimately, ensuring that patients receive immediate medical treatment takes precedence over any other social welfare need.

---

[1] Of course, this is not to say that all decentralization policies have problems. There have been good examples of where state and municipal governments have effectively implemented newly decentralized health policy responsibilities; on this note, see Tendler (1997).

Responding to Contested Epidemics in the United States

In the US, there is a long history of political contestation and delayed national government response to health epidemics. Beginning with polio, syphilis, and TB during the 20th century, the only time presidents and congressional leaders responded was when these health threats challenged the national security, such as military readiness, and economic growth (Brand, 1985; Levenstein, 1993; Mullen, 1989). Although malnutrition and syphilis were ignored by the national government prior to the two world wars, once these diseases affected the military's ability to recruit personnel, new federal agencies and health programs were immediately created in order to work with the states to eradicate these diseases (Brandt, 1985; Levenstein, 1993; Mullen, 1989). Yet, when the national security was not at stake, historically a political leader's personal experience, their fears and empathy for others helped to prompt a national response. After years of essentially ignoring the polio epidemic, for example, President Franklin D. Roosevelt's (1933–1945) affliction with this disease eventually motivated him to increase funding for vaccination while providing resources and technical support to the states (Oshinsky, 2006).

Decades later, when the AIDS and obesity epidemics emerged, presidents and congressional lawmakers also had no interest in immediately responding (Altman, 1986; Shilts, 2007). Notwithstanding US Public Health Service (PHS) officials' warning about these heath threats and pushing for a more centralized response, their recommendations were never taken seriously (Altman, 1986; Shilts, 2007). For these presidents and much of Congress, I argue that the absence of AIDS and obesity's perceived threat to the national security, such as military readiness and economic growth, the dearth of convincing epidemiological data as well as the absence of presidential and/or other leaders' personal experiences with these ailments failed to instigate a response. Furthermore, the powerful influence of evangelical and private sector interest groups opposing AIDS and obesity legislation, respectively, further incentivized the president and Congress to refrain from responding (Perrow and Guillen, 1990). Once again, the bureaucrats were the only ones pushing for a centralized response; nevertheless, their calls were never heard, as presidential and congressional politics always trumped bureaucratic interests (Altman, 1986).

Further complicating matters was the design and performance of bureaucratic institutions. During the early part of the 20th century, the rise of the professionalized scientific bureaucracy engendered by the 1980s the highly fragmented and competitive US PHS, which included the Centers for Disease Control and Prevention (CDC), National Institutes of Health (NIH), National Cancer Institute (NCI), and others (Panem, 1988). These agencies competed with each other over the right to conduct research and to provide policy advice (Altman, 1986; Panem, 1988; Shilts, 2007); yet, this was much more the case for AIDS when compared to obesity, as the latter did not pose as much of a scientific mystery and perceived national threat. When it came to AIDS, a great deal of policy overlap and responsibility emerged (Panem, 1988). In a context of fiscal constraints and bureaucratic downsizing, PHS fragmentation and competition over funding substantially delayed attempts to establish a national response (Altman, 1986; Panem, 1988; Shilts, 2007).

Amidst this challenging institutional context, civil society responded. When it came to AIDS, society's initial response emerged in the cities of New York and San Francisco in 1982, where several gay community-based AIDS NGOs arose to work with city health officials in order to increase awareness and provide social services, while pressuring local and federal agencies for assistance (Cohen and Elder, 1989). Despite efforts to mobilize and pressure the HHS and CDC for a response, NGOs' policy ideas and efforts ultimately fell on deaf ears (Cohen and Elder, 1989). I argue that when it came to obesity, those civil society groups initially responding to the epidemic were essentially divided in their response, failing to create a well-organized, collective movement pressuring local and federal agencies for assistance. Social health movements, such as the National Association to Advance Fat Acceptance (NAAFA), which formed as early as 1969, never criticized and pressured the government for a response (White, 2010). Instead, NAAFA decided to work on its own, increasing social awareness and social acceptance while focusing on non-discrimination

(White, 2010). Other civic organizations, such as the American Heart Association, focused on the individual's poor eating habits in an attempt to avoid the growth of non-communicable diseases, such as heart disease and cancer (Kersh and Morone, 2002).

Empathizing with civil society and fearing ongoing death, the international community eventually began to pressure the US for a more aggressive response to AIDS and obesity (Bliss, 2012; Norum *et al.*, 2009). International agencies, such as the WHO, UNAIDS, scientists, activists, and the media underscored the absence of effective national programs (Bliss, 2012; Norum *et al.*, 2009). However, these international criticisms and pressures had essentially no policy influence. When it came to AIDS, Presidents Ronald Reagan (1981–1989) and George H.W. Bush (1989–1993) essentially ignored these pressures and proceeded to respond at their own pace, gradually increasing funding for research, the CDC and NIH, yet with no clear and centralized bureaucratic and policy agenda — notwithstanding repeated pressures from their very own presidential AIDS advisory committees to do so (Behrman, 2004). And despite the WHO's pressures on the George W. Bush administration in 2004 to regulate the fatty food industry in order to curb the spread of obesity, not only did Bush ignore these pressures, but he even issued an executive order forbidding any CDC officials from working with the WHO on these issues. Instead, Bush decided to handle the obesity situation on his own (McKenna, 2004; Norum, 2010).

In the absence of AIDS and obesity's threat to the national security, then, the government's response ultimately depended on the president and other leaders' personal interests. With respect to AIDS, the government's response increased with the arrival of President William Clinton in 1992 (McKinney and Pepper, 1999). Campaigning on the AIDS issue, in 1993 Clinton created the Office of National AIDS Policy (ONAP) in the White House while doubling the federal budget for AIDS prevention and treatment (The Body, 2001). The institutional challenges hampering the government's initial response to AIDS, such as PHS fragmentation and competition, had also subsided.

When it came to obesity, I argue similarly that the government began to respond but only after Presidents Bush and Obama and high-ranking health officials felt personally threatened by the epidemic (Obama, 2010; Vulliamy, 2002). Similar to what occurred with Roosevelt and polio in the past, these politicians and health officials' concerns of personal or family members' weight gain, as well as its associated ailments, generated a sense of empathy and concern for others, prompting them to do something about the situation (Obama, 2010; Vulliamy, 2002). While no centralized reforms were pursued, these personal interests and concerns have helped to increase awareness and to place obesity on the national agenda. However, the fear that obesity is now negatively affecting the youth's ability to enlist in the military has prompted government officials to believe that obesity is slowly becoming a national security threat (Park, 2010). Going forward, and as we saw with malnutrition during the two world wars, obesity may motivate the government to create new federal agencies and more aggressive policy initiatives.

Yet another factor limiting the government's response to AIDS and obesity had to do with how it worked with civil society. That is, while AIDS and obesity NGOs as well as social health movements eventually grew in size and number, at no point did PHS officials try to work with them in order to bolster the bureaucracy's legitimacy and influence when seeking to acquire resources from Congress (NASTAD, 2005). In this context NGOs and social health movements have been viewed more as sources of information, receivers of federal assistance, rather than genuine partners in serving the bureaucracy's administrative and policy needs. While this may sound counter-intuitive — that is, a democratic state only listening to civil society's needs and working with it for its selfish expansionist reasons — as I will explain shortly, this strategic usage of civil society can lead to ongoing centralized bureaucratic and policy reforms. In the long run, and as we will see in Brazil, this can also benefit civil society.

Finally, in an age of heightened international efforts to combat AIDS and other diseases, I argue that the US government's obsession with helping the developing world eradicate AIDS distracted the government from focusing on its domestic policy needs. Nowhere was this more evident than under the George W. Bush administration (2001–2009). Motivated by his personal Christian beliefs, encouraged by influential, likeminded evangelical interest groups, and supported by the bipartisan views of civil society, in 2003 President Bush created the largest federal bureaucracy ever created in response to AIDS: PEPFAR (President's Emergency Plan for AIDS Relief) (Hindman and Schroedel, 2010). Housed within the White House, through PEPFAR Bush substantially increased funding for the provision of antiretroviral (ARV) medication to developing nations (mainly Africa) as well as prevention programs (Hindman and Schroedel, 2010). While admirable and certainly necessary, Bush's global focus nevertheless took his attention away from ongoing domestic policy needs. In fact, funding for domestic AIDS prevention policies *decreased* under Bush, infuriating AIDS activists beyond measure, while no corresponding hike in spending for AIDS treatment emerged (Platt and Platt, 2013). While President Obama has simultaneously supported new domestic and international initiatives, in a context of ongoing economic recession, it has been difficult to implement and expand policy.

Responding the Brazilian Way

The initial years of Brazil's response to AIDS and TB essentially mimicked the US's delayed response to AIDS and obesity. Transitioning from a dictatorship to a democracy in 1986, initially the president and senior Ministry of Health (MOH) officials believed that there was not enough credible epidemiological evidence supporting the presence of a serious public health threat (Parker, 2003). The president and MOH officials also perceived TB to be an old disease that had been permanently eradicated during the 1950s, when Brazil had a strong vertical TB program (Santos Filho, 2006). At the same time, the new democratic government was fully committed to healthcare decentralization (Weyland, 1995), a health system response that emerged from the military government (Beyrer *et al.*, 2005; Weyland, 1995). In this context, it was nearly impossible to justify an immediate centralized bureaucratic and policy response to AIDS and TB. Nevertheless, and similar to what we saw in the US, there were other health officials that thought otherwise, seeing the AIDS and TB situation as urgent, while repeatedly pressuring for an immediate centralized response (Da Costa Marques, 2003); yet these officials were often criticized and ignored (Da Costa Marques, 2003; Galvão, 2000).

During this period, civil society also began to respond. Mainly organized by gay community-based organizations in the cities of São Paulo and Rio de Janeiro, beginning in 1985 AIDS NGOs formed to provide social support for the AIDS afflicted, to increase public awareness, and to pressure the government for a centralized response (Parker, 2003). However, because of the absence of TB's scientific appeal and because TB was mainly affiliated with the poor, the social movement for TB was much slower, forming as late as 2003 (Santos Filho, 2006). But even when these TB social movements organized themselves and pressured the government for a response, MOH officials were not fully committed to incorporating their policy recommendations (Basilia, 2009; Gelasi, 2009). During the first few years of the AIDS and TB epidemics, then, and similar again to what we saw in the US, and in spite of their aggressive mobilization tactics, civil society had absolutely no influence on the national government's response.

Because of this, by the early 1990s Brazil joined the US in being exposed to a high level of international criticisms and pressures. In contrast to the US, however, Brazil's presidents reacted differently to this situation. Instead of ignoring them and pursuing reforms on their own, I argue that Presidents Fernando H. Cardoso (1994–2002) and Luis Ignacio "Lula" da Silva (2002–2010) saw these pressures as a golden opportunity to increase Brazil's international reputation as a modern state capable of eradicating disease. Through the introduction of new bureaucratic and policy reforms, by 1995 President Cardoso became committed to showing the world that Brazil could join the other advanced industrialized nations in successfully curtailing the spread of AIDS and TB. Brazil's presidents also wanted to reveal that they were committed to the emergence of international health norms, such as access to healthcare and medical treatment as a human right, as well as joint partnerships with the international community.

With respect to AIDS, by the mid-1990s, and with the assistance of a generous loan from the World Bank in 1994 (Beyrer *et al.*, 2005), Brazil's MOH essentially doubled its financial commitment to prevention programs, while creating a federal law in 1996 guaranteeing every Brazilian the "constitutional" right to obtain ARV medication from the government — something that would be unheard of in the US (Beyrer *et al.*, 2005; Lieberman, 2009). Since the late 1990s, moreover, the national AIDS program has continued to introduce new prevention programs focusing on the gay community and women (the most at-risk groups), while allocating more funding for ARV medication (Beyrer *et al.*, 2005; Lieberman, 2009). By the early 2000s, domestic budgetary outlays far outpaced the amount of funding received from the World Bank and other donors. Furthermore, realizing that healthcare decentralization through the universal SUS healthcare system was problematic, mainly due to a shortfall of funding at the municipal level, in 2003 the national AIDS program also created the Política de Incentivo Fundo-a-Fundo policy (Barboza, 2006). This policy provides conditional fiscal transfers to mayors as long as they comply with the national AIDS program's policy recommendations (Barboza, 2006). In addition to contracting NGOs to monitor municipal government compliance with these mandates and the effective usage of Política de Incentivo transfers, these policy innovations have helped the national AIDS program to maintain its centralized influence amidst broader commitments to healthcare decentralization.

While international criticisms and pressures for a more effective response to TB arose several years later, eventually the president and the MOH responded in a similar manner (Santos Filho, 2006). In addition to maintaining its preexisting commitment to purchase and distribute medications, the national TB program began to work with civil society (Santos Filho and Gomes, 2007), to provide not only prevention programs but also new streams of funding for partnerships with social health movements, such as the TB Forums, which is a network of NGOs and community-based organizations located in the cities of Rio de Janeiro and São Paulo.

Nevertheless, while Brazil's international reputation-building interests certainly proved to be a necessary catalyst for reform, I argue that it was insufficient for *ongoing* centralized bureaucratic and policy reforms to occur. In order to consistently increase the federal budget and introduce new policy innovations, especially in periods of fiscal duress, other strategies were needed. Specifically, national AIDS and TB officials also needed to strategically use and work closely with civil society: that is, the presence of proactive social health movements, such as the *sanitarista* movement,[2] and NGOs that health officials could partner with and use to increase their legitimacy, justification, and influence in obtaining ongoing financial and political support for their programs — or what I call *civic supporters*, a concept that I will explain in greater detail shortly. By the mid-1990s, these civic supporters acted as a helpful resource for officials because they increased officials' legitimacy and policy influence. This was due to the fact that the policy ideas the *sanitaristas* and AIDS NGOs were advocating, that is, an immediate, centralized bureaucratic and policy response to epidemics, were credible in the eyes of politicians; moreover, this concerned the idea's long policy history, stemming from the early 20th century, and proven track record (Hochman, 1998).

The *sanitaristas* and NGOs were also resourceful in furthering health officials' legitimacy because they represented a long tradition of social health movements committed to working closely with the bureaucracy in response to disease (Carrara, 1999). This tradition was highly revered and supported by politicians because of the government's new democratic commitment to the inclusion of civil society into the policymaking process, a notion that was enshrined into the 1988 democratic constitution (Ciconello, 2008). Recognizing the importance of these civic supporters, after years of the national AIDS program essentially ignoring them, AIDS officials began to pursue a closer partnership with them in order to increase their legitimacy and influence when garnering support for their policies.

Nevertheless, when compared to AIDS, national TB officials in Brazil did not have access to these civic supporters. This was mainly due to the gradual decline in social movements for TB since the 1950s (Santos Filho, 2006), which mainly occurred because of the

---

[2]Emerging in the 1960s as a pro-leftist social movement, the *sanitaristas* were comprised of medical doctors, state-level politicians, activists, patients, and the clergy; they collectively pressured the military governments (1964–1985) for a more universal, equitable, and decentralized healthcare system.

rapid decline in TB mortality, as well as a lack of political attention and support for TB victims (Basilia, 2009). Consequently, when TB reemerged as an epidemic by the late-1990s, due mainly to co-infection with HIV (Santos Filho, 2006), national TB officials were not able to acquire nearly as much political and financial support to expand their national TB program and provide adequate assistance to the states.

The BRICS Nations and What They Can Learn From Brazil

However, are Brazil's successful responses to contested epidemics only applicable to Brazil? Or can other nations learn from Brazil and potentially adopt the government's bureaucratic and policy approach? When compared to Brazil's emerging BRICS counterparts, namely Russia, India, China, and South Africa, it seems that political leaders can potentially learn some lessons from Brazil. In Chapter 7 of this book, I explore this issue in depth, illustrating how and why Brazil's simultaneous commitment to bolstering its international reputation in health as well as health officials' usage of civic supporters could help the BRICS respond to diseases such as AIDS, obesity, and TB. Nevertheless, the extent to which Brazil's approach is transferable to these nations is questioned. Given Brazil's unique history in state–civil society relations in response to epidemics, as well as its unique relationship with the international community, it seems that transferring its experiences to the other BRICS nations may not be as easy as we thought.

Theoretical Considerations

My in-depth comparison of the US and Brazil not only reveals intriguing empirical findings but it also challenges some of the literature's emphasis on the conditions under which democracies respond to health epidemics. In contrast to what others have claimed, findings from the US and Brazil suggest that it is not the presence of an elected

national legislature, political representation, accountability, and electoral incentives that motivates presidents and legislatures to respond
immediately to new health threats (McGuire, 2010; Putzel, 2004;
Ruger, 2005; Sen 1999; Whiteside, 1999), nor does the presence of
well-organized NGOs, social health movements, and their pressures
on the government incentivize such a response (Altman, 1986; Barnett
and Whiteside, 2006; Boone and Batsell, 2001; Gauri and Lieberman,
2006; Lieberman, 2009; Parker, 2003; Rau, 2006). Instead, the cases
of the US and Brazil reveal that it is the interests of presidents, their
personal beliefs and ambitions (especially at the global level), as well as
threats to the national security that instigate a national response.

In the US, historically presidents and their legislatures never pursued a centralized response until epidemics such as malnutrition and
syphilis threatened the national security, specifically military recruitment, or the economy. Decades later, in the absence of AIDS and
obesity's security threats, there were no incentives to engage in a
centralized bureaucratic and policy response. Instead, the government's response to AIDS and obesity only became a priority when
US presidents were personally interested and felt threatened by their
presence. In Brazil, on the other hand, presidents and lawmakers
responded to AIDS and TB not because civil society and local governments were clamoring for assistance, but because these politicians
wanted to increase their international reputation.

Brazil's response to AIDS and TB indeed suggests that the incentives for a centralized response to epidemics often reside not at the
domestic but at the *international* level. When the WHO and the
scientific community began to criticize Brazil for its weak response to
AIDS and TB, Presidents Cardoso and Lula saw this as a great opportunity to increase their support for a massive scale up in financial and
human resource assistance to the MOH's national AIDS and TB
programs. These leaders were mainly motivated by their interest in
building Brazil's international reputation by creating new federal programs and initiatives aiding the states in their response. Policymaking
was therefore a *means* to alternative foreign policy ends.

This finding nevertheless suggests that scholars have not done an
adequate job of *combining* the literature discussing the domestic policy

influence of international criticisms and pressures with the literature discussing how and why nations create health policies for alternative foreign policy objectives. Some have recently highlighted how pressures from the WHO, the World Bank, and the Global Fund to Fight AIDS, Tuberculosis and Malaria can incentivize domestic political leaders to introduce new health policy measures because of the financial conditionalities and expectations that these multilateral lenders impose (Lieberman, 2009; Huang, 2006, 2010; Olunzi and Macrae, 1995). Lieberman (2009) also claims that representatives of international financial agencies engage in a form of peer pressure at international meetings and conferences in order to persuade policymakers in the developing world into adopting their policy recommendations. Alternatively, the Global Health Diplomacy literature emphasizes how political leaders often create more aggressive public health policies as a way to increase their international reputation and "soft power" influence (Nye, 2005), that is, garnering international attention and praise for their policies while using this attention in order to increase their influence in international discussions within multilateral organizations, such as the WHO's World Health Assembly (Chan *et al.*, 2010; Feinsilver, 2008; Feldbaum *et al.*, 2010; Feldbaum and Michaud, 2010; Fidler, 2009; Labonté and Gagnon, 2010).

However, the case of Brazil's response to AIDS and TB suggests that scholars can — and indeed should — combine these two strands of literature. This approach provides further insight into when and why political leaders not only pursue reforms, but also why they sustain them over time. As we will see in Brazil, not only did pressures from the WHO, the World Bank, and the scientific community incentivize Presidents Cardoso and Lula to pursue bureaucratic and policy reforms, but they also did this with an eye to increasing Brazil's international reputation. Over the years, these reputation-building interests not only help to sustain and deepen domestic reforms, but it would eventually motivate Brazil to help other nations combat AIDS.

At the level of civil society, as mentioned earlier, while empirical findings from the US and Brazil suggests that civil society was not important in prompting an immediate government response to epidemics, findings from Brazil nevertheless suggest that civil society can play a different, more important role. And that civil society's role and influence increases *after* the government has responded on its own.

Indeed, scholars have recently found that NGOs and social health movements can play important roles in the post-reform period (Garcia and Parker, 2011). Specifically, after ignoring pressures from civil society during the first few years of an epidemic, government officials may decide to eventually work with NGOs and social movements in order to help monitor municipal health policies (Rich and Gómez, 2012), provide materials on AIDS prevention in hard to reach areas (Garcia and Parker, 2011), and hold local governments accountable to the MOH and the local electorate (Rich and Gómez, 2012). Ministries of health may also strategically use their partnerships with NGOs and social health movements in order to obtain ongoing financial support from international financial donors that prioritize strong state–civil society partnerships in public health — such as the Global Fund to Fight AIDS, Tuberculosis and Malaria.

Nevertheless, findings from Brazil suggest that these scholars have overlooked yet another important role that NGOs and social health movements play in strengthening a government's response to epidemics. That is, researchers seem to have overlooked the fact that contemporary NGOs and social health movements can help officials in their efforts to sustain and deepen their policy reforms. Thus, in contrast to the aforementioned interest group literature, where civil society pressures the state and the latter works to secure their needs, in this book, it is civil society that eventually *works for the state* in helping achieve its policy objectives. In this sense, NGOs and social health movements become helpful civic supporters.

I define civic supporters as the presence of multiple, well-organized NGOs and social health movements advocating historically proven policy ideas of a centralized bureaucratic and policy response to epidemics while representing similar types of civic organizations and social movements in the past. The emergence of effective civic supporters requires the presence of multiple, well-organized, funded, and globally integrated NGOs and/or social health movements that provide officials with an influential network of civil society actors supporting their cause. The historically proven policy ideas that civic supporters proffer focus on the fact that the central government should immediately respond to epidemics whenever they emerge; that the government should create a strong public health bureaucracy in response; that the government should guarantee universal access to healthcare treatment while providing assistance the states; and finally, that civil society and public health officials work together in order to contain the spread of disease. When compared to more contemporary ideas guiding initial policy responses to epidemics, such as decentralization, these older, historically based policy ideas emphasizing centralization may have more credibility. This is because they have a long, proven track record of success, as well as wider popularity within government and civil society.

As we will see in Brazil, when the AIDS epidemic emerged, health officials sought out and strategically used these civic supporters in order to increase their legitimacy and influence when seeking ongoing political and financial support from Congress. Working with civic supporters increased these officials' legitimacy because the aforementioned historical policy ideas that these supporters advocated had a proven track record of success, dating back to the early 20th century, and because these civic supporters resembled similar, highly regarded social health movements in the past, such as the Liga contra a Tuberculose and the Sifilógrafo movements, which responded to TB and syphilis, respectively, during the early 20th century. Moreover, these were movements that initially engendered these historical policy ideas and that worked closely with public health officials to implement them.

However, these civic supporters were not present for other health sectors in Brazil, such as TB — nor were they ever present in the US. Despite Brazil's presidents increasing their support for bureaucratic and policy reforms after the emergence of international criticisms and pressures, in contrast to AIDS, there were no civic supporters that national TB officials could use to increase their legitimacy and influence when seeking ongoing reforms. The eventual disappearance of the aforementioned Liga contra a Tuberculose, which occurred mainly in response to the discovery of a TB vaccine by the 1950s, the absence of an opportunity for scientific discovery, as well as the diseases' association with the poor generated few incentives for medical and scientific elites to help the poor create NGOs and social health movements during the 1980s. While a social health movement for TB began to emerge in 2003, it was very small, poorly funded and poorly organized, in turn leaving a weak and unappealing support network that national TB officials could use to bolster their legitimacy and influence. As a result, when compared to the AIDS sector, the national TB program has not been able to acquire nearly as much support for its initiatives.

Methodology

In this study, I employed a qualitative methodological approach to research. With regards to my comparative case study design, I used what is known as a Most Similar Systems Design (MSSD) (Faure, 1994; Landman, 2008; Przeworksi and Teune, 1970). Often used when conducting comparisons within similar types of geographic regions, MSSD entails the selection of case studies based on similar contextual variables, such as culture, demographics, socioeconomic conditions, and the design of political and economic systems, while nevertheless highlighting key differences in causality and outcomes, a distinct methodological advantage associated with this approach (Faure, 1994; Gerring, 2007; Landman, 2008).

In this study, the US and Brazil were selected because they are perceived as similar types of nations: i.e., historically, both were agricultural, slave-based trading economies; both emerged as federations with strong state governors possessing considerable autonomy and influence by the 19th century; beginning in the early 20th century, both nations also exhibited massive waves of immigration, mainly from Europe and Asia; and as mentioned earlier, both nations have high degrees of income inequality, while having the largest populations and geographic territories in the western hemisphere. And since the late 1980s, Brazil joined the US in becoming a free market system with a high level of decentralization and local government responsibilities, especially in terms of healthcare. Of course, one could argue that these nations are considerably different given that per capita income has, on average, been higher in the US and that from 1964 to 1986, Brazil was not a democracy but rather and military dictatorship committing human rights violations. Despite these differences, prior to military rule and especially after Brazil's return to democracy in 1986, when focusing on electoral institutions, federalism, decentralization, as well as the presence of free markets, there appears to be more similarities than differences between the US and Brazil. Nevertheless, both nations eventually differed in how they responded to contested epidemics, with Brazil outpacing the US in its centralized bureaucratic and policy response.

Next, the US and Brazil were compared in order to highlight their historical and contextual uniqueness in institutional and policy responses to epidemics. Similar to what Skocpol and Sommers (1980) once described as a "comparative history as contrast of contexts", the purpose of my comparison was to highlight the unique historical, political, and social factors accounting for key differences in causality and outcomes between two similar case studies. Northrop (2012) has argued that these types of historical comparisons are important for underscoring unique causal explanations and complexity in cross-cultural history. Through this kind of comparison, one may increase the visibility and understanding of a particular case study, while underscoring their ongoing cultural, institutional, and economic obstacles to success (Bendix, 1964; Northrop, 2012; Skocpol and Sommers, 1980). According to this approach, moreover, conceptual and empirical themes and questions — such as how Brazil did better than the US when responding to epidemics — serve as guides illuminating key differences between case studies (Skocpol and Sommers, 1980). Conceptual themes, moreover, are not to be tested with the historical case studies in order to devise a generalizable claim. Rather, maintaining the historical integrity and causal details of each case is perceived as more important (Northrop, 2012; Skocpol and Sommers, 1980).

However, what was my reason for examining government responses to syphilis, TB, polio, malnutrition, AIDS, and obesity? I choose these epidemics for the following reasons: First, to examine government response to sexually transmitted and non-sexually transmitted diseases, thus controlling for the negative impact of stigma on political elite perceptions and response;[3] second, because these epidemics were highly contested by politicians and health officials during the first few years of their emergence, thus leading to a delayed government response; and finally, to display diversity in the types of cases examined, i.e., to go beyond the popularized study of AIDS[4] to address other epidemics that have claimed just as many, if not more, lives.

With regards to data, this study relied on several different types of qualitative and quantitative sources. With regards to qualitative evidence, these sources ranged from archival newspaper clippings and articles obtained from NGOs and research institutions in Brazil and the US, as well as more recently published articles, books, and policy reports. I also relied on newspaper clippings obtained from on-line news engines, such as Access World News, World News Connection, and Google. Because these news sources also translate foreign languages into English, they were particularly helpful when conducting research in nations where I could not read the language, such as Russia and China. Next, interviews were conducted with public health officials, activists, and researchers in English and Portuguese. Conducted in the US and Brazil, interviewees were chosen based on their extensive policy experience and knowledge of the topic. Interviewees were not selected for their specific points of view, as this would have certainly biased the interview data. With respect to quantitative data, this study relied on archival and contemporary epidemiological data obtained from public health institutions in the US and Brazil. Budgetary data on federal government expenditures were also obtained from on-line databases in the congresses and departments of health in both countries.

---

[3] That is, assuming that the stigma associated with AIDS leads to discrimination and inaction, based on moral beliefs of sexual immorality, as a plethora of the literature suggests, then the absence of this stigma for other diseases should lead to a more aggressive government response.

[4] Most of the scholarly research on the politics of government response to epidemics has tended to focus on AIDS. This in large part stems from the greater amount of attention AIDS has received in recent years when compared to other diseases. In part this is mainly due to the stigma, political, and social conflict surrounding AIDS, the rapid increase in AIDS cases and deaths throughout the 1990s, and higher levels of international funding for AIDS relative to other diseases.

A Roadmap

In the next chapter, I discuss the US's and Brazil's historic response to contested epidemics, the conditions under which both countries eventually responded, as well as the historical origins of social health movements, centralized bureaucratic and policy ideas, and state–civil society partnerships. I then provide in-depth case studies of the US's response to AIDS and obesity followed by Brazil's response to AIDS and TB, as well as a comparison of Brazil to the other BRICS nations. This book concludes with an analysis of the key empirical and theoretical lessons learned. In light of my position that Brazil eventually outpaced the US in its policy response, at the end of the concluding chapter I then consider what lessons the Brazilians may have for the US and what US domestic and global health policies would look like if the US were to take Brazil's policy recommendations seriously.

References

Aggleton, P. (2001). HIV/AIDS in Europe: The Challenge for Health Promotion Research, *Health Education Research*, **16**, 403–409.

Allard, S. (2009). *Out of Reach: Place, Poverty, and the New American Welfare State*, Yale University Press, New Haven.

Altman, D. (1986). *AIDS in the Mind of America*, Doubleday Press, New York.

Anderson, T. (2009). HIV/AIDS in Cuba: Lessons and Challenges, *Pan American Journal of Public Health*, **26**, 78–86.

Arretche, M. (2003). Federalism, Intergovernmental Relations and Social Policies in Brazil. Paper prepared for the seminar Comparative Analysis of Intergovernmental Management Mechanisms and Formulation of alternatives for the Brazilian Case, Brazil, September 17 and 18. Published by the Forum of Federations.

Baldwin, P. (2007). *Disease and Democracy: The Industrialized World Faces AIDS*, University of California Press, Berkeley.

Barboza, R. (2006). *Gestão do Programa Estadual DST/Aid de São Paulo: Uma Análise do Processo de descentralizacão das Acões no Período de 1994 a 2003*. Master's thesis, University of São Paulo.

Barnett, T. and Whiteside, A. (2006). *AIDS in the Twenty-First Century*, Palgrave Macmillan Press, New York.

Basilia, C. (2009). Personal interview. November 15.

Behrman, G. (2004). *The Invisible People: How the U.S. Has Slept Through the Global AIDS Epidemic, the Greatest Humanitarian Catastrophe of our Time*, The Free Press, New York.

Bendix, R. (1964). *Nation Building and Citizenship*, University of California Press, Berkeley.

Beyrer, C., Gauri V., and Vaillancourt, D. (2005). *Evaluation of the World Bank's Assistance in Responding to the AIDS Epidemic: Brazil Case Study*, The World Bank Group, Washington DC.

Bliss, K. (2012). *From Atlanta to Washington: History and Politics of the International AIDS Conferences, 1985-present*, Center for Strategic and International Studies, Washington, DC.

Blumenthal, D. and Morone, J. (2009). *The Heart of Power: Health and Politics in the Oval Office*, University of California Press, Berkeley.

Boone, C. and Batsell, J. (2001). Politics and AIDS in Africa: Research Agendas in Political Science and International Relations. *Africa Today*, **48**, 3–33.

Bor, J. (2007). The Political Economy of AIDS Leadership in Developing Countries: An Exploratory Analysis, *Social Science & Medicine*, **64**, 1585–1599.

Brandt, A. (1985). *No Magic Bullet: A Social History of Venereal Disease in the United States since 1880*, Oxford University Press, New York.

Carrara, S. (1999). 'A AIDS e a História das Doencas Venéreas no Brasil', in Parker, R., Bastos, C., Galvão, J., and Pedrosa, J. (eds), *A AIDS no Brasil*, ABIA Press, Rio de Janeiro, 273–306.

Cervo, L. (2011). *Inserção Internacional: Formação dos Conceitos Brasileiros*, Editora Saraiva, São Paulo.

Chan, L., Chen L., and Xu J. (2010). China's Engagement with Global Health Diplomacy: Was SARS a Watershed? *PLoS Medicine*, 7, 1–6.

CIA (Central Intelligence Committee) (2013). The World Factbook. Available on-line: https://www.cia.gov/library/publications/the-world-factbook/rankorder/2172rank.html. Accessed March 13, 2014.

Ciconello, A. (2008). 'Social participation as a democracy-consolidating process in Brazil', *From Poverty to Power: How Active Citizens and Effective States can Change the World*, Case Study, Oxfam International, Boston, 2–12.

Clemens, W. (2000). *America and the World, 1898–2015: Achievements, Failures, and Alternative Futures*, St. Martin's Press, New York.

Cohen, I. and Elder, A. (1989). Major Cities and Disease Crisis: A Comparative Perspective, *Social Science History*, **13**, 25–63.

Da Costa Marques, M. (2003). *A História de Uma Epidemia Moderna: A Emergencia Política da AIDS/HIV No Brasil*, RiMa/Eduem Press, São Paulo.

Dauvergne, P. and Farias, D. (2012). The Rise of Brazil as a Global Development Power, *Third World Quarterly*, **33**, 903–917.

Faure, A.M. (1994). Some Methodological Problems in Comparative Politics, *Journal of Theoretical Politics*, **6**, 307–322.

Feinsilver, J. (2008). Oil-for-Doctors: Cuban Medical Diplomacy Gets a Little Help from a Venezuelan Friend, *Nueva Sociedad*, **216**, 1–15.

Feldbaum, H., Lee, K., and Michaud, J. (2010). Global Health and Foreign Policy, *Epidemiological Review*, **32**, 82–92.

Feldbaum, H. and Michaud, J. (2010). Health Diplomacy and the Enduring Relevance of Foreign Policy Interests, *PLoS Medicine*, **7**, 1–6.

Fidler, D. (2009). Vital Signs: Health and Foreign Policy, *The World Today*, **65**, 27–29.

Galvão, J. (2000). *AIDS no Brasil: A Agenda de Construção de Uma Epidemia*, ABIA Publishers, São Paulo.

Garcia, E. (2012). *O Sexto Membro Permanente o Brasil e a Criação da ONU*, Contraponto Editora Ltda, Rio de Janeiro.

Garcia, J. and Parker, R. (2011). Resource Mobilization for Health Advocacy: Afro-Brazilian Religious Organizations and HIV Prevention and Control, *Social Science & Medicine*, **72**, 1930–1938.

Gauri, V. and Khaleghian, P. (2002). Immunization in Developing Countries: Its Political and Organizational Determinants, *World Development*, **30**, 2109–2132.

Gauri, V. and Lieberman, E. (2006). Boundary Politics and HIV/AIDS Policy in Brazil and South Africa, *Studies in Comparative International Development*, **41**, 47–73.

Gelasi, V. (2009). Personal interview. October 13.

Gerring, J. (2007). *Case Study Research: Principles and Practices*, Cambridge University Press, New York.

Hacker, J. (2004). Dismantling the Health Care State? Political Institutions, Public Policies and the Comparative Politics of Health Reform, *British Journal of Political Science*, **34**, 693–724.

Hindman, A. and Schroedel, J. (2010). *U.S. Response to HIV/AIDS in Africa: Bush as a Human Rights leader?* Unpublished manuscript, Claremont Graduate University.

Huang, Y. (2006). The Politics of HIV/AIDS in China, *Asian Perspective*, **30**, 95–125.

Huang, Y. (2010). Pursuing Health as Foreign Policy: The Case of China, *Indiana Journal of Global Legal Studies*, **17**, 105–146.

Hochman, G. (1998). *A Era do Saneamento: As Bases da Política de Saúde Pública no Brasil*, Editora Hucitec-Anpocs, São Paulo.

Immergut, E. (1992). *Health Politics, Interests, and Institutions in Western Europe*, Cambridge University Press, New York.

Kaiser Family Foundation (2011). *Financing the Response to AIDS in Low- and Middle-Income Countries: International Assistance from Donor Governments in 2010*, Policy Report, August 11.

Kepp, M. (2008). Cracks Appear in Brazil's Primary Health-Care Programme, *The Lancet*, **372**, 877.

Kersh, R. and Morone, J. (2002). The Politics of Obesity: Seven Steps to Government Action, *Health Affairs*, **21**, 142–153.

Kerwin, J. (2003). *Rulemaking: How Government Agencies Write Law and Make Policy*, Congressional Quarterly Press, Washington, DC.

Labonté, R. and Gagnon, M. (2010). Framing Health and Foreign Policy: Lesson for Global Health Diplomacy, *Globalization and Health*, **6**, 1–19.

Landman, T. (2008). *Issues and Methods in Comparative Politics: An Introduction*, Routledge Press, New York.

Levenstein, H. (1993). *Paradox of Plenty: A Social History of Eating in Modern America*, Oxford University Press, New York.

Lieberman, E. (2009). *Boundaries of Contagion: How Ethnic Politics have shaped Government Responses to AIDS*, Princeton University Press, Princeton.

Marmor, T., Feeman R., and Okma, K. (2005). Comparative Perspectives and Policy Learning in the World of Health Care, *Journal of Comparative Policy Analysis*, **7**, 331–448.

McGuire, J. (2010). *Health, Wealth, and Democracy in East Asia and Latin America*, Cambridge University Press, New York.

McKenna, M. (2004). Government to limit access to CDC experts, *Ventura County Star*, July 1, 14.

McKinney, M. and Pepper, B. (1999). 'From Hope to Heartbreak: Bill Clinton and the Rhetoric of AIDS', in Elwood, W. (ed.), *Power in the Blood: A Handbook of AIDS, Politics, and Communication*, Routledge Press, Florence, pp. 77–91.

Mullen, F. (1989). *Plagues and Politics: the Story of the United States Public Health Service*, Basic Books Press, New York.

NASTAD (National Alliance of State and Territorial AIDS Directors) (2005). *A Turning Point: Confronting HIV/AIDS in African American Communities*, NASTAD Press, Washington DC.

Northrop, D. (2012). *A Companion to World History*, Blackwell Publishing, Malden.

Norum, K. (2010). Personal interview. June 16.

Norum, K., Waxman, A., Selikowitz, H., Bauman, A., Puska, P., Rigby, N., James, P., and Yach, D. (2009). 'The WHO Global Strategy on Diet, Physical Activity and Health', in Tellnes, G. (ed.), *Urbanisation and Health: New Challenges in Health Promotion and Prevention*, Oslo Academic Press, Norway.

Oshinsky, D. (2006). *Polio: An American Story*, Oxford University Press, New York.

Nathanson, C. (1996). Disease Prevention as Social Change: Towards a Theory of Public Health, *Population and Development Review*, 22, 609–637.

Nye, J. (2005). *Soft Power: The Means to Success in World Politics*, Public Affairs Press, New York.

Obama, M. (2010). Michelle on a Mission: How we can Empower Parents, Schools, and the Community to Battle Childhood Obesity, *Newsweek*, March 22, 40–48.

Olunzi, S. and Macrae, J. (1995). Whose Policy is it Anyway? International and National Influences on Health Policy Development in Uganda, *Health Policy & Planning*, 10, 122–132.

Panem, S. (1988). *The AIDS Bureaucracy*, Harvard University Press, Cambridge.

Park, M. (2010). Ex-military Leaders: Young Adults 'Too Fat to Fight, *CNN*, April 20. Available on-line: http://www.cnn.com/2010/HEALTH/04/20/military.fat.fight/index.html. Accessed April 20, 2010.

Parker, R. (2003). Building the Foundations for the Response to HIV/AIDS in Brazil: The Development of HIV/AIDS Policy, 1982–1996, *Divulgação em Saúde para Debate*, 27, 143–183.

Patterson, A. (ed.) (2005). *The Politics of AIDS in Africa*, Ashgate Publishers, Aldershot.

Perrow, C. and Guillen, M. (1990). *The AIDS Disaster: The Failure of Organizations in New York and the Nation*, Yale University Press, New Haven.

Platt, M. and Platt, M. (2013). *From GRID to Gridlock: The Relationship between Scientific Biomedical Breakthroughs and HIV/AIDS Policy in the US Congress.* Unpublished manuscript, Harvard University, Department of Government.

Price-Smith, A. (2002). *The Health of Nations: Infectious Disease, Environmental Change, and their Effects on National Security and Development*, MIT Press, Cambridge.

Price-Smith, A., Tauber, S., and Bhat, A. (2004). State Capacity and HIV Incidence Reduction in the Developing World: Preliminary Empirical Evidence, *Seton Hall Journal of Diplomacy*, Summer/Fall, 149–160.

Pritchett, L. and Woolcock, M. (2004). Solutions when *the* Solution is the Problem: Arraying the Disarray in Development, *World Development*, **32**, 191–212.

Prud'homme, R. (1995). The Dangers of Decentralization, *The World Bank Observer*, **10**, 201–220.

Przeworksi, A. and Teune, H. (1970). *The Logic of Comparative Social Inquiry*, Wiley-Interscience Press, Hoboken.

Putzel, J. (2004). The Politics of Action on AIDS: A Case Study of Uganda, *Public Administration and Development*, **24**, 19–30.

Rau, B. (2006). The Politics of Civil Society in Confronting HIV/AIDS. *International Affairs*, **82**, 285–295.

Rich, J. and Gómez, E. (2012). Centralizing Decentralized Governance in Brazil, *Publius: The Journal of Federalism*, **42**, 636–661.

Rodden, J. (2006). 'The Political Economy of Federalism', in Weingast, B. and Whitman, D. (eds), *Oxford Handbook of Political Economy*, Oxford University Press, New York, 357–372.

Rosenbrock, R. and Wright, M. (Eds). (2000). *Partnership and Pragmatism: Germany's Response to AIDS Prevention and Care*, Routledge Press, London.

Ruger, J. (2005). Democracy and Health. *Quarterly Journal of Medicine*, **98**, 229–304.

Santos Filho, E. (2006). *Política de Tuberculose no Brasil: Uma Perspectiva da Sociedade Civil*, Public Health Watch, George Soros Foundation/Open Society Institute.

Santos Filho, E. and Gomes, Z. (2007). Strategies for Tuberculosis Control in Brazil: Networking and Civil Society Participation, *Revista Saúde Pública*, **41**, 1–6.

Sen, A. (1999). *Development as Freedom*, Knopf Press, New York.

Shilts, R. (2007). *And the Band Played On: Politics, People, and the AIDS Epidemic*, St. Martin's Press, New York.

Skidmore, T. (2007). *Politics in Brazil (1930–1964): An Experiment in Democracy*, Oxford University Press, New York.

Skocpol, T. and Sommers, M. (1980). The Uses of Comparative History in Macro-Social Theory, *Comparative Studies in Society and History*, **22**, 174–197.

Sparer, M., France, G., and Clinton, C. (2011). Inching Toward Incrementalism: Federalism, Devolution, and Health Policy in the United States and the United Kingdom, *Journal of Health Politics, Policy & Law*, **36**, 33–57.

Tendler, J. (1997). *Getting Good Government in the Tropics*, The Johns Hopkins University Press, Baltimore.

The Body (2001). Presidential Advisory Council on HIV/AIDS Issues First Recommendations to President Bush, July 20.

The National Advisory Committee (2000). *Rural Public Health: Issues and Considerations*, National Advisory Committee Press, Rockville.

United Nations (2008). *Demographic Yearbook — Population by Sex, Rate of Population Increase, Surface Area and Density*, United Nations Press, New York.

UNAIDS (1999). *UNAIDS and Nongovernmental Organizations*, UNAIDS, Geneva.

United States Census Bureau (2013). Population Estimates. Available on-line: http://www.census.gov/popest/about/terms.html. Accessed July 17, 2013.

Vallgarda, S. (2007). Problematizations and Path Dependency: HIV/AIDS Policies in Denmark and Sweden, *Medical History*, **51**, 99–112.

Vulliamy, E. (2002). Bush Declares War on Fat America, *The Guardian*, June 23, 1.

Weyland, K. (1995). Social Movements and the State: The Politics of Health Reform in Brazil, *World Development*, **23**, 1699–1712.

Weyland, K. (2007). *Bounded Rationality and Policy Diffusion: Social Sector Reform in Latin America*, Princeton University Press, Princeton.

White, F. (2010). Personal interview. June 25.

Whiteside, A. (1999). *The Threat of HIV/AIDS to Democracy and Governance.* USAID briefing paper. USAID Press, Washington DC.

World Bank (2013). Population database. Available on-line: http://data. worldbank.org/indicator/SP.POP.TOTL. Accessed March 13, 2014.

World Health Organization (1992). *Forty-Fifth World Health Assembly: Global Strategy for the Prevention and Control of AIDS*, World Health Organization, Geneva.

Chapter 2

20th Century Responses to Contested Epidemics in the United States and Brazil

Throughout the 19th and early 20th century, policymakers in the US and Brazil confronted a host of *contested epidemics*. Syphilis, tuberculosis (TB), polio, and malnutrition, for example, emerged to challenge government commitments to safeguarding civil society and meeting their healthcare needs. Yet, in both nations, governments did not immediately respond to these epidemics. This inaction was mainly the product of intensive inter-elite contestation and conflicting views between presidents, legislative representatives, and the bureaucracy over the prevalence and seriousness of these health threats. In several instances this contestation was also shaped by the president's belief that some epidemics simply did not pose serious national health threats, a view influenced by the presence of multiple diseases and the absence of convincing epidemiological data.

In both countries a centralized bureaucratic and policy response eventually emerged. However, this occurred mainly when epidemics threatened one of the core aspects of national security, such as military readiness and/or economic development, or when political leaders were personally afflicted and had an interest in responding. Responses were never the product of vehement civic protests and demands for government intervention.

With time, however, Brazil's motivation for responding to epidemics began to differ from the US's. As an emerging nation eager to make its way in the world, eventually international criticisms and pressures became important motivational factors for eliciting a centralized response. By the 1940s, Brazil's presidents, health officials, and social health movements became more cooperative with the international community, while strategically using a more aggressive centralized response as a way to enhance the government's international reputation. In contrast, the international community instigated no such incentives in the US; instead, presidents and health officials responded on their own, motivated either by national security threats or their personal experiences with disease.

This chapter, however, also shows that social health movements can play an important role in working with the bureaucracy for a response. As we will see in Brazil, while centralized health policy ideas and pressures from social health movements were not effective in motivating the government to respond, society's ideas dovetailed nicely with those health officials seeking a centralized response. These social movements also worked closely with the international community to pressure the government for a more timely response. By attending international conferences, sharing data, and discussing Brazil's achievements in the areas of science and medicine, these social movements increased their international and domestic prestige; and because of this, they provided health officials with the *civic supporters* needed to increase these officials' legitimacy and influence when striving to obtain political support for a centralized response. While unsuccessful in convincing the government to engage in these endeavors, this state–civil society partnership did, nevertheless, establish precedents and more importantly, centralized bureaucratic and policy ideas and partnerships that future bureaucrats could use for their benefit — as we will see in response to AIDS in Chapter 4.

In contrast, in the US these state–civil society dynamics never emerged during the early 20th century. Despite the emergence of several contested health epidemics during this period, such as polio, malnutrition, and syphilis, no well-organized, globally integrated social health movement emerged proffering the need for a centralized response. While local health movements and community responses existed, they were often isolated and working on their own. And while health officials did suggest a centralized response, policy ideas that mainly emerged from western Europe, in contrast to what we saw in

Brazil, these officials never tried to establish strong partnerships with social health movements. Because of this, no civic supporters and historical precedents of state–civil society partnerships ever emerged, in turn posing challenges for future bureaucratic efforts to combat epidemics — as we will see with AIDS and obesity in Chapters 3 and 5.

The Origins of Public Health Institutions in the US and Brazil

Public health institutions in the US and Brazil started off on different paths. Historically, these institutions were more decentralized in the US and centralized in Brazil. In the US, beginning in the early 18th century, the states and local governments bore the brunt of health policy responsibility, mainly through municipal health boards and in some instances, merchant marine hospitals. The national government occasionally intervened through congressional acts in order to regulate diseases in port areas. In April 1798, President John Adams signed a congressional act stating that sickly seamen returning to port areas should receive aid from nearby merchant marine hospitals. Adams appointed the directors of these hospitals, which in turn signaled a high level of presidential commitment to disease eradication (Mullan, 1989). The act also led to the creation of the Marine Hospital Fund, which was managed by these directors. The Fund essentially called for a 20% tax on the income of seamen to pay for these services (Mullen, 1989). In 1799, at the request of the secretary of the treasury, Oliver Welcott, a large marine hospital opened in Boston, followed by New Port, Rhode Island, and Norfolk, Virginia, in 1802 (Mullen, 1989).

Many of these hospitals were poorly staffed and in some instances abandoned, used by civil war soldiers as barracks. Before the civil war started, only 8 of the 26 marine hospitals were in operation. In 1870, in an effort to strengthen the marine hospital system, new legislation was proposed to create a more centralized Marine Hospital Service (MHS), to be controlled by bureaucrats in Washington DC through a supervising surgeon general, namely John Woodworth. After considering the inefficiencies associated with a decentralized approach to marine hospital care, and after considering the limited number of state and municipal health hospitals at the time (only one official state hospital was in operation, i.e., the Massachusetts state hospital, which opened in 1869), Woodworth successfully made the case for a more centralized approach to public health, followed by the introduction of merit-based exams and a uniformed — seemingly militant — service (Mullan, 1989). Although state and municipal hospitals gradually grew in size and assumed most of the responsibility for providing public health services, Surgeon General Woodworth's newly centralized MHS tried to gradually assert its control over the states.

The federal imposition of quarantines marked the first impulse of the MHS's tendency to create a centralized bureaucratic and policy response to epidemics. While the Treasury Department played a key role in helping the states impose quarantines in port areas during the early 19th century (Williams, 1951), by 1878 the MHS obtained even greater authority to impose quarantines onto the states through the Quarantine Act of 1878, which sought to curb the spread of disease and safeguard the flow of commerce (Mullen, 1989; Williams, 1951).

It must be noted, however, that the main intention of the surgeon general and the marine hospitals was not only to protect military personnel but also private business, for both these elements comprised key aspects of US national security. When health epidemics did not pose these security threats, state and city hospitals were expected to provide public health services on their own, even if they were poorly funded, staffed, and riddled with corruption. Over the years, there seemed to emerge a tension between the state and municipal health departments and the surgeon general's marine hospitals, as the latter sought to intervene not only for public health issues but also for those epidemics deemed as threats to national security.

By the early 20th century, however, the public health system converged into a more decentralized form of disease control. This was concretized with the replacement of the MHS with the US Public Health Service (PHS) in 1912. The PHS officially recognized the states' autonomy in rendering health services. From then on, the PHS's role was relegated to intervention but only at the behest of state and municipal health officials. This penned agreement notwithstanding, the

PHS periodically intervened through quarantine and other policies whenever the president and Congress perceived new epidemics as threatening port areas, merchant and naval personnel, and the flow of commerce (Mullen, 1989; Williams, 1951).

The president and Congress' obsession with safeguarding the economy and military readiness was so extreme that by 1922, ownership of the PHS was transferred from the Department of the Treasury to the Federal Security Agency (Williams, 1951). This effort essentially solidified the government's interest in pursuing a centralized bureaucratic and policy response whenever epidemics posed direct threats to national security. We will see this centralized impulse reemerge with the government's response to syphilis and malnutrition during the early 20th century as well as childhood obesity decades later.

Birth of a Competitive Public Health Bureaucracy

It was also during the 20th century that we saw the birth of the modern public health bureaucracy in the US. While the turn to a rational, scientific state emerged with the Pendleton Act of 1848, which required meritocratic procedures for recruitment into federal agencies, it was mainly after the great depression and the First World War that the notion of a centralized modern bureaucracy working on social welfare issues arose (Rosemblum and McCurdy, 2007). Due in part to President Franklin D. Roosevelt's "New Deal" initiatives, the mid-20th century witnessed the emergence of a myriad of federal agencies working on economic and social welfare programs (Rosemblum and McCurdy, 2007). It was during this state-building period that the PHS emerged as a scientific agency eager to monitor, classify, and respond to public health threats.

This context also led to the creation of public health institutions which, although highly competitive, were instigated through a fear of agency survival. In response to the escalation of a malaria outbreak during the 1930s near military barracks in the southern part of the US, in 1942 the PHS created the Malaria Control in War Areas Unit (MCWAU). Later renamed the Centers for Disease Control and Prevention (CDC) in 1946, the CDC's purpose was to protect military soldiers preparing for battle in Europe (Ethridge, 1992). CDC officials nevertheless feared that as soon as the Second World War ended, their department would be eliminated (Ethridge, 1992). To help ensure its survival, in 1951 CDC officials pursued new initiatives that would help convince Congress of its ongoing importance. That year, the Epidemic Intelligence Service (EIS) was created. EIS was a cadre of elite scientists dedicated to finding, labeling, and reporting new health threats. With the EIS's help, CDC officials immediately embarked on a strategy to use the emergence of health threats as a *means* to agency survival. By strategically labeling each epidemic as a threat to US national security, CDC officials believed that they could garner more congressional support, resources, and, above all, survive (Astor, 1983).

For example, in response to the polio outbreak, the CDC strategically used the epidemic's emergence as a means to rejuvenate the agency's prestige, to distinguish itself from other agencies and to garner more attention and financial support. Astor (1983) puts it nicely:

> ... the increasing incidence of poliomyelitis early in the decade and the Asian flu pandemic of 1957 gave the Atlanta institution an opportunity to prove itself. In a five-year period, the CDC moved from a position of relative obscurity in public health to one with major responsibilities for epidemic control. (Etheridge, 1992: p. 67).

By the 1960s, this strategy paid off. Under President Lyndon Johnson, the amount of money given to the CDC substantially increased (Etheridge, 1992). In response to the CDC's impressive work on polio, and in part because of Johnson's commitment to social welfare through his "Great Society" endeavor (i.e., a series of welfare policies that were created in order to help people get out of poverty), he began to request and allocate funding to the CDC's family planning programs and its lead-based poisoning projects (Etheridge, 1992).

Yet the CDC's strategies quickly developed into a habit of competing with other agencies whenever new health threats emerged. The goal was to convince the president and Congress that the CDC was the primary agency responsible for reporting and containing the spread of disease, not the National Institutes of Health (NIH) or any other research division. The NIH was perceived mainly as a research institution, without the responsibility of tracking and reporting cases, as well as working with the states to implement policy (Ethridge, 1992). The fact that the NIH was receiving more financial support when compared to the CDC also contributed to tensions between the two agencies (Ethridge, 1992). However, as the pioneers of science and discovery, the NIH stood its ground, arguing that their role in disease eradication was just as, if not more, important than the CDC's.

These turf battles had long-run implications. In an effort to once again distinguish itself, the CDC immediately emerged to stake its claim over tracking the HIV virus and policy response. This upset other agency heads, such as researchers in the NIH, who rejected the CDC's attempted ownership over AIDS and consequently refrained from cooperating with the CDC in response. Compounding these territorial disputes was the presence of an economic recession, where budgetary support for PHS expansion waned. As we will see in the following chapter, the end result was the emergence of a high degree of inter-agency competition, lack of cooperation, and a delayed government response to AIDS.

Global Health Leadership

Throughout the 19th and early 20th century, the US also became highly visible and involved in global health. The government's intention was essentially two-fold: first, to become the world leader in providing bilateral assistance to developing nations in order to eradicate disease — as well as poverty and malnutrition; and second, to encourage the participation of philanthropic institutions in helping developing nations achieve the same.

Historically, the PHS was committed to helping developing nations eradicate disease. Even before the PHS's creation in 1912, commissioned marine hospital officers were sent to other countries in order to study foreign diseases and to help contain their spread. Officers were also dispatched to foreign consulates to help ensure that vessels departing for the US were thoroughly inspected (Bennett and DiLorenzo, 2000; Coming, 1970). Not only was this perceived as altruistic bilateral assistance, but it was also perceived as a necessity for ensuring US national security. Later on, during the Second World War and at the height of PHS's expansion, the latter created the office of International Health Relations, which worked closely with the countries of Liberia, Greece, and Iran to develop their public health systems (Murran, 1989). And in 1946, at the International Health Conference organized by the UN in New York, Surgeon General Thomas Parran was elected as president of the conference. At this event, Parran helped to write the World Health Organization's (WHO) first constitution and to shape its primary obligations and duties (Murran, 1989).

During the 1950s, the PHS also led the global campaign to eradicate malaria in several Western and Central African nations. It worked closely with the USAID (United States Agency for International Development) to finance several malaria-eradication programs and worked with the WHO to ensure that nations, such as Brazil, were responding (Ethridge, 1992). During the 1960s, the CDC also proudly led the fight against the smallpox epidemic in Africa and Asia, as well as Brazil (Ethridge, 1992).

But it was with smallpox that the CDC started to reveal its commitment to global health leadership. The CDC director at the time, Dr. William Foege, made several trips to Asia in order to convince health officials that they needed to redouble their efforts against smallpox (Ethridge, 1992). In 1973, Foege also went to India to direct the last and final phase of the WHO's smallpox-eradication program. Through these efforts, Foege and the CDC helped to lead the fight against not only smallpox but a host of other diseases across Africa, East Asia, Central and South America (Ethridge, 1992).

Throughout the early-to-mid 20th century, the US government also encouraged philanthropic organizations to provide assistance to developing nations. Private philanthropy not only played a key role in helping build public health infrastructure, but other social welfare services as well, such as malnutrition and education (Lovett, 2005). In Brazil, for example, the Rockefeller Foundation helped establish several rural outposts for the eradication of yellow fever, malaria, and other diseases (Hochman, 1998). Other philanthropists emerged, such as

Mrs. Irene Diamond (subsequent co-partner with her husband, Aaron Diamond, of the Aaron Diamond Foundation), to give thousands of dollars for combating malaria and other diseases. Rockefeller and Diamond were the Bill & Melinda Gates and Warren Buffetts of their day. Together they helped finance several health initiatives throughout Latin America and Africa (McNeil, 2006).

Nevertheless, it is important to note that during this period, the PHS was not as receptive to international criticisms and policy recommendations. When compared to most nations, the US was more isolationist in nature and believed in establishing its own solutions to its own health problems, readily imposing its policy prescriptions onto other countries through bilateral policy measures (Kickbusch, 2002). Because of the US's unwavering dedication to providing bilateral assistance, and because the government arguably had the most financial, technical, and infrastructural resources for health in the world, the PHS always viewed itself as a global leader rather than follower and receiver of international assistance. Over the years, this engendered a government that had no incentive to engage in an aggressive, centralized bureaucratic and policy response in the hopes of increasing its international reputation. Further, as the case studies in this chapter illustrate, because of this the US's isolated public health system instigated a bureaucratic and policy response that was, and continues to be, shaped mostly by domestic political interests.

Over the years, scholars note that the US has become even more isolationist in terms of international health cooperation (Kickbusch, 2002). Moreover, this has occurred despite the emergence of an increasingly integrated global health community (Kickbusch, 2002). Notwithstanding the rise of a new international consensus that nations should work together in order to share resources, knowledge, and eradicate disease, since the 1980s the US has refrained from working in close partnership with other nations to achieve these goals (Kickbusch, 2002). As we will see later in this chapter and in Chapter 5, the only time the US has worked in close partnership with other nations is when it has been in its own medical and economic interests, or when the military, political leaders, and its citizens (in this order) have felt threatened by the emergence of a new disease (Kickbusch, 2002). This kind of biased response has motivated recent scholars to encourage the US to work more closely with the WHO, UNAIDS, and other international health organizations, such as the Global Fund to Fight AIDS, Tuberculosis and Malaria (Kickbusch, 2002; Yach and Bettcher, 1998). Despite these recommendations, and as we will soon see with the recent response to AIDS and obesity, the US continues to refrain from working closely with the international community in its domestic response to contested epidemics.

Brazil

When compared to the US, the history of constructing public health institutions in Brazil is rather different. In contrast to the US, the Brazilian government initially created and maintained a centralized approach to disease eradication. Shortly after political independence in 1822, governing elites responded to epidemics such as yellow fever, malaria, and smallpox by creating a highly centralized public health agency: namely, the Departmento Geral de Saúde Público (DGSP), which existed until the end of the first Republican government (1889–1930). Designed with the intent of monitoring and curbing the spread of disease, the DGSP was also linked to the Ministry of Justice in the interior. The DGSP acted as a highly autonomous bureaucracy, freely intervening at the state level in order to achieve its policy objectives (Hochman, 1998).

What is important to note is that throughout this period, the emperor and his medical staff were highly autonomous and isolated from political interests and those of civil society. Because epidemics were perceived as posing a serious threat to economic development, the emperor did not want the DGSP to be influenced by the interests of powerful governors and agricultural elites (Hochman, 1998). Civic organizations also had absolutely no influence over the policymaking process (Vascondelos, 2004). The only social actors that did were medical doctors, professors, and intellectuals (Lima and Britto, 1996). But even then their influence was limited, relegated to minimal policy suggestions on how to improve medical access and treatment.

Even with the arrival of a new government in 1930, this pattern of centralized bureaucratic control persisted. Led by a charismatic politician,

Getúlio Vargas, the government increased the amount of fiscal resources going to the Ministerio de Educação e Saúde Público (MESP, which replaced the DGSP in 1931), bolstered its centralized authority, while creating in 1942 the Servicio Especial de Saúde Publico (SESP). SESP was created in order to guarantee healthcare services for all workers (Acurcio, 2004). Like his predecessors, Vargas tried to maintain and strengthen the federal campaign to eradicate disease, thus helping to ensure economic modernization and prosperity.

During the early 19th century, the Brazilian government also developed a strong collaborative relationship with international health organizations and governments. At the height of the yellow fever, syphilis, and tuberculosis epidemics, the DGSP sent several medical doctors to western Europe, especially France, to share research and to learn more about Western approaches to disease eradication.[1] This was done mainly through their attendance at international conferences. At these venues, Brazil's medical community was also able to share their scientific knowledge and to discuss their approach to disease eradication (Peard, 1999). In large part this stemmed from the government and the scientific community's interest in revealing to the international community Brazil's ability to overcome disease, modernize, and prosper (Peard, 1999). In essence, this marked the genesis of Brazil's interest in increasing its international reputation as a modern state capable of eradicating disease.

During this period the Brazilian medical community also worked closely with several international philanthropists. The campaign to eradicate yellow fever and malaria witnessed, for example, several Catholic organizations, such as the Santa Casa de Misericórdia, medical and healthcare professionals working with the Rockefeller Foundation, the Irene Diamond Foundation, and the Red Cross to obtain financial assistance and acquire infrastructural resources (Stepan, 1976). It was a period of medical and scientific experimentation, breakthrough, and collaboration with the global philanthropic movement (Stepan, 1976).

---

[1] One only needs to look at the excessive amount of French health policy books in the archival stacks of the Fundação Fio Cruz (Brazil's largest public health archival library) to get a sense of Brazil's close relationship with France during the early 20th century. In fact, most of the books that I found on early syphilis and tuberculosis eradication, as well as general public health administration, were written in French.

Unlike the US, since the 1930s Brazil's Ministry of Health and the medical community were also quite receptive to international recommendations for how to construct a more effective public health system. In addition to receiving medical advice, the aforementioned philanthropies were also important for providing recommendations to the DGSP on how to construct rural outposts for malaria treatment (Hochman, 1998). This helped the DGSP expand its presence in rural areas (Hochman, 1998). It was the first time that any international organization provided technical advice on how to expand and strengthen public health administration in Brazil.

The United States

Contesting polio (1900–1957)

At the turn to the 20th century, polio was perhaps the most contested epidemic of its day. The number of polio cases and deaths spiked in the summer months of 1916, mainly in New York, gradually spreading across the states, increasing again during the post-Second World War period at a fast pace. From 1945 to 1949, an average of over 20,000 cases were reported each year (Smith, 1990: 86). The epidemic mainly hit young children in congested urban centers.

Polio was the first major epidemic that the PHS confronted. Several theories existed for polio's cause and spread, ranging from the filth and dirt brought over from European immigrants (mainly Italian), to the pesky little black flies that flew in and out of kitchen windows. New York's health department, as well as PHS officials, were aghast with the myriad of theories attributed to polio's spread, each contributing to the notion that polio's origins were unknown and that it was not as serious as they expected (Gould, 1995). Despite the federal government's awareness of the outbreak, the government did not immediately respond.

This occurred for several reasons. First, the president and Congress did not perceive polio as posing an eminent threat to US national security (Rogers, 1992). And second, no major political or bureaucratic official was affected by it, thus failing to kindle any personal interest in the matter. In contrast, PHS officials were eager to respond (Rogers, 1992). Motivated by scientific objectivity and professionalism, the burgeoning number of polio cases in poor inner city areas, most notably New York, prompted efforts to work closely with local health officials in order to understand polio's causes and to find a cure (Rogers, 1992). PHS pressures for a centralized response notwithstanding, unless convinced otherwise the president and Congress relied on a decentralized approach to polio eradication (Rogers, 1992).

The federal government did not start to pay attention to polio until it affected the life of a particular individual: Franklin D. Roosevelt (Rogers, 1992; Oshinsky, 2005). A former New York state senator (1910–1913) and assistant secretary of the navy under Woodrow Wilson (1913–1920), as well as vice presidential democratic nominee in 1920, prior to his election into the presidency, Roosevelt was a highly regarded politico. Rogers (1992) notes that the government's attention to polio was essentially non-existent until after Roosevelt was diagnosed with it in 1929. Contracted during his annual retreat to his summer home in Campobello Island, New Brunswick, Canada, within a matter of weeks Roosevelt became paralyzed from the waist down. Polio immediately affected every aspect of his life, however clandestine and discrete he hoped to keep it (Gallagher, 1999).

But more importantly, polio immediately affected Roosevelt's persona, making him humble and empathetic to those suffering from the disease. For even prior to his illness, Roosevelt began to worry about his children and others in the quiet neighborhoods of his vacation home in Campobello. Roosevelt once commented: "The infantile paralysis in NY and vicinity is appalling. *Please* kill all the flies I let. I think it really important" (Roosevelt quoted in Gould, 1995: p. 25).

But Roosevelt's worries heightened all the more shortly after becoming ill. Francis Perkins (1946) writes of Roosevelt that "the pain and suffering had purged the slightly arrogant attitude" and that the "lack of humility" and "the streak of self righteousness" waned, supplanted with a sense of empathy and understanding for others (Blumenthal and Morone, 2009: p. 26; Perkins, 1946; Rogers, 1992). Lew Howe, perhaps Roosevelt's most trusted political adviser at the time, once commented that Roosevelt "... began to see the other fellow's point of view. He thought of others who were ill and afflicted and in want" (Howe quoted in Smith, 1990: p. 51). Fennis Far (1972: pp. 127–128) goes on to claim that: "There can be no doubt of it, those months of pain put Franklin Roosevelt into the human race, and the permanent crippling that resulted from his disease kept him there … he had become conscious of other people, of weak people, of human frailty" (Blumenthal and Morone, 2009: p. 26).

Roosevelt's personal experience with polio changed his perception of the epidemic. Prior to his illness, he was essentially apathetic to the issue, relegating policy responsibilities to city health officials starved of resources and attention (Rogers, 1992). It was only after his condition worsened that he began to pay close attention to the epidemic. Moreover, his illness changed society's perceptions of polio and the stigma surrounding it (Rogers, 1992). Polio was no longer perceived as a poor, filthy man's disease. It was now viewed as an illness that anyone could get, even a high-powered politician.

Roosevelt's experience and interests in his disease transformed polio policy. His personal experiences motivated him to pursue a series of national health campaigns aimed at increasing awareness and eradicating polio. However, Roosevelt's involvement took the form of government co-sponsorship. That is, realizing that he could not create a federal agency and/or initiate new programs on his own, instead he sought to create and work with a philanthropic foundation focused exclusively on polio (Oshinsky, 2005). In 1938, Roosevelt worked with a long-time friend and law partner, Basil O'Connor, to create the National Foundation of Infantile Paralysis. Housed in the Waldorf Astoria hotel in New York, the Foundation was a private endeavor, such that it was not financed by the government and was not affiliated with the PHS, although it obtained the full attention and support of Roosevelt.

Nevertheless, Roosevelt acted as if he ran the Foundation himself. He poured swaths of time and money into it. He also obtained the interest of other philanthropists donating thousands of dollars to the cause. Within two years, the Foundation surpassed in wealth any other philanthropic organization at the time, such as the National

Tuberculosis Association (founded in 1904), the National Society of Crippled Children (now known as the Easter Seal Society, founded in 1919), and the American Heart Association (formed in 1924) (Offit, 2005; Smith, 1990). Managed by skilled and dedicated workers, the Foundation was able to raise a lot of money: $1.8 million in donations by 1938, increasing to almost $3 million in 1941, $5 million in 1942, $6.5 million in 1943, over $12 million in 1944, and nearly $20 million in 1945 (Smith, 1990: 82). This was an astronomical amount of money for a newly created charity foundation.

Roosevelt's unwavering commitment to the Foundation motivated him to work closely with O'Connor on a host of initiatives. Within just a few years, they transformed the Foundation into a large, well-organized hierarchical organization, with a central office in New York and a host of regional offices scattered throughout the nation (Oshinsky, 2005).

But even prior to the Foundation's creation, Roosevelt had worked with O'Connor on several fund-raising campaigns, including the infamous presidential birthday balls, which raked in thousands of dollars (Oshinsky, 2005). Roosevelt and O'Connor also worked very closely with Hollywood. Roosevelt's friend, Eddie Cantor, was a famous movie star and used his cinematic influence to persuade moviegoers to donate one dime to the Foundation's campaign. This gave birth to the March of Dimes, which exists to this day. The March of Dimes did a brilliant job of raising awareness, instigating fear and awareness, while broadcasting their message through radio announcements and publications in order to inspire Americans to work together in fighting the good fight (Wilson, 1990). March of Dimes posters were found in a host of magazines and billboards, serving to spark a spirit of patriotism and militancy to fight for the children, to protect them from the deadly polio virus.

The Foundation also helped to provide medical treatment and to fund bio-medical research and innovation. It stood as a model for what philanthropic organizations could achieve. In addition to working with local volunteer communities (many of which were women's clubs) in order to provide treatment services to polio victims (Wilson, 1990), the Foundation became the largest grantee for polio research, far surpassing the NIH's budget. In fact, it was the Foundation that ended up financing Dr. Jonas Salk's research and discovery of the polio vaccine in 1957 (Oshinsky, 2005).

Roosevelt's personal experience with polio therefore motivated him to create a unique quasi-governmental response to the epidemic. The Foundation had become so popular and influential that citizens began to view it as a government institution, giving it the "unquestionable approval usually reserved for motherhood and the flag" (Smith, 1990: 64). Although the Foundation was not an official government agency, it certainly behaved as one. For no other national initiative bore as big a Roosevelt fingerprint, his direction and guidance. Roosevelt's personal conviction provided the political, financial, and popular support needed to strengthen the plight against polio. However, Roosevelt soon realized that a centralized, state-guided response was much needed.

Roosevelt's personal interest in polio did more than create a new federal campaign; it also motivated him to provide recommendations to the general public. Roosevelt called on all family members to take on a more responsible approach to protecting themselves and their loved ones. Roosevelt, O'Connor, and their staff continuously reminded families that they were personally obligated to protect themselves and their children (Oshinsky, 2005; Rogers, 1992).

Civil society responds

During the first few years of the 1916 polio outbreak, the social health movements and initiatives that emerged in response were essentially divided. On one hand, the New Public Health Movement, comprised of medical doctors, scientists, and PHS officials, arose to propose the importance of cleanliness and sanitation as a preventative measure. Advocating a "germ theory" of polio's spread, this movement was focused on education and awareness, emphasizing that municipal governments, schools, businesses, and families should rid their inhabitants from dirt, filth, and the little black flies that carried the virus (Rogers, 1992). With regards to health policy, the New Public Health Movement emphasized giving PHS and municipal health officials the authority to impose quarantines and to sanitize public areas (Rogers, 1992). However, the movement had no interest in strengthening the PHS's direct involvement at the local level (Rogers, 1992). Instead, PHS officials sought to empower municipal health officials while the latter successfully pleaded with state and city governments to provide them with policymaking autonomy and funding (Rogers, 1992).

On the other hand, a social health movement and voluntary organizations comprised of parents, concerned citizens, and family members began to emerge. Their views and policy interests, however, conflicted with the New Public Health Movement's interests (Rogers, 1992). Instead of emphasizing quarantine and sanitation, these social movements and civic groups emphasized family responsibility in safeguarding their children, keeping them at home, cleaning their hands, diligently watching where they went and who they spent time with (Gould, 1995; Rogers, 1992). Families — especially mothers — took charge in forming voluntary community organizations to study polio and discuss how they should respond (Gould, 1995; Rogers, 1992). And even before Roosevelt became infected with polio, after 16 cases broke out in his small quaint town of Oyster Bay, New York, he proposed and worked closely with municipal council members to establish the Committee of 21, which looked into the matter and took preventative measures (Gould, 1995). The Committee of 21 was soon joined by yet another voluntary group in the same community, the Committee for the Suppression of Infantile Paralysis, which was mainly composed of Italian and Polish immigrants. Research universities also created their own investigative committees, such as the Harvard Infantile Paralysis Commission, founded in 1916 (Gould, 1995). But these groups were not interested in the PHS's centralized policy intervention (Gould, 1995). Families were in fact suspicious of the PHS and the New Public Health Movement's emphasis on germ theory, sanitation, and bacterial science (Gould, 1995). Through their respective committees, families preferred to respond on their own; for they believed that their loving kindness and commitment to safeguarding their children was the best defense against polio.

Complicating matters further was the fact that the PHS was also far from interested in either creating an agency subdivision focused exclusively on polio or increasing funding to the states. The most assistance that the PHS provided during this period was to dispatch scores of PHS field agents to New York and other cities in order to facilitate the imposition of quarantines (Rogers, 1992). Believing that it was European immigrants living in congested urban centers that spread the virus (Rogers, 1992), PHS field agents worked closely with local health officials to quarantine this group. Additionally, the PHS seemed to ignore policy ideas and requests put forward by the citizens. Rogers (1992) documents scores of letters from concerned family members and volunteer groups that were *rejected* by PHS officials. This reinforced the suggestion that the PHS had no interest in forming a close partnership with civil society.

Two problems therefore emerged during the polio epidemic. First, there was no well-organized effort by social health movements to propose the idea and advocate for a centralized PHS response. Second, no partnership in response to polio ever emerged between PHS officials and civil society. Social health movements and foundations wrestled with the disease on their own, mainly by way of funding and experimenting with vaccines (Rogers, 1992). The closest the government came to forging such a partnership was with the National Foundation. But even then, it was Roosevelt's presence that represented the government, not the PHS.

Contesting malnutrition (1900–1947)

Perhaps the best precursor to the obesity epidemic of the 21st century was the early 20th century response to malnutrition. The US's first encounter with this epidemic occurred during the early 1900s. During this period, food shortages and malnutrition posed a serious public health threat. While obesity was also an issue (Stearns, 1997), though mainly among the affluent classes and new immigrants crafting fatty menus (the Italians, for example, where well known for their smoky sausages, soups, and pastas), malnutrition was most problematic among the urban poor. Lovett (2005) writes that during this period, New York's health department became increasingly concerned about how it would respond to child malnourishment, which was estimated to be 23% in 1906 (Levitt, 2005; Spargo, 1906). Food shortages and redistribution posed yet another challenge. In response, the government asked families to cut back on the consumption of scarce foods, such as flour, meat, sugar, and butter (McIntosh, 1995). But despite the federal government's awareness of the problem, it did not immediately respond, either through the creation of new federal agencies, the strengthening of existing ones, or the provision of financial and technical assistance to the states (McIntosh, 1995).

There was a good reason for this: among politicians and bureaucrats, malnutrition was a highly contested epidemic. Most politicians and presidents, up through Roosevelt, as well as PHS bureaucrats did not believe that there was credible statistical evidence alluding to a serious national health threat (Levenstein, 1993). The main problem was that there was a lack of consensus on how malnutrition was being defined and measured; because of this, a dearth of accurate and reliable statistical data emerged (Levenstein, 1993). Levenstein (1993) writes that this federal perception emerged even when politicians knew that there was an ongoing malnutrition problem, especially in large cities and the rural south.

This is not to say that the entire government was apathetic towards the issue. Prior to the First World War, the US Department of Agriculture and the US Children's Bureau argued that malnutrition was a serious problem and that the government should respond (Lovett, 2005); these agencies were in fact quite proactive in helping organize health clinics while disseminating information about malnutrition, mainly through educational pamphlets and films on children's health (Lovett, 2005). In response to food shortages and a sudden rise in prices for milk and dairy, the Senate also called for the provision of subsidies for milk and other food products, including relief measures such as cooperatives, subsidized stores, public kitchens, and school lunch programs (Levenstein, 1993; Lovett, 2005). And finally, during the Second World War, even Roosevelt's secretary of labor, Francis Perkins, insisted that Roosevelt respond through new federal programs, especially for children (Levenstein, 1993). However, Perkins' plea fell on deaf ears (Levenstein, 1993).

Despite these efforts, prior to the First World War, the presidents, Congress, and the PHS had no interest in creating a federal agency — or even a bureaucratic subdivision — to address the growing malnutrition problem, nor were there any efforts to expand and strengthen the US Department of Agriculture (Levenstein, 2003b; Lovett, 2005). Moreover, there was no steady stream of funding to schools for healthy lunches (Lovett, 2005). The only organization working to provide these services was the Commonwealth Fund, which was a philanthropic organization financed by Standard Oil. But this did not occur until 1918 (Lovett, 2005). Until the 1930s, the Commonwealth Fund was the most proactive organization providing educational and technical assistance to the cities to combat malnutrition.

A centralized bureaucratic and policy response eventually emerged. But rather than being a product of political and civil society pressures, the impetus for reform lied in the government's perceived threat to one of the core aspects of US national security: military readiness.

In fact, the White House's first response to malnutrition emerged when in 1917 President Woodrow Wilson appointed Herbert Hoover, who later became US president, as the "Food Czar" of the National Food Administration (NFA). This was done in order to ensure that military soldiers were adequately nourished for the war in Europe, as well as providing food for the poor in several European nations (Levenstein, 1993). NFA was focused entirely on the war; however, when it came to meeting the needs of the urban poor, Presidents Wilson, Hoover, and even Roosevelt relied on local charities, such as the Commonwealth Fund and the Red Cross, as well as poorly funded and administered municipal health departments (Levenstein, 1993).

Furthermore, the only executive order issued in response to malnourishment was targeted at Hoover and the NFA: it mandated an increase in the NFA's autonomy and influence. Newly empowered, the NFA began to ask families to make, save, and donate food for hungry troops overseas (Levenstein, 1993; Lovett, 2005). In an effort to further encourage these efforts, in 1918 Hoover created the "Food Will Win the War Campaign." This campaign was explicitly designed to encourage families to ration food in order to donate food to US troops and starving families in Europe. Slogans such as "Meatless Mondays" and "Wheatless Wednesdays" were often used to encourage families to ration food for these purposes. In essence, the Food Will Win the War Campaign was designed to conjure up a sense of self-sacrifice and commitment, to generate a spirit of communitarianism, solidarity, and pride.

During the interwar period, however, the government's centralized response came to an abrupt end. In fact, from 1931–1934, federal assistance for those suffering from malnourishment, mainly in the form of grants in aid to local health departments, declined, as did local government spending for malnourishment and public health in general (Levenstein, 1993).

But once again, war prompted state building. The catchy phrase that Hoover proffered in 1917, i.e., "Food will win the war!," was used by the Farm Security and War Food Administration (WFA) during the Second World War. As in the past, this phrase was used to encourage farmers to produce and ration food in order to maintain a steady supply of rations for soldiers in Europe (Thomas, N/D). In 1941, in response to a record number 41% of enlistees rejected for military service due to malnutrition, the Food and Nutrition Board (FNB) of the National Research Council (NRC) was established to advise the government on better nutrition as it pertained to national defense. Military generals rallied to get Congress to pass new legislation that would enhance school lunch programs and to provide better nutrients for future enlistees (Levenstein, 1993; McIntosh, 1995). Charged by Roosevelt with the task of developing a set of dietary guidelines, the FNB developed the first set of recommended dietary allowances (RDAs) for the nation (McIntosh, 1995).

Next, in 1941 Roosevelt created the WFA. The WFA was responsible for convening experts and providing advice on the kinds of food soldiers should consume, as well as controlling food policy for Roosevelt's New Deal programs (Levenstein, 1993). Henceforth, any domestic initiative for food policy was driven by Roosevelt's concern for the war. For example, Roosevelt gave Paul McNutt, director of the Defense Health and Welfare Services (DHWS) agency, complete authority to expand the DHWS and to create a special division on nutrition, which served to further buttress the DHWS's needs (Levenstein, 1993).

While the government was focused on the war, non-governmental organizations (NGOs) were focused on better nutrition and food processing. There was a growing movement in society and the medical community in favor of regulating the food industry, specifically its content and advertising. This was viewed as important because it helped to potentially decrease the consumption of foods contributing to malnutrition. It was believed that if consumers knew the fat content of their foods, or its precise nutritional value, that they would choose foods that were more nutritious. Collectively pressuring the government for increased food processing and marketing regulations was perceived as an effective policy response.

These efforts nevertheless fell short of influencing the food industry, which was an oligopoly owned by manufacturers such as General Mills and Standard Brands. In 1911, spearheaded by Arthur Kallet and Frederick Schlink of the Consumers Research Inc., as well as other concerned citizens, a new social movement emerged to pressure senators for an amendment to the Food and Drug Act of 1906 (Levenstein, 1993). The goal was to increase the regulation on food additive processing. In response, the food corporations joined the United Medicine Manufacturers of America in organizing a powerful lobby against this proposed legislation. Among the provisions they found most objectionable was a proposal that false and misleading advertising be penalized (the 1906 Act banned only false labeling), something that would jeopardize their exaggerated health and nutritional claims.

Consumer Research Inc. and the growing social movement in favor of federal regulation never succeeded in countering this response. For, in addition to the food industry's strong partnership with a federal government in favor of increased food production for war purposes, even the American Medical Association (AMA) was supporting the food industry's plight to destroy this regulatory movement (Levenstein, 1993). While the passage of an amendment would eventually emerge several years later, this resistance foretold of future difficulties in the government's ability — or better yet, willingness — to increase its regulation of the food industry. As we will see in Chapter 5, this problem reemerged under the George W. Bush administration and its unwillingness to regulate the fast food industry in response to obesity.

Civil society responds

During the 1920s and 1930s, civil society's interest and policy recommendation for a centralized response to malnutrition never emerged. In fact, no well-organized group of NGOs or even social health movements arose to put forth the idea that the PHS should immediately intervene to address malnutrition (Levenstein, 1993; Schwartz, 1969). Motivated to work on their own and guided by the belief that they knew the best response and needs of malnourished groups, small charity organizations, volunteers, philanthropists, and Parent Teacher Associations (PTA) each did their part in providing food relief, nutritious foods, and dietary information (Levenstein, 1993). These groups were known to provide school lunches — though to a limited extent because of funding shortfalls (Levenstein, 1993). For example, a wealthy businessman in the city of Philadelphia set up the country's first free school breakfast program. But eventually, this program had to close down because of insufficient funding (Levenstein, 1993; Schwartz, 1969). Various civic organizations and charity groups also tried distributing food to the poor. These groups, as well as the media and private physician organizations, such as the Field Foundation, worked to draw public attention to malnourishment and hunger in the cities and the rural south (Eisinger, 1998).

All of these efforts were nevertheless done without any federal assistance, as federal and local government officials believed that giving away food surplus encouraged laziness and dependence on the government (Levenstein, 1993). And because malnutrition was perceived as a problem found mainly among the marginalized poor, the federal government during the 1930s had no interest in creating a national campaign to address the issue (Levenstein, 1993). Plagued by poor statistics and inadequate evidence, malnutrition was perceived by most federal officials as unworthy of a centralized response.

Angry farmers chimed in claiming that every pound of food given away equated to a loss of revenue. They worked with federal administrators to block proposals for a national food relief program (Levenstein, 1993). The Hoover administration's Department of Agriculture, and even its head under Roosevelt, Henry Wallace, as well as Harry Hopkins, director of federal relief programs (and a close friend of Roosevelt), instructed all administrators not to provide free food to the poor (Levenstein, 1993; Schwartz, 1969). Instead, they suggested monetary assistance in exchange for work (Levenstein, 1993). The only federal program that emerged to provide assistance was Roosevelt's Federal Surplus Relief Corporation in 1933, which handed out pork to families because of an overabundance of pigs and their wasteful disposal. The Corporation was managed by Harry Perkins, who was, however, strongly opposed to providing direct relief to the malnourished and unemployed (Levenstein, 1993). As a result, the Corporation was poorly managed and was soon shut down (Levenstein, 1993).

The upshot to this response from civil society and the government to malnutrition was that no partnership ever emerged between them for a centralized response. Civil society never proposed any ideas for a centralized response to malnutrition, while the government was only interested in centralization when it threatened national security. Similar to what we saw with polio, then, no civic supporters ever emerged for malnutrition — an outcome that failed to provide advantageous precedents for future public health officials.

Brazil

Contesting TB (1900–1945)

A product of urbanization and increased immigration, TB emerged as a major health problem in Brazil's largest cities during the early 20th century. However, TB's emergence did not elicit an immediate government response, as policymakers believed that it did not pose a serious national threat. In contrast to diseases such as yellow fever, malaria, samparo, and syphilis, TB was not riddled throughout the nation (Antunes *et al.*, 2000; Nascimento, 1997; Nascimento, 1991). It was instead concentrated in tightly congested urban centers, such as in the cities of Rio de Janeiro and São Paulo.

During this period the government confronted a myriad of public health threats (Nascimento, 1991). This convinced presidents and senior health officials that TB should not receive special attention. Notwithstanding the fact that TB was spreading at a faster rate and killing more people in major cities, and despite ongoing pressures from public health officials to respond immediately, government officials were still not convinced that TB warranted immediate federal attention (Nascimento, 1991).

Rather than expanding the DGSP in response to TB, Presidents Afonso Pena (1906–1909) and Nilo Peçanha (1909–1910) issued several national decrees requiring the increased sanitation of municipalities (Netto and Pereira, 1991). Led by mayors, such as Pereira Passos, the mayor of Rio (who was an engineer by training), and medical doctors such as Dr. Oswaldo Cruz, then director of the DGSP, from 1890 to 1910 Presidents Pena and Peçanha mandated the cleanup of Rio's cities, port areas, and housing (Netto and Pereira, 1991). From 1876 to 1886, five decrees were issued as well as a ministerial suggestion (known as *avisos*) for the DGSP sanitary police (Netto and Pereira, 1991).

What is even more alarming is that government inattentiveness emerged at a time when pressures from civil society for a response reached an apogee. From 1870 to the 1920s, at the height of the TB epidemic (Antunes and Waldman, 1999), a host of influential medical and intellectual elites arose to educate the government and civil society about the importance of responding to TB. On June 4, 1900, medical elites and intellectuals in Rio and São Paulo formed the Liga contra a Tuberculose (the Leagues against Tuberculosis, henceforth, Liga) in order to increase public awareness about the epidemic while providing treatment services through the creation of several health sanitariums (Filho, 2001; Nascimento, 1991). These Liga also worked closely with the Santa Casa de Misericórdia, which were lay Catholic brotherhood organizations (spanning back to conquest in the 1500s) that were the first to provide housing and treatment for the poor suffering from TB and other diseases. The Liga were thus the first and only responders to TB at the height of the epidemic (Filho, 2001; Nascimento, 1991).

During this period the Liga were also closely aligned with a burgeoning global health movement seeking a more aggressive response to TB. In 1900, Liga members started attending international conferences in Europe and even organized an international conference in

Rio, such as the X Congresso Internacional de Higine e Demografica (International Conference for Hygiene and Demography). Liga members started educating the government about the successful efforts of western European nations in combating TB through the centralized expansion of the public health bureaucracy and increased intervention at the state level (Nascimento, 1991). The Liga started emulating prevention and treatment programs in western Europe, while highlighting the fact that these nations also had civic organizations committed to combating TB (Ribeiro, 1956). Alluding to experiences in western Europe was done in order to convince presidents and Congress that they should emulate Europe's (especially Scandinavia's) centralized approach to TB control, rather than relying on decentralization and the work of Liga members and charity institutions (Nascimento, 1991). Through these initiatives, Liga members were also able to inform the international health community of their unwavering commitment to eradicating the epidemic while at the same time pressuring the government to respond through aggressive centralized reforms (Filho, 2001; Nascimento, 2005).

In addition, through these initiatives the Liga increased their popularity and legitimacy within government and society. Their reputation further increased when the Liga started organizing several conferences, public lectures, and the publication of their findings in several conference proceedings (Nascimento, 1997; 2005). The Liga community quickly emerged as an ally and resource for those public health bureaucrats agreeing with them on the need to strengthen the national government's response to TB.

But even this was not enough. Despite their reputation, between 1900 and 1920 the Liga still proved incapable of convincing presidents and Congress to intervene. Even the government's most prized medical doctor, urban engineer, and director of the national public health program, Dr. Oswaldo Cruz, could not influence the government's position. Cruz was closely aligned with the Liga movement and worked with them to pressure the government for a centralized response (Nascimento, 1997, 2005). In 1906, realizing that TB was now the largest killer in Rio and in São Paulo, Cruz proposed the construction of a new federal agency within the DGSP committed to combating the epidemic (Nascimento, 2005). The agency was to centralize all aspects of TB prevention and treatment, thereby ending the overburdened, underpaid work of the Santa Casas and the Liga. But the government completely ignored Cruz's request (Nascimento, 1997; 2005).

In an effort to placate Cruz and the Liga movement, the president appointed a highly experienced epidemiologist to the DGSP, Dr. Carlos Seidle. Seidle was chosen for his extensive experience with TB research and commitment to finding a cure (Nascimento, 1991, 1997). He was also a well-known academic and maintained a close relationship with university intellectuals and Liga members.

However, the appointment of Seidle instigated even more bureaucratic and Liga pressures for the creation of a federal response to TB. In an effort to quell growing opposition and to address what was, by then, an obvious public health problem, the government finally responded. In 1920, President Epitácio Lindolfo da Silva Pessoa authorized the creation of the Inspectoria de Profilia da Tuberculose in the city of Rio de Janeiro — then the nation's capital. This was the first federal agency ever created in response to TB (Hijjar *et al.*, 2007). The agency was responsible for working with municipal health departments for greater TB prevention (mainly through education) and treatment services.

However, it quickly became apparent that the Inspectoria was inefficient and incapable of adequately responding to TB (Antunes *et al.*, 2000). It lacked the resources, manpower, and above all, the president and Congress' ongoing attention and support (Antunes *et al.*, 1999). In essence, the Inspectoria appeared to be a cosmetic institution; that is, it was intended to look good, and to placate the interests of civil society and the bureaucracy rather than effectively intervene at the local level. As we will soon see with the more recent resurgence of TB in Chapter 6, as well as AIDS in Chapter 4, the government would initially respond to these epidemics in a similar manner.

It took a brief period of isolation from the international community, the emergence of TB's threat to the national security, followed shortly thereafter by Brazil's reintegration into world politics to elicit an effective centralized response to TB. This response began to emerge with the arrival of President Getúlio Vargas in 1930. A charismatic politician unwaveringly committed to transforming Brazil into a modern state, Vargas was genuinely concerned with the TB problem as well as any other health issues potentially thwarting economic development and national security (McCann, 2006). Like other nations at the time, this was a period of government isolation from the international community. The isolationist Vargas was also committed to creating a government that was more centralized in nature and autonomous from the regional political forces that he accused of paralyzing the government during the First Republic. During his first few years in office, his centralized approach to TB also reflected his broader commitment to state building as a means to enhanced policy effectiveness.

During the 1930s, Vargas' concern with national security and development motivated him to implement a series of bureaucratic reforms ensuring a more rapid response to TB. Soon after entering office, Vargas worked with the DGSP to establish hundreds of sanitarian outposts (Vargas, 1938). His commitment to doing this and funding prevention and treatment programs increased after 1938 when he instituted the Estado do Novo (The New State; Vargas, 1938). Vargas believed that unless TB was controlled by the federal bureaucracy, the disease would undermine the labor force and harm the economy.

Vargas' subsequent reintegration into the international community, mainly by way of his active participation as an ally in the Second World War, motivated him to become more concerned about his international partnerships and reputation. Through his active involvement in foreign military campaigns, Vargas positioned Brazil as an emerging nation with international military, political, and economic clout. Vargas' interest in enhancing Brazil's international reputation as a nation that could simultaneously develop the economy and eradicate disease also increased during this period (Gómez, 2008). His concern with Brazil's international reputation had a positive influence on his perceived need to strengthen Brazil's public health institutions (Gómez, 2008).

As the leader of an emerging and influential nation, Vargas was very attentive and responsive to any international criticisms of Brazil's response to TB and healthcare in general. In addition to receiving criticisms from western Europe and the Liga movement, Vargas also received them from the US. In 1941, for example, he was criticized by a famous American hygienist, Dr. Charles Wilson, for having a "backwards" healthcare system and for Vargas' repeated inability to successfully respond to TB. Wilson would go on to claim that the US was outpacing Brazil in its response to TB (Filho, 2004). This incensed Vargas beyond measure (Filho, 2004). Though upset, Vargas accepted these criticisms and used them as a new opportunity to pursue a more aggressive, centralized response.

First, in 1941, Vargas created an agency whose sole purpose was to monitor and respond to TB: that is, the Servicio Nacional de Tuberculoses (SNT), which was housed within the MESP. Next, in 1946 Vargas created a new federal campaign to eradicate TB, the Campanha Nacional contra Tuberculoses (CNCT). Falling under the purview of the SNT, the CNCT initiative was highly autonomous and had ample resources; in fact, it was often referred to as a "great wonder" and excellent example of federal intervention in public health (Hijjar *et al.*, 2007). The CNCT created an aggressive vertical program for TB prevention and treatment. The CNCT established medical sanitarium posts throughout the cities and countryside (Hijjar *et al.*, 2007). In contrast to his presidential predecessors, Vargas wanted to ensure that his government could effectively monitor and manage every aspect of TB policy. Moreover, the increased centralization of administrative authority for public health was a bold move at the time, since it completely abolished the government's prior decision in 1926 to give the city of São Paulo complete control over all aspects of healthcare policy (Filho, 2001; Hijjar *et al.*, 2007). (At the time, São Paulo was the only city allowed to govern its own healthcare system.)

The CNCT marked the birth of Brazil's first national TB program. Under subsequent democratic and military regimes, it continued to grow and at one point usurped approximately 50% of the total public health budget (Santos Filho, 2006). It also benefited from garnering multiple sources of revenue, mainly from the Ministry of Health and the Ministry of Education, while receiving contributions from several governors (Ruffino-Netto and Figueiredo de Souza, 2001). While the CNCT continued to expand under the military, the last few years of military authoritarian rule (1974–1985) saw a gradual devolution of healthcare administration and policy to the states, followed by a hasty devolution of health policy responsibility to the municipalities in 1988. By 1990, and as I discuss in Chapter 6, in the absence of pressures from civil society and the Ministry of Health's interest in maintaining a centralized response, the national TB program was completely dismantled. It was supplanted with the decentralized SUS program (Sistema Única de Saúde), introducing new administrative inefficiencies and a lack of government responsiveness with the resurgence of TB in the 1980s.

And finally, although there was a new social health movement, the Liga Contra a Tuberculose, which unified doctors, intellectuals, and activists, the Liga' pressures, as well as its close partnership with public health officials, was not the key factor motivating Vargas to engage in an effective centralized response. In fact, with the eventual discovery of a cure for TB through the introduction of chemotheretic treatment by the 1950s, the Liga movement eventually died out. Especially as the number of TB cases rapidly declined due to advances in medicine and living standards improved — brought about mainly through import substitution industrialization of the 1960s and 1970s — medical and intellectual elites lost their interest in helping sustain the Liga movement. As we will see in Chapter 6, the end result is that, in contrast to what we will see in Chapter 4 with the government's response to AIDS, the resurgence of TB did not benefit from an enduring social health movement that was well equipped and motivated to immediately fight for the needs of those afflicted by TB — mainly the poor.

Civil society responds

Although the partnership between the Liga, public health officials, and their calls for reform did not lead to an immediate centralized response, two advantageous precedents emerged from this partnership that would have long-run positive implications for public health officials. First, these efforts established a bureaucratic tradition of working in close partnership with social health movements whenever new epidemics emerged — unlike what we saw in the US. By establishing partnerships with social health movements based on similar policy ideas and beliefs in a centralized response to epidemics, bureaucrats were able to establish a tradition of working closely with these movements in order to amplify their legitimacy and influence.

This partnership between bureaucrats and civil society was solidified through the sharing of the following policy ideas: (1) that the government should immediately intervene and provide healthcare treatment to all citizens in periods of health crisis; (2) that the government should build new federal agencies to facilitate intervention through increased resources and technical expertise to the states; and (3) that the government should provide universal prevention and treatment services. Wedded through similar policy ideas and beliefs in a centralized bureaucratic and policy response to epidemics, this partnership provided future health officials with the civic supporters needed to strengthen their legitimacy and influence when seeking a centralized response to epidemics.

Finally, these historic partnerships established a precedent for future health officials: that they should work closely with social health movements and NGOs in order to increase their legitimacy, influence, and ability to effectively respond. This is especially the case when social health movements and NGOs have ties to the international community and as a result are perceived as legitimate and influential at both domestic and international levels.

The United States

Contesting syphilis

As with polio and malnutrition, during the early 20th century the US was also delayed in its response to sexually transmitted diseases (STDs), such as syphilis. Despite the fast-paced growth of syphilis cases throughout the nation, the president, Congress, and the PHS failed to respond, relying instead on a decentralized approach to containing the epidemic. In so doing, and as mentioned earlier, the government was adhering to its preexisting commitment to creating a decentralized approach to public health, which began with the creation of the US PHS in 1912.

But, as the number of rejected applicants for military enlistment began to increase due to syphilis, the government began to perceive the situation differently. Any stigma and discrimination within government towards those with syphilis was quickly supplanted with a purely medical, scientific point of view. Cutler and Arnold (2000: p. 496) claim that "at the outset of World War I, when VD [venereal disease] was a leading cause of incapacitation or rejection for active duty, public concern was sufficient to override the previous moralistic judgmental inhibitions against VD control efforts." Because this essentially meant a potentially rapid decline in the number of enlistees capable of fighting in Europe, the president and Congress began to realize that it needed to respond by creating new federal agencies and programs. It was only under these circumstances that the government began to draw up and implement plans for centralized intervention while providing a steady flow of financial and technical resources to the states (Brown, 1970; Ness, 1942).

Ness (1942) writes that during the First World War the president, the Congress, the secretary of war, and social health movements agreed that they should start working together to create new federal agencies and programs in response to syphilis (Ness, 1942). They also agreed to provide funding to the states, going so far as to provide support for sex education programs.

As Table 1.1 illustrates, a brief review of the number of congressional acts and federal programs enacted by Congress during the two world wars lends credence to the notion that the government's response was primarily influenced by national security concerns.

For example, in 1918 Congress responded to syphilis with the passage of the Chamberlin–Kahn Act, also known as the Army Appropriation Act of 1918, which mandated the creation of the Division of Venereal Diseases (DVD) within the US PHS. The fear that STDs would spread among enlistees on US bases, and thus undermine the military's readiness capabilities, prompted the provision of approximately $2 million to the PHS work with state health departments in order to curb the spread of this "social disease" (Mullan, 1989). In an effort to reduce the number of enlistees infected with syphilis, the Chamberlin–Kahn Act also authorized the allocation of direct grants in aid to those states committed to implementing anti-VD programs.

Table 1.1   US Congressional acts and government programs in response to syphilis

Year	Congressional acts and programs
1918	*Chamberlin–Kahn Act*
	Act creates the Division of Venereal Diseases in the US PHS; it provides information about the maintenance and upkeep of syphilis programs at the state level; it also provides grants to the states for syphilis control. In addition to controlling the spread of syphilis, this Act was introduced in order to reduce the number of infected enlistees into the military.
1918	*US Inter-Departmental Hygiene Board*
	This was an educational campaign against syphilis and other VDs; Congress provides grants to universities to conduct VD research and teaching.
1937	*National Venereal Diseases Control Act*
	Federal and state authorities map out a plan of attack against VD; Congress provides funds for medical and public health attack; this Act also provides money to the states for syphilis and other VD control.
1938	*La Follett–Bulwinkle Bill (Congressional Act)*
	Congressional funds provided to the states; expansion of Division of Venereal Diseases of the PHS to improve research, treatment schedules, patient follow up, record keeping, and program analysis.
1939	*Eight Point Agreement Program*
	Program where the Department of War and Navy and the Federal Security Agency work in close cooperation with the PHS to monitor syphilis' spread while prohibiting prostitution activities near military bases.
1940	*Social Protection Program, Defense Health and Welfare Services of the Federal Security Agency*
	Program created 24 field officers throughout the country to work with other agencies, such as law enforcement, public assistance, recreation, child protection, and health agencies to monitor syphilis; program entailed repression of commercial prostitution in order to protect soldiers; provision of social services and treatment for prostitutes; 24 field agents also worked with local governments to enforce these policies.
1941	*May Act*
	Made prostitution illegal near military bases.
1952	*Speed-Zone Epidemiology*
	First major federal campaign to control gonorrhea spread. Through this initiative, the PHS worked closely with the states and urban health departments.

Source: My own calculations based on several sources.

Furthermore, in 1918 Congress created the US Inter-Departmental Hygiene Board. The Board's responsibility was to distribute sex education pamphlets, create anti-VD placards and even use the movie industry to increase public awareness about syphilis (Brown, 1970). And in 1919, Congress appropriated $200,000 for administrative expansion and $400,000 to the Inter-Departmental Social Hygiene Board for medical research (Parran, 1937).

For the first time, the PHS, through the DVD, also provided financial and technical assistance to the states. As Culter and Arnold (2000) maintain: "Because of the overriding concerns with the war effort it was possible under the leadership of the US PHS in 1917 to initiate a cooperative control program among state and local health departments and the private sector, including medical practitioners, the hospital system, and voluntary agencies." One example of the PHS's assistance to the states came in 1918, when it provided an estimated $1 million in grant assistance to the states (*Science Illustrated*, 1949). The DVD also dispatched 24 PHS agents to work with the governors in order to ensure that their programs were being effectively implemented (Parran, 1937).

The center's aggressive response soon led to policy diffusion throughout the states. By 1920, 88 laws were enacted by 35 states in order to increase prevention and treatment for syphilis. In essence there quickly emerged a sub-national commitment to combating syphilis (Lock, 1939).

But what the federal government did shortly after the First World War provides even further credence to the notion that national security was its primary concern (Brandt, 1985; Ness, 1942; Parran, 1937; Thompson, 1987). Shortly after the war ended, the president authorized Congress to withdraw its support for the DVD (Brandt, 1985; Mullan, 1989; Ness, 1942). The government no longer viewed syphilis as a national security threat and therefore had no incentive to sustain DVD programs (Lock, 1939). Furthermore, shortly after the war, Brandt (1985) claims that Congress also decided not to reauthorize funding for the US Inter-Departmental Hygiene Board. This sent a clear message that in the absence of a national security threat, the government no longer prioritized about the ongoing syphilis problem (Brandt, 1985).

After the First World War, Congress also stopped providing financial assistance to the states. By 1935, the Chamberlin–Kahn Act was terminated. Congress went from allocating $1 million in 1918, to $100,000 in 1921, then to a meager $58,000 by 1936 (*Science Illustrated*, 1949). This downsize in federal funding was attributed to the "return to normalcy," mainly because the national security threat was gone and the government no longer felt compelled to help state and local governments respond to syphilis (*Science Illustrated*, 1949). This reduction in government spending for programs coupled with a rapid decline in financial aid to the states generated fewer incentives for local governments to maintain their anti-VD programs (Parran, 1936).

Reinforcing Congress' decision to stop funding syphilis and other VD programs was the change in the general mode of the people after the First World War. As some scholars note, there emerged a sudden disinterest in syphilis, and consequently apathy towards the disease and its programs:

> A change in the attitude of the people was observed with the return of the troops after World War I. This change was reflected in Congress. Once the Versailles Treaty was signed the people of the United States assumed that Germans had been beaten for all time. When the U.S. Army was demobilized a similar assumption was made regarding the defeat of the spirochete and the gonococcus, and the VD problem was forgotten. In the third year of existence of the new Division of Venereal Diseases, the grant-in-aid program dwindled to $1,000,000 and thereafter was discontinued altogether. The activities of the Public Health Service in venereal disease control were reduced to research investigations. Venereal disease control was in the doldrums and remained there for about fifteen years. (Vonderlehr and Heller, 1946: 5–8; quote taken from Cutler and Arnold, 2000: 497).

The end of the federal campaign instigated a flurry of criticisms. Most of these criticisms did not come from society, but from the

PHS. PHS officials emerging from progressive schools of thought took a more secular, professional approach to STDs. They did not attribute STDs to race or class. Instead, they viewed diseases such as syphilis through a purely scientific lens and, more importantly, as a national threat worthy of an immediate government response. These bureaucrats did not care about war; they cared about people.

Such views were harbored by perhaps the biggest proponent for a centralized bureaucratic and policy response to syphilis: Surgeon General Thomas G. Parran (1936–1948). A medical doctor by training, Parran was the only political appointee to critique the government's short-term centralized response to syphilis. Serving as surgeon general during the First World War, Parran criticized the government for failing to maintain its VD propaganda campaign (through the US Inter-Departmental Hygiene Board) and various educational campaigns implemented during the two world wars. Often disliked for his candid, somewhat brusque criticism of Roosevelt's policies, Parran published his views in a book that he wrote while serving as surgeon general entitled *Shadow on the Land: Syphilis*:

> For the country as a whole we have carried on guerilla warfare against syphilis, with spirited skirmishes and valiant forays in some of the states which sow casualties to their credit. There never has been a coordinated drive against it by all the states, with the exception of the wartime effort which died a-borning. It is for this reason, I believe, that there is no evidence to be found of a general decline in the attack rate of syphilis for the country as a whole. We have indications of improvement, but they are few and scattering. Nowhere here can be seen the dramatic reversal of trend of the Scandinavian countries in which as the result of long continued, popularly supported government action, syphilis has become a rare disease. ... Unfortunately, the enthusiasm that had gone up like a rocket [i.e., for a national, centralized response to syphilis] came down like a stick. The national spirit swung like a pendulum from "anything to win the war" to aversion for the war status. Discipline was replaced by the license of the roaring twenties. President Hardin's phrase "getting back to normalcy" was the excuse for dumping useful effort and bureaucratic regimentation on the same

rubbish heap. Congress apparently thought the spirochetes of syphilis were 'demobilized' with the army. More accurately, no further thought whatever was given to syphilis, and this first national public health effort came to an untimely end (Parran, 1937: p. 67 and p. 85).

It is evident from these writings that Parran believed that Roosevelt should not have stopped building the DVD, nor should he have decreased the amount of money going to the states. While in office Parran held firm to his belief that syphilis was a serious national health threat, and that as such the federal government needed to sustain its centralized response (Mullan, 1989). In fact, in *Shadow on the Land*, Parran wrote two chapters comparing the US's response to syphilis to the Scandinavian states' successful centralized response. He praised Scandinavia's ongoing commitment to strengthening their national public health administration, national anti-VD programs and their unwavering commitment to financing state and local government policies. Parran struck this comparison in order to accentuate the problems that the US government had in maintaining its commitment to reform — in a similar vein, I have compared the US to Brazil for this very reason.

Parran also worked closely with stigmatized groups in society. Noticing that the black community, especially in the south, had the largest number of syphilis cases as well as inadequate medical attention, Parran began to work closely with these communities and philanthropies to increase sex education and medical treatment. For example, he worked with the Julius Rosenwald Fund in Mississippi, a philanthropic organization concerned with the health of African Americans, in order to co-sponsor several new projects increasing the capacity of municipal hospitals to treat syphilis patients and to provide them with educational materials (Mullan, 1989). Jones (1981) also notes that Parran strove to strengthen the Julius Rosenwald Fund's partnership with the PHS. Parran was also committed to increasing the recruitment of African Americans into the medical and nursing profession, an initiative that the Julius Rosenwald Fund was already committed to.

By the mid-1930s, civil society also began to increase its interest and response to syphilis. Parran's efforts to transform syphilis into a national issue helped to kindle society's interest in centralized government intervention (Locke, 1939). According to Locke (1939), a gallop poll[2] taken in 1939 revealed that most citizens were in favor of increased federal assistance in containing the spread of syphilis. Society's awareness was aided by the media's heightened attention to the issue. Brown (1970) maintains that in 1935, there were only five newspaper articles written about syphilis in *The New York Times*, within the next five years, this count rose to 255 (Brown, 1970).

Notwithstanding Parran's ongoing efforts to convince the government of maintaining its centralized response, his policy suggestions ultimately fell on deaf ears. Even Roosevelt, generally considered to be liberal, began to complain about Parran's bickering in his book, *Shadow on the Land* (Brandt, 1985: p. 163). At one point, Roosevelt stated that: "If the Surgeon General of the Army or the Surgeon General of the Navy [referring to Parran] had written this book before taking all prior steps called for, he would have been liable to immediate court martial" (Roosevelt quoted in Brandt, 1985: p. 163). Parran's superior, Paul McNutt, director of the Federal Security Agency, upon considering Parran's recommendations for a centralized response, took sides with Roosevelt, claiming that: "There will be no repetition of such unethical and untactful procedure" (McNutt quoted in Brandt, 1985: p. 163). Parran quickly found himself making more enemies than friends.

Nevertheless, in 1935, thanks in part to Parran's criticisms and the broader realization within government that something needed to be done, Title VI of the Social Security Act of 1935 authorized $8 million in grants-in-aid to state health departments for its VD programs,

---

[2] A gallop poll survey at the time indicated that civil society was in favor of government intervention for VD control. The questions and answers were as follows: "Are you in favor of the PHS distributing information concerning VD's spread? 90 yes, 10 no. Should the PHS set up clinics for the treatment of VD? 88 yes, 12 no. Should Congress appropriate $25,000,000 to help control VD? 79 yes, 21 no. In strict confidence and at no expense to you, would you like to be given by your physician a blood test for syphilis? 87 yes, 13 no. Would you favor a law requiring doctors to give every expectant mother a blood test for syphilis? 88 yes, 12 no. Do you think Congress should appropriate money to aid states in fighting VD? 86 yes, 14 no. Would you be willing to pay higher taxes for this purpose? 69 yes, 31 no." (Brown, 1970).

as well as $2 million a year for scientific research (Cutler and Arnold, 2000). And, in 1937, Roosevelt and Congress agreed to create the National Venereal Control Act. This marked yet another step in the government's centralized response to syphilis, a commitment that was nevertheless instigated by syphilis' threat to national security. Through the National Venereal Control Act, federal and state governments agreed to map out a new plan for responding to syphilis, while Congress agreed to allocate more money to the states (Brandt, 1985; Etheridge, 1992). However, this was only a prelude to the massive state building that occurred during the Second World War, which further revealed the government's primary interest: safeguarding military readiness.

Indeed, as Cutler and Arnold (2000: 501) note: "The entry of the US into WWII had served as a catalyst to the national [VD] program, again because of the high rates of rejection of draftees due to syphilis and because of the high rates of absence from duty of military manpower resulting from syphilis and gonorrhea." Medical doctors and the social hygiene movement alluded to studies indicating that many of the new army enlistees were testing positive for primary and secondary syphilis. By 1940, the army absorbed 98.9% of all the military selectees (across all service branches) with syphilis and other venereal diseases (Cutler and Arnold, 2000). Approximately 0.25 of all black enlistees had syphilis, while only 1.7 white enlistees were infected (Cutler and Arnold, 2000). Once again, syphilis had emerged to threaten the national security (Ness, 1942). And once again, the government responded with a flurry of centralized bureaucratic and policy reforms.

First, in 1939, and building on the 1937 National Venereal Disease Control Act, the president and Congress agreed to create the Eight Point Agreement Plan. Under this plan, a new phase of inter-agency cooperation emerged between the Department of the War, Department of the Navy, the Federal Security Agency and the US PHS in order to increase centralized surveillance and response to syphilis and other venereal diseases near military camps (Ness, 1942). Through this plan, moreover, prostitution was prohibited near military compounds.

Any prostitutes found in the area were either imprisoned or confined to Rapid Treatment Centers for one to two weeks (Brown, 1970).

At the same time, in 1939 Congress passed the La Follett–Bulwinkle Bill. Through this bill, the Congress restarted its financial assistance to the states in order to increase medical research and treatment for syphilis. Scores of PHS personnel were also sent to state and local health departments in order to make sure that there was an adequate level of human resources — doctors and nurses — for syphilis and VD programs (Cutler and Arnold, 2000). The PHS also made plans to work through the Conference of State and Territorial Health Officers for a nationwide program protecting national wellbeing and health (Cutler and Arnold, 2000). Furthermore, and similar to what occurred with the Chamberlin–Kahn Act of 1918, the La Follett–Bulwinkle bill authorized an increase in budgetary outlays for the expansion of the DVD within the PHS. And two years later, in 1941, Congress created the May Act of 1941. The May Act added to the Eight Point Agreement Plan by making it illegal to engage in prostitution activities near military bases. Moreover, through this Act the federal government required that local police monitor and enforce the law, though many, including Parran, believed that it was never effectively enforced (Brandt, 1985).

The government, through the Federal Security Agency, also created the Social Protection Program. Through this program the Federal Security Agency created over 20 federal security field agents assigned to working with a myriad of state and municipal social welfare agencies to monitor prostitution activity and where necessary, invoke the May Act. The program sought to enforce the government's commitment to regulating prostitution and working with local officials to imprison prostitutes and provide medical treatment. In essence, it was an effort by the Federal Security Administration to enforce the May Act and to ensure that local governments were in full compliance.

Thus, as we saw during the First World War, syphilis' threat to the national security generated a heightened interest and commitment to engaging in a centralized bureaucratic and policy response. Cutler and Arnold (2000: 502) capture these circumstances nicely: "World War II brought about national recognition of the adverse effects of

VD, particularly syphilis, and permitted the plans that leaders such as Parran and others had developed to be realized."

Civil society responds

During the non-war periods, in contrast to what we saw with the response to polio and malnutrition, civil society responded and worked with the PHS in putting forth the idea of the federal government creating federal programs and providing assistance to the states. Private philanthropists, such as the Julius Rosenwald Fund and the Rockefeller Foundation, were major proponents of creating federal programs and funding to combat syphilis at the local level (Jones, 1981; McBride, 1991). At the same time, social health movements, such as the Booker T. Washington National Coalition for Black Health Awareness, formed in 1910 and, through their sponsorship of the Black Health Improvement Week, began to work with PHS officials to construct a partnership pressuring the PHS for financial and technical assistance (Jones, 1981; McBride, 1991). As Jones (1981: 35) puts it: "During the 1920s, the Public Health Service became the movement's [i.e., Booker T. Washington Coalition's] working arm, and financial backing came from the Juilus Rosenwald Fund ..." By the 1920s, the PHS entered into a partnership with these philanthropists and social health movements in order to pressure the federal government for a centralized response, one based on progressive principles of science and education (Jones, 1981). Despite these efforts, as long as the president and Congress' interests were fixated on national security, the PHS and civil society's efforts would not be influential.

In contrast, the policy ideas, and bureaucratic and civil society partnerships that were most successful were those that focused on national security during the two world wars. In fact, when it came to convincing the president and Congress that syphilis posed a direct threat to national security via challenges to military enlistment, a strong, cooperative partnership emerged between high-ranking officials in the Department of War and the military, on one hand, and the social hygienists and physicians in society, on the other (Jones, 1981). The social hygienists emerged during the late 19th century, during the progressive era, and were comprised of doctors, scientists, intellectuals, clergymen, educators, lawyers, social workers, businessmen, and philanthropists seeking to regulate and control venereal diseases, prostitution, and promote sex education through morality-based principles (Jones, 1981). In essence, the social hygienists believed that sexual behavior could be controlled and reformed by reeducating the public about the importance of adopting a single moral code of proper sexual behavior, for men and woman (Jones, 1981). Department of War officials, PHS officials and the social hygienists worked together to successfully persuade the president and Congress that syphilis was negatively affecting military enlistment while working with lawmakers to create new legislation (Jones, 1981). In fact, so close was the social hygienist movement's partnership with the PHS that the PHS eventually "functioned as little more than an appendage of the American Social Hygiene Association" (Jones, 1981: 50).

Brandt (1985) writes that during the First and Second World War, the social hygienists frequently met with the secretary of war and Congress to provide data illustrating that syphilis was negatively affecting the health of potential military enlistees and that if nothing was done, the military could very well experience a decline in its fighting capabilities (Brandt, 1985; Jones, 1981). Through these efforts, the secretary of war finally obtained the president and Congress' support to introduce new policy initiatives. A new partnership emerged between politicians, PHS bureaucrats, and the social hygienists for the creation of centralized bureaucratic and policy initiatives.

This partnership led to the creation of the US Inter-Departmental Social Hygiene Board in 1918, an initiative designed to increase public awareness about syphilis and other venereal diseases. The social hygienists continued to work with the government, in turn reinforcing the president, Congress, and the military's perceptions that aggressively responding to syphilis was important for safeguarding the strength and expansion of military forces. Yet, with the aforementioned decline of congressional support for VD programs during the interwar period, the social hygienist movement's policy ideas and influence waned, in turn reinforcing the fact that, once again, the federal government was mainly concerned with syphilis' threat to national security. Thus, civic supporters were briefly present and influential, but only when policy-makers were interested in syphilis' threat to the military.

Brazil

Contesting syphilis

In a similar manner to the US, Brazil's federal government did not initially perceive syphilis as posing a serious national health threat. Notwithstanding an increase in syphilis growth rates throughout the late 19th century, the government did not create a federal program in response to syphilis until 1914, several years after the epidemic emerged[3] (Cararra, 1999). This delayed response was mainly attributed to the fact that syphilis was perceived as something "natural," that is, a social disease that was expected to spread and thrive in Brazil's tropics. To understand this, one must recall Brazil's unique history of venereal disease: specifically the widely held perception within government and society that Brazil was "born out of the devil," that it was "sinful in nature," awash in peccadillos leading to the wild-fire spread of venereal diseases (Carrara, 1996). Men were known to boast of their syphilis condition. Others considered the disease as the mark of a true manly man. As the Brazilian historian Gilberto Freye once put it: Brazil was "syphilized" since the very beginning (Freye, 1946).

Because of these views, prior to the First World War, the president felt no urgency to respond to syphilis. This lack of urgency was further compounded by the absence of syphilis' threat to military and economic security. Moreover, the director of the DGSP and most of its bureaucrats were apathetic to the burgeoning growth of syphilis

---

[3] Early 20th century epidemiological data for all forms of syphilis prevalence and deaths does not exist. I took three trips to Brazil trying to locate this data in Rio and São Paulo. Colleagues inform me that this data was never recorded by the government because of the inaccuracy of DGSP and MESP surveys and because it was perceived as such a widespread, common disease that medical elites were frankly not interested in carefully monitoring its spread. After the introduction of penicillin therapy in 1943, however, the government did start to monitor and publish syphilis case rates, mainly to display its effectiveness in combating the epidemic.

cases and deaths (Carrara, 1996; 1999). In essence this also stemmed from the fact that the DGSP had to respond to a host of public health threats. Syphilis was just one of a myriad of diseases these bureaucrats were grappling with, failing to convince them that they needed to give syphilis special attention (Carrara, 1996, 1999).

Civil society's views towards syphilis were rather different, however. From 1900 until the end of the Second World War, there emerged an aggressive social health movement pressuring the government for an immediate federal response. Led by doctors, public health workers, and university professors, the social movement favoring this response was called the Sifilógrafos movement (Carrara, 1996). The Sifilógrafos believed that syphilis posed a serious national threat and that the government should respond by strengthening the DGSP and, later, the MESP under Vargas. The Sifilógrafos also believed that that there was nothing immoral about syphilis and that society should not be afraid to openly discuss syphilis and seek medical attention (Miranda, 1936). DGSP and MESP officials involved in this movement also believed that syphilis was not associated with the black and indigenous race, thus avoiding the discrimination associated with syphilis as seen in the US (Carrara, 2004). Syphilis was mainly associated with the white upper class, brought over by promiscuous Portuguese colonizers during the 16th century (Carrara, 1997).

The Sifilógrafos also pressured the federal government to introduce new sex education and prevention campaigns. Sex education was seen as essential for syphilis prevention (Vieira, 1930; Primeira Conferencia Nacional de Defesa contra a Sífilis, 1941). The Sifilógrafos eventually persuaded the government to disseminate new sex education pamphlets, to sponsor sex education information commercials in movie theaters, post messages on public billboards, and work with state and local governments to provide sex education in schools (Fernandes, 1931; Carrara, 1996; Miranda, 1936; Zéo, 1941). And finally, the Sifilógrafos were a major proponent of the federal government financing and providing free medical treatment. The Sifilógrafos noticed that other nations were doing this, especially in western Europe, and felt compelled to pressurize the government to do the same (Araujo, 1939).

Above all, the major policy idea that the Sifilógrafos were pressing for was the increased centralization of bureaucratic control over syphilis prevention and treatment policy. They believed that it was the government's responsibility to immediately respond to epidemics through this type of centralized response (Carrara, 1992; 1996). This entailed expanding the DGSP and MESP, providing financial and technical resources to the states, and working closely with them to implement prevention and treatment policy (Carrara, 1992; 1996). The Sifilógrafos were quick to point out that western Europe had already created a successful, centralized response to syphilis; in fact, they often made reference to this in public health journals (d'Esaguy, 1938).

Prior to and throughout the First World War, the Sifilógrafos were also eager to get involved at the international level (Carrara, 1997). They had a distinct interest in showing the world that Brazil was committed to eradicating syphilis; and there were several reasons for doing so. First, as an emerging nation, the Sifilógrafos wanted to show that Brazil had the medical and infrastructural capacity to quickly eradicate syphilis through scientific breakthrough and policy reform (Carrara, 1997). To prove their point, the Sifilógrafos participated in a host of international health conferences sponsored by other (mainly western European) governments (Primeira Conferencia Nacional de Defesa contra a Sífilis, 1941). They often traveled to Europe to discuss their research and prevention policies. At one point, a Brazilian doctor, Dr. Gustavo Werneck, made such a good impression that in 1911 he was awarded an honorary medal at a conference in France for his efforts to eradicate syphilis (Primeira Conferencia Nacional de Defesa contra a Sífilis, 1941).

The Sifilógrafos also wanted to distinguish themselves from western Europe by showing that their approach to eradiating syphilis derived from a purely scientific, secular perspective (Carrara, 1996). At the time, France was well known for having a moralistic, regulatory, and somewhat condemnatory approach to syphilis control — mainly through the imprisonment of prostitutes. The Sifilógrafos wanted to demonstrate their alternative approach, which was focused on sex education and prevention (Carrara, 1999). They were also tired of the international community's presumption that Brazilian culture encouraged sexual promiscuity, contributing to syphilis' spread. The Sifilógrafos were out to prove a point: that Brazil could overcome disease, modernize, and prosper.

The president and DGSP bureaucrats certainly appreciated these efforts. As policymakers positioning themselves as an emerging power, they were equally as committed to displaying Brazil's commitment to syphilis eradication. To that end, the DGSP sponsored several of the Sifilógrafos' trips to Europe (Carrara, 1996, 1997). And, even though the president was more focused on expanding the state and economic development, he relied on the Sifilógrafos and state health departments as primary responders and had incentives to support the Sifilógrafos' work. Doing so sent a clear message to the world: that the government was fully committed and capable of eradicating disease. The Sifilógrafos' active involvement in the international community and their growing reputation helped them to convince the president that syphilis was a serious problem and that he needed to respond. However, the Sifilógrafos' growing popularity, influence, and pressures were still insufficient for convincing the president to engage in a centralized response.

Because of their active participation and influence at the global level, however, the Sifilógrafos' domestic reputation increased (Primeira Conferencia Nacional de Defesa contra a Sífilis, 1941). This facilitated their ability to establish and strengthen their ties with public health bureaucrats in the DGSP and the MESP who shared similar centralized policy ideas. The Sifilógrafos' connections with the international community also increased the reputation and influence of those DGSP and MESP bureaucrats working with them (Carrara, 1999). This motivated these bureaucrats to maintain and strengthen their partnership with the Sifilógrafos (Carrara, 1999). But it is also important to emphasize that many DGSP and MESP bureaucrats hailed from the Sifilógrafo movement, which further contributed to the latter's credibility while solidifying their shared policy beliefs (Carrara, 1999).

Scholars also confirm the fact that the partnership between the Sifilógrafos and the international community emerged before the government responded to syphilis. In his detailed account of the civic movements that emerged in response to syphilis and, later, HIV/ AIDS, Carrara (1999) explains that the Sifilógrafo movement arose in tandem with the new global health movement focusing on the eradication of syphilis, and that this occurred prior to the government's policy response. Carrara (1999) also maintains that the Sifilógrafos were highly involved in politics and used their connections with the international community strategically in order to convince a seemingly apathetic government of the need to reform its public health infrastructure (Carrara, 1999). These efforts added greatly to the Sifilógrafos' credibility and appealed to those DGSP and MESP bureaucrats seeking to build a reform coalition.

Nevertheless, it is important to emphasize that despite the bureaucracy's growing partnership with the Sifilógrafos, this was still not enough to influence the president's views and response. In fact, it was not until 1920 that the government's centralization efforts began in earnest. That year, a change in presidential perceptions and interest in pursuing a centralized response stemmed primarily from the rise of international criticisms, pressures, and the opportunity to once again demonstrate to the world that Brazil had the capacity to develop and prosper. Similar to what we saw with the government's response to TB, during this period the president received a lot of criticism from the international community, mainly from doctors and scientists in other nations (Filho, 2001). They were mainly concerned with the poor quality of Brazil's public health system (Filho, 2001, 2004). Other nations' criticisms were often manifested in the media and conference proceedings. International philanthropists, such as the Rockefeller Foundation and Irene Diamond Foundation, also contributed to these pressures.

These criticisms and pressures created incentives for President Epitácio Pessoa (1919–1922) to show the world that Brazil could effectively curb the spread of syphilis and other diseases through new bureaucratic and policy reforms (Gómez, 2008). In so doing, Pessoa believed that he could increase the government's international reputation (Gómez, 2008).

For example, in 1920, the government embarked on a series of centralized bureaucratic and policy reforms. First, the president and

Congress decided to create a new public health agency that completely nationalized the response to syphilis. That year, the government created the Inspectoria de Profilaxia de Lepra e das Doencas (IPLD) (Primeira Conferencia Nacional de Defesa contra a Sífilis, 1941). The IPLD was dedicated to centralizing the funding of syphilis prevention and treatment services. It was highly autonomous and drew heavily from congressional coffers (Primeira Conferencia Nacional de Defesa contra a Sífilis, 1941). It was well staffed and had unwavering presidential and congressional support. The mere fact that it was a federal agency focusing on syphilis and other venereal diseases sent a clear message that the government was finally committed to eradicating syphilis.

In addition to the IPLD's provision of funding to the states, President Pessoa also issued several executive decrees requiring that state health agencies provide new health services for syphilis. In 1920, the government issued Lei art #5, which mandated that state governments provide free treatment and educational services to the municipalities. Furthermore, any state agency that did not adhere to this decree was fined from (R$, Réis) 100.00 up to 500.00 (R$, Réis) (Primeira Conferencia Nacional de Defesa contra a Sífilis, 1941: p. 168). Consequently, a host of state governments began to create new anti-venereal centers focusing on syphilis eradication. Approximately 709 centers for the treatment of syphilis were created throughout the states, with 55 created near the nation's capital. Because of these efforts, public health experts at the time claimed that the number of syphilis cases declined by 50% (Mota, 1941).

The IPLD also started working closely with the private sector. In 1920, it began to work with the largest medical charity at the time, the Fundação Gafrée-Guinle. Founded in 1920 by the Guinle family with a generous gift of 16.000:00$000 (*dezesseis mil conts*), the Fundação was a private hospital and clinic committed to conducting lab research in addition to increasing public awareness and education about syphilis. Next to the Sifilógrafos, the Fundação was the most vocal proponent of sex education in schools and private industry. It worked closely with academia and the Sifilógrafos and repeatedly approached Congress for more funding. After several failed attempts to obtain a formal dual-financing contract from Congress (due mainly to co-financing disputes), in 1923 Congress agreed to provide additional funding for ten clinics that the Fundação established in the rural areas (Mota, 1941). With this funding, the Fundação could concentrate and commit its resources to treating patients.

Because many of the state and municipal health agencies at the time were understaffed and poorly financed, the Fundação was important for helping the government treat patients. It took in the lion's share of syphilis patients in the city of Rio de Janeiro, in addition to funding the provision of medical treatment (mainly needle injections). The federal government sustained its partnership with the Fundação until syphilis was eradicated with the introduction of penicillin treatment by the mid-to-late 1940s.

Efforts to build federal agencies and policies continued. While the federal government had already created the highly centralized IPLD in 1920, with the arrival of President Getúlio Vargas in 1930, the government further centralized all aspects of health insurance and public health. In 1938, in an effort to strengthen the MESP, Vargas incorporated the IPLD into the MESP. Vargas was a true state builder. He was a centralizer. He had a disdain for the fragmentation of federal agencies and fervently believed that all public health policies should be placed under one roof (Hauchman, 1998).

In contrast to President Pessoa's intentions, initially Vargas' motivation to create the MESP was not prompted by international criticisms, pressures, and efforts to increase Brazil's international reputation. As mentioned earlier, this is because Vargas' presidency marked the beginning of Brazil's isolation from the international community, underscoring a strong sense of nationalism and commitment to economic development — tenants that were present throughout the world during this period. In this context, Vargas was more concerned with national security issues, such as military capacity and economic growth, as well as the centralization of political power (McCann, 2006). If anything, during this period syphilis' threat to Brazil's national security, measured especially in terms of its potential effects on economic development, was the key motivational force guiding Vargas' intentions to expand the MESP.

Nevertheless, and similar again to what we saw with Vargas' response to tuberculosis, his response to international criticisms and pressures eventually changed when Vargas began to reinsert Brazil into the international community. This occurred through his involvement in foreign military campaigns. By 1942, at the height of the global campaign against Germany, Vargas broke from his isolationist tendencies and began to reintegrate Brazil into geopolitics. This occurred not only to help rid the world of Nazi fascism but also to safeguard Brazilian citizens from foreign-born disease. Indeed, in 1944 Vargas sent one of his best medical doctors, Dr. Geraldo de Paula Souza, to work with Dr. Szeming Sze of China and Dr. Karl Evang of Norway to create the WHO (Ruttan, 1996). From that point on, Vargas became concerned with his international reputation and image as a president committed to eradicating syphilis and other diseases. Similar to what we saw with his response to TB, these reputation-building incentives motivated Vargas to press harder for an expansion of the MESP and other federal programs focused on eradicating syphilis.

Civil society responds

Similar to what we saw with the emergence of TB during the early 19th century, notwithstanding the formation of a close partnership between the Sifilógrafos and public health bureaucrats over the need for a centralized response, this partnership did not have an impact on the governing elites' policy response. Instead, governing elites' interests and response was shaped by other factors, such as national security concerns or the arrival of international criticisms and pressures. Despite this state-civil societal partnership's inability to influence reforms, several occurrences emerged facilitating the rise of civic supporters during this historical period.

Similar to what we saw with the response to TB, galvanizing the partnership between the Sifilógrafos and public health bureaucrats was the sharing of their similar ideas and beliefs in a centralized response to epidemics. First proffered by the Sifilógrafos, these ideas were based on the following beliefs: first, that bureaucratic and policy centralization should be immediately pursued whenever epidemics emerge; second, that the government should provide universal prevention and treatment services; third, that the Sifilógrafos, as well as other social health movements, and public health bureaucrats should establish close partnerships in order to ensure that a centralized response emerged and persists; and finally, that social health movements and public health bureaucrats should work in close partnership with the international community.

The Sifilógrafos and public health bureaucrats therefore came together to proffer centralized policy ideas in response to syphilis. Although this partnership proved incapable of pressuring the government for a centralized response, these efforts nevertheless set the groundwork for the emergence of civic supporters decades later.

Conclusion

Notwithstanding historical differences in public health systems and institutions — decentralized in the US and centralized in Brazil — both governments were similar in that they did not immediately respond to their contested epidemics. When isolating themselves from participating in international health politics and policy, as seen in the US and briefly under President Vargas in Brazil, domestic national security threats became of chief concern, leading to aggressive, centralized bureaucratic and policy responses.

However, Brazil eventually pursued a different path. By the 1940s, Brazil reintegrated itself into world politics and, in contrast, to the US, became more concerned with establishing its international reputation as a nation capable of eradicating disease. Centralized bureaucratic and policy responses were kindled by efforts to reform bureaucratic institutions and policy as a means to achieving these reputation-building ends; and yet, no such response emerged in the US. As we will see in all of the following chapters, these differences in government response to international criticisms and pressures persisted, ultimately engendering different government responses to recently contested epidemics.

In the US, historically the government's response was also influenced by the personal interest and experience of political leaders. For instance, Roosevelt's experience with polio motivated him to not only increase public awareness and discussions about the epidemic, in turn helping subdue the stigma surrounding the disease, but he also established a quasi-governmental response through the National Foundation of Infantile Paralysis. While an official, government-sponsored bureaucratic and policy response was never pursued, Roosevelt's personal experiences and empathy for others helped place polio onto the national agenda.

The benefits of a political leader's personal interest in epidemics did not stop with Roosevelt, however. For, as we will see in Chapter 5, this dynamic reemerged with the government's response to arguably the most contested epidemic of our time: obesity. As I discuss in Chapter 5, recent presidents, first ladies, agency directors, and even governors have expressed their personal battle with weight gain, identifying and empathizing with others struggling with this health challenge; moreover, these personal interests and responses have helped to put obesity onto the national agenda, while inching the government closer to a centralized response.

Finally, the US and Brazil differed in their historic emergence of civic supporters. In response to tuberculosis and syphilis in Brazil, social health movements emerged to proffer ideas of centralized bureaucratic and policy responses to contested epidemics. These social health movements developed strong partnerships with public health bureaucrats with the hopes of seeing their policy ideas come to fruition. To that end, these movements and bureaucrats forged strong partnerships, molded together through similar policy beliefs in centralized bureaucratic and policy responses to epidemics. Although they were not successful in pressuring the government for an immediate response to epidemics, these social movements and their policy ideas nevertheless established the groundwork necessary for the emergence of civic supporters decades later, in response to AIDS and, to a certain extent, TB. Conversely, in the US, in response to polio and malnutrition, although perhaps with the exception of the government's brief response to syphilis during wartime efforts, these types of social health movements, centralization ideas, and partnerships with public health bureaucrats never emerged. As a result, and in contrast to what we saw in Brazil, this did not set the groundwork for the emergence of future civic supporters in response to the US's recently contested epidemics, such as AIDS and obesity.

References

Acurcio, F. (2004). *Evolução Histórica das Políticas de Saúde no Brasil.* Unpublished manuscript, Profesor do Depto de Farmácia — UFMG Doutor em Epidemiologia Médico, Brazil.

Antunes, J. and Waldman, E. (1999). *Tuberculosis in the Twentieth Century: Time-Series Mortality in São Paulo, Brazil, 1900–1997.* Unpublished manuscript.

Antunes, J., Waldman E., and Morales, M. (2000). A Tuberculose Através do Seculo: Icons Canonicos e Signos do Combate á Enfermidade, *Cienca Saude Coletiva*, 5, 367–379.

Araujo, O. (1939). As Tendencias Modernas no Luta Contra as Doencas Venerais, *Jornal de Sífilis e Urologia*, 111.

Associated Press (2005). Obesity Takes its Toll on the Military: Officials Increasingly Worried about Troops being too Fit to Fight, July 5. Available on-line: http://www.nbcnews.com/id/8423112/#.UpSgNxbonHg. Accessed March 14, 2014.

Astor, G. (1983). *The Disease Detectives: Deadly Medical Mysteries and the People who Solved Them*, Plume Books, New York.

Bennett, J. and DiLorenzo, T. (2000). *From Pathology to Politics: Public Health in America*, Transaction Publishers, New Brunswick.

Blumenthal, D. and Morone, J. (2009). *The Heart of Power: Health and Politics in the Oval Office*, University of California Press, Berkeley.

Brandt, A. (1985). *No Magic Bullet: A Social History of Venereal Disease in the United States since 1880*, Oxford University Press, New York.

Brown, W. (1970). *Syphilis and Other Venereal Diseases*, Harvard University Press, Cambridge.

Carrara, S. (1992). *O Tribute a Venus: a Luta Anti-venera no Brasil de Fins do Seculo XIX ate os Anos de 1940*, Ph.D. dissertation, Programa de Pos-Graduação em Antropologia Social do Museu Nacional/UFRJ.

Carrara, S. (1996). *Tributo a Venus: A Luta Contra a Sífilis no Brasil, da Passagem do Século aos Anos 40*, Casa Oswald Cruz Publications, Rio de Janeiro.

Carrara, S. (1997). A Geopolítica Simbólica da Sífilis: Um Ensaio de Antropologia Histórica, *Historia, Ciencias, Saúde*, **3**, 391–408.

Carrara, S. (1999). 'A AIDS e a História das Doenças Venéreas no Brasil', in Parker, R., Bastos, C., Galvão, J., and Pedrosa, J. (eds), *A AIDS no Brasil*, ABIA Press, Rio de Janeiro, 273–306.

Carrara, S. (2004). 'Estratégias Antícoloniais: Sífilis, Raça e identidade nacional no Brasil do Entre-Guerras', in Hochman, G. and Armus, D (eds), *Cuidar, Controlar, Curar: Ensaios Históricos Sobre Saúde e Doenca na América Latina e Caribe*, Casa Oswald Cruz Publications, Rio de Janeiro.

Coming, H. (1970). 'The United States Quarantine System during the Past Fifty Years', in Mazyck, P. (ed.), *A Half Century of Public Health*, Arno Press, New York, p. 120.

Cutler, J. and Arnold, R. (2000). 'Venereal Disease Control by Health Departments in the Past', in Reverby, S. (ed.), *Tuskegee's Truths: Rethinking the Tuskegee Syphilis Study*, University of North Carolina, Chapel Hill, pp. 495–506.

d'Esaguy, A. (1938). As Doencas Venereas, *Jornal da Sífilis e Urologia*, **106**.

Eisinger, P. (1998). *Toward an End to Hunger in America*, Brookings Institution Press, Washington DC.

Etheridge, E. (1992). *Sentinel for Health: A History of the Centers for Disease Control*, University of California Press, Berkeley.

Far, F. (1972). *FDR*, Arlington House Publishers, New Rochelle.

Fernandes, R. (1931). Syphilis, Doenca Social, *Jornal da Sífilis e Urologia*, **22**.

Filho, C. (2001). *História Social da Tuberculose e do Tuberculoso: 1900–1950*, Editora FIOCRUZ, Rio de Janeiro.

Filho, C. (2004). *História da Saúde Pública no Brasil*, Edtora Ática, São Paulo.

Freye, G. (1946). *Casa Grande & Senzala*, José Olympio Publications, Rio de Janeiro.

Gallagher, H. (1999). *FDR's Splendid Deception: The Moving Story of Roosevelt's Massive Disability — and the Intense Efforts to Conceal it from the Public*, Vandamere Press, St. Petersburgh.

Gómez, E. (2008). *Responding to Contested Epidemics: Democracy, International Pressures, and the Civic Sources of Institutional Change in the United States and Brazil*. PhD Dissertation, Department of Political Science, Brown University.

Gould, T. (1995). *A Summer Plague: Polio and its Survivors*, Yale University Press, New Haven.

Hijjar, M., Gerhardt, G., Teixeira, G., and Procópio, M. (2007). Retrospect of Tuberculosis Control, *Rev Saúde Publica*, **41**, 1–9.

Hochman, G. (1998). *A Era do Saneamento: As Bases da Política de Saúde Pública no Brasil*, Editora Hucitec-Anpocs, São Paulo.

Jones, J. (1981). *Bad Blood: The Tuskegee Syphilis Experiment*, Free Press, New York.

Kickbusch, I. (2002). Influence and Opportunity: Reflections on the U.S. Role in Global Public Health, *Health Affairs*, **21**, 131–141.

Levenstein, H. (1993). *Paradox of Plenty: A Social History of Eating in Modern America*, Oxford University Press, New York.

Locke, H. (1939). Changing Attitudes Toward Venereal Diseases, *American Sociological Review*, **4**, 836–843.

Lovett, L. (2005). The Popeye Principle: Selling Child Health in the First Nutrition Crisis, *Journal of Health Politics, Policy & Law*, **30**, 803–838.

Lima, N. and Britto, N. (1996). 'Salud y Nación: Propuesta para el Saneamiento Rural. Un Estudio de la Revista Saúde (1918–1919)', in Cueto, M. (ed.), *Salud, Cultura y Sociedad en América Latina: Nuevas pespectivas históricas*, Organización Panamericana de la Salud, Lima, pp. 135–158.

McBride, D. (1991). *From TB to AIDS: Epidemics among Urban Blacks since 1900*, State University of New York Press, Albany.

McCann, F. (2006). 'The Military Dictatorship: Getúlio, Góes, and Dutra', in Hentschke, J. (ed.), *Vargas and Brazil: New Perspectives*, Palgrave Macmilan Press, New York, pp. 109–142.

McIntosh, E. (1995). *American Food Habits in Historical Perspective*, Praeger Press, Westport.

McNeil, D. (2006). Buffett's Billions Will Aid Fight Against Disease, *The New York Times*, June 27, p. 1.

Miranda, V. (1936). A Educação Sexual e os Males, *Jornal da Sífilis e Urologia*, **78**.

Mullen, F. (1989). *Plagues and Politics: the Story of the United States Public Health Service*, Basic Books, New York.

Nascimento, D. (1997). A Doença e o Poder Público ou o Poder das Doenças: Elementos Para Uma Análise em Torno do Estado no Combate á Tuberculose, unpublished manuscript.

Nascimento, D. (1991). Tuberculose: De Questão a Questão de Estado a Liga Brasileira Contra a Tuberculose, Maestrado em Saúde Coletiva (Masters Thesis), Instituto de Medicina Social, Universidade do Estado do Rio de Janeiro.

Nascimento, D. (2005). *As Pestes do Séclo XX: Tuberculose e Aids no Brasil, uma História Comparada*, Ediotora Fiocruz, Rio de Janeiro.

Ness, E. (1942). Venereal Disease Control in Defense, *The Annals of the American Academy*, **220**, 89–93.

Netto, A. and Pereira, J. (1981). Mortalidade por Tuberculose e Condições de Vida: O Caso Rio de Janeiro, *Saúde em Debate*, **12**, 27–34.

Offit, P. (2005). *The Cutter Incident: How America's First Polio Vaccine Led to the Growing Vaccine Crisis*, Yale University Press, New Haven.

Oshinsky, D. (2005). *Polio: An American Story*, Oxford University Press, New York.

Parran, T. (1937). *Shadow on the Land: Syphilis*, Reynal & Hitchcook, New York.

Peard, J. (1999). *Race, Place, and Medicine: The Idea of the Tropics in Nineteenth-Century Brazilian Medicine*, Duke University Press, Raleigh.

Primeira Conferencia Nacional de Defesa contra a Sífilis (1941). Imprensa Nacional, Rio de Janeiro.

Ribeiro, L. (1956). *A Luta Contra a Tuberculose no Brasil: Apontamentos Para Sua Historia*, Serviço Nacional de Tuberculose, Rio de Janeiro.

Rogers, N. (1992). *Dirt and Disease: Polio Before FDR*, Rutgers University Press, New Brunswick.

Rosemblum, D. and McCurdy, H. (eds) (2007). *Revisiting Waldo's Administrative State: Constancy and change in Public Administration*, Georgetown University Press, Washington, DC.

Ruffino-Netto, A. and Figueiredo de Souza, A. (2001). Evolution of the Health Sector and Tuberculosis Control in Brazil, *Pan American Journal of Public Health*, **9**, 306–310.

Ruttan, V. (1996). *United States Development Assistance Policy: The Domestic Politics of Foreign Economic Aid*, The Johns Hopkins University Press, Baltimore.

Santos Filho, E. (2006). *Política de Tuberculose no Brasil: Uma Perspectiva da Sociedade Civil*, Public Health Watch, George Soros Foundation/Open Society Institute.

Schwartz, B. (1969). 'Unemployment Relief in Philadelphia, 1930–32', *Pennsylvania Magazine of History and Biography*, **42**, reprinted in Sternsher, B. (ed.), (1970). *Hitting Home: The Great Depression in Town and Country*, Quadrangle Press, Chicago, pp. 73–77.

Science Illustrated (1949). The New Attack on Venereal Diseases, 30–32.

Smith, J. (1990). *Patenting the Sun: Polio and the Salk Vaccine*, William Morrow and Company, Inc., New York.

Spargo, J. (1906). *Underfed School Children: The Problem and the Remedy*, Charles H. Kerr Publishers, Chicago.

Stearns, P. (1997). *Fat History: Bodies and Beauty in the Modern West*, New York University Press, New York.

Stepan, N. (1976). *Beginnings of Brazilian Science: Oswaldo Cruz, Medical Research and Policy, 1890–1920*, Science History Publications, New York.

Thomas, G. (N/D). 'Food Will Win the War — And Shape the Peace that Follows,' *Air Group 4: 'Casablanca to Tokyo'*. Available on-line: http://www.airgroup4.com/food.htm. Accessed March 15, 2014.

Thompson, L. (1987). The AIDS-Syphilis Parallel: Similarities and Differences, *The Washington Post*, March 31, Health Section, p. Z13.

Vargas, G. (1938). *A Nova Política do Brasil*, Livraria José Olympio, Rio de Janeiro.

Vasconcelos, M. (2005). *Participação Popular e Educação nos Primórdios da Saúde Pública Brasileira*. Unpublished manuscript, UFPB, Brazil.

Vieira, F. and Reis, A. (1930). A Educacão Sexual Como Medida de Proteção á Infancia, *Jornal de Sífilis e Urologia*, **25**.

Vonderlehr, R. and Heller, J.R. (1946). *The Control of Venereal Disease*, Reynal & Hitchcock, New York.

Williams, R. (1951). *The United States Public Health Service, 1798–1950*, United States Public Health Service, Washington, DC.

Wilson, D. (1990). *Living with Polio: The Epidemic and its Survivors*, The University of Chicago Press, Hyde Park.

Yach, D. and Bettcher, D. (1998). The Globalization of Public Health, I: Threats and Opportunities, *American Journal of Public Health*, **88**, 735–744.

Zéo, A. (1941). A Propaganda e Educação Anti-Venérea no Meio Familiar e Escolar — Medidas Indispensaveis na Campangha de Profilaxia da Sífilis, *Primeira Conferencia Nacional de Defesa contra a Sífilis*, Imprensa Nacional, Rio de Janeiro.

Chapter 3

Contesting AIDS in the United States

Similar to what we saw with malnutrition, syphilis, and polio in the past, by the early 1980s AIDS emerged in the US as a health epidemic potentially posing a great risk to society. Prevailing theories would seem to suggest that the US's longstanding democratic electoral institutions, political accountability, the representation of the needs of civil society through national congressional committees, as well as the presence of the latest technology, resources, and a highly skilled healthcare worker force would lead to an immediate, aggressive response to the epidemic (Aggleton, 2001; Altman, 1986; Baldwin, 2007; Nathanson, 1996; Price-Smith, 2002; Price-Smith *et al.*, 2004; Rosenbrock and Wright, 2000; Ruger, 2005; Sen, 1999; Vallgarda, 2007). Similarly, one would expect the US to respond more aggressively than Brazil, especially in light of the fact that Brazil did not enjoy these favorable preconditions throughout the early years of the AIDS epidemic (Lieberman, 2009; Parker, 2003). Nevertheless, as I explain in this chapter, despite these seemingly favorable preconditions, political and bureaucratic elites in the US did not immediately respond to AIDS, nor was their subsequent response very successful.

Initially the importance of AIDS and its perceived threat to the nation was highly contested between politicians, bureaucrats, and civil society. This contributed to a delayed national government response.[1] Moreover, during the first years of the epidemic, the president's belief

---

[1]This is not to say that state and municipal governments were also delayed in their response. When compared to the national government, New York and California, especially at the municipal level, were more timely in their response (Altman, 1986; Fox, 1986, 1992). However, the focus of this book is on the national government's response and its assistance to the states.

that AIDS did not pose a credible national health threat, the perceived absence of AIDS's threat to the national security, and the penetration of well-organized conservative religious interest groups engendered a lack of presidential and, for the most part, congressional interest in pursuing a centralized response. Further, this occurred despite the HHS (Department of Health and Human Services) and PHS (Public Health Service) vehemently pushing for a centralized response, while AIDS activists frequently testified before Congress, pleading for help. But neither the bureaucracy nor civil society could convince the White House and congress to immediately respond.

But institutions also mattered, that is, the presence of a fragmented and uncoordinated PHS structure, comprised of the Centers for Disease Control (CDC), National Institutes of Health (NIH), and the National Cancer Institute (NCI) hampered policy research and implementation. In a context of limited funding and fiscal retrenchment, fears of agency downsizing prompted intense inter-agency competition and a lack of cooperation. The rich tradition of bureaucratic survival and usage of new diseases as a means to justify and obtain more resources as well as political support once again emerged to delay the government's response to an epidemic.

By the early 1990s, international health agencies, scientists, and activists heavily criticized the government for its lackluster policy response. But these international criticisms and pressures had no influence on the president and congress' policy decisions; instead, these policymakers responded on their own, and at their own pace. In contrast to what we saw with malnutrition and syphilis during the two world wars, in the absence of AIDS's threat to national security, these leaders had no incentive to pursue a centralized response — notwithstanding ongoing local government financial and policy needs (Altman, 1986; Shilts, 2011). Furthermore, no political leaders and/ or bureaucrats were personally affected by the epidemic, which failed to instigate a personal interest in reform. It was only when President Clinton was elected in 1993 that strong political leadership and a government commitment to AIDS finally emerged. In contrast to his predecessors, Clinton strove to increase national AIDS policy coordination and implementation through the creation of the Office of National AIDS Policy (ONAP) in 1993, while increasing funding for domestic programs. While Clinton kept his campaign promise and created ONAP, many soon criticized him for failing to ensure that it had effective leadership and influence.

Equally, if not more, problematic during this period was the inability of HHS and CDC officials to work closely with, and strategically use, civil society. That is, there were no *civic supporters* that national AIDS officials could use to increase their legitimacy and influence when seeking ongoing financial and political support for their programs. As I explained in Chapter 1, civic supporters emerge when contemporary non-governmental organizations (NGOs) and/or social health movements proffer historically proven policy ideas of immediately pursuing a centralized bureaucratic and policy response to epidemics; these civic supporters also resemble similar social health movements and civic organizations in the past. Civic supporters are helpful because, given their popularity in government and society, they can provide health officials with the legitimacy and influence needed to garner more political and financial support. However, when it came to AIDS, these civic supporters never arose: that is, NGOs never advocated these centrist policy ideas, often preferring to work on their own and/or with limited support from state governments. Moreover, even if these civic supporters had proffered centrist policy ideas, as we saw in the previous chapter, these ideas were never advocated by non-governmental entities in the past; as a result, these ideas failed to have a proven, successful track record.

A strong government response to AIDS was also hampered by the White House's increased focused on global AIDS. When George W. Bush entered office in 2000, a critical juncture of propitious international and domestic political and social conditions motivated Bush and congressional leaders to emphasize helping other nations combat the epidemic; with this goal in mind, within two years Bush succeeded in creating the world's largest bureaucracy dedicated to combating AIDS: PEPFAR (President's Emergency Plan for AIDS Relief). PEPFAR as well as the White House's and Congress' increased contributions to multilateral agencies, such as the Global Fund to Fight AIDS, Tuberculosis and Malaria, eventually distracted the government from focusing on increasing domestic funding and policy initiatives. Furthermore, this occurred despite escalating AIDS cases and deaths in several US cities — a silent epidemic motivating CNN reporters to draw similar parallels with the epidemic's spread in several African nations (CNN, 2008; Hoye, 2012). Recognizing Bush's limited domestic response, in contrast, the Barack Obama administration entered office with a focus on increasing the domestic response to AIDS while maintaining Bush's global initiatives. Despite his efforts, an ongoing economic recession has limited Obama's ability to accomplish these objectives.

The Initial Years of the AIDS Epidemic

In the summer of 1981, a mysterious virus emerged in Los Angeles. A few young gay men become fatally ill, first to pneumonia, then to a rare form of skin cancer called Kaposi's sarcoma — which was more commonly seen among the elderly. By 1982, scores of gay men in Los Angeles and New York had tested positive for Kaposi's sarcoma, pneumonia, and other related diseases.

Official news of a viral outbreak contributed to growing fears and uncertainty. In major cities municipal officials instructed police officers and public health workers to refrain from helping anyone suspected of carrying the HIV virus (Altman, 1986; US News & World Report, 1983). Local health officials were quick to blame the gay community and to impose a phalanx of laws prohibiting any social activity perceived as contributing to the virus' spread — such as bathhouses, gay clubs, and restaurants (*US News & World Report*, 1985a; Trafford *et al.*, 1985).

Despite the CDC's warnings and MMWR (Morbidity and Mortality Weekly Report) reports indicating that a new epidemic had emerged, the White House did not immediately respond. In fact, by 1983, when publicly questioned about AIDS, the White House admitted to not knowing anything about it. Consider, for example, the response of the White House Press Secretary, Mr. Larry Speakes, when questioned by a reporter about AIDS at an official White House press hearing on October 15, 1983:[2]

Q: Larry, does the President have any reaction to the announcement [by] the Centers for Disease Control in Atlanta, that AIDS is now an epidemic and [that we] have over 600 cases?

MR. SPEAKES: What's AIDS?

Q: Over a third of them have died. It's known as "gay plague." (Laughter.) No, it is. I mean it's a pretty serious thing that one in every three people that get this have died. And I wondered if the President is aware of it?

MR. SPEAKES: I don't have it. Do you? (Laughter.)

Q: No, I don't.

MR. SPEAKES: You didn't answer my question.

Q: Well, I just wondered, does the President?

MR. SPEAKES: How do you know? (Laughter.)

Q: In other words, the White House looks on this as a great joke?

MR. SPEAKES: No, I don't know anything about it, Lester.

Q: Does the President, does anyone in the White House know about this epidemic, Larry?

MR. SPEAKES: I don't think so. I don't think there's been any ...

Q: Nobody knows?

MR. SPEAKES: There has been no personal experience here, Lester.

Q: No, I mean, I thought you were keeping ...

MR. SPEAKES: I checked thoroughly with Dr. Ruge this morning and he's had no (laughter) ... no patients suffering from AIDS or whatever it is.

---

[2] This transcript was obtained from Jon Cohen's book, *Shots in the Dark: The Wayward Search for an AIDS Vaccine*, 2001, Chapter 1, pp. 3–4.

Q: The President doesn't have gay plague, is that what you're saying or what?

MR. SPEAKES: No, I didn't say that.

Q: Didn't say that?

This pressroom exchange accurately depicts the White House's initial perception of AIDS; that is, that it was a mysterious disease, relegated to a small group of gay individuals, unworthy of presidential attention. For the White House, AIDS was far from a national priority. It was "their" problem.

Congress was also not very responsive. This was mainly attributed to the fact that the House and Senate were divided over whether or not AIDS posed a serious risk to society, worthy of an immediate response. While the House was dominated by the Democrats' sympathy to the AIDS community, and while the Democrats created venues for activists to explain the situation, such as legislative hearings (Altman, 1986), the Republican-dominated senate did no such thing (Talbot and Bush, 1985). These partisan divisions stymied any efforts to create a bipartisan consensus for the need to provide more resources to the HHS and PHS while providing assistance to the states.

In contrast, public health officials saw the AIDS situation as urgent, in need of government assistance and complete bipartisan support (Brandt, 2006; Rich, 1985; *US News & World Report*, 1985a; *Frontline*, 2006; Russell, 1983). HHS Secretary Margaret Heckler (1983–1985), HHS Undersecretary Edward Brandt, as well as CDC officials immediately pressured the Reagan administration and Congress for an aggressive response. Heckler mentioned to reporters that she wanted to "conquer" AIDS (Herek, 1990; Rich, 1985; Shilts, 2007). In contrast to the White House and Congress, health officials were motivated by the epidemiological reality that an epidemic was at hand, and that every person, regardless of their lifestyles and religious beliefs, should be helped (Curran, 2006; Herek, 1990; Rich, 1985; Shilts, 2007).

In fact, even President Reagan's surgeon general, Dr. Everett Koop, disagreed with Reagan and the Republican party's views, ignoring any of the stigma associated with AIDS. Koop once emphatically claimed that "I am the surgeon general of the heterosexuals and the homosexuals, of the young and the old, of the moral [and] immortal ... I don't have the luxury of deciding which side I want to be on" (Koop quoted in Whitman, 1987). In essence, Koop wanted a more aggressive federal response, regardless of the social stigma surrounding AIDS (Fox *et al.*, 1989).

However, there were several reasons why the White House and Congress did not agree with these health officials. First, the White House and Congress believed that there simply was not enough credible evidence suggesting that AIDS was quickly developing into a serious national health threat. Notwithstanding an escalating rate in the percentage change of AIDS cases reported each year, this growth was mainly occurring in select cities, such as New York and Los Angeles, and was concentrated among the gay community. Despite CDC reports by December 1983 indicating that the virus had spread to intravenous drug users and heterosexuals, it was still perceived by the White House as a gay disease (Padgug and Oppenheimer, 1992).

Second, unlike the presidential and bureaucratic response to syphilis during the Second World War, AIDS did not immediately threaten the fundamentals of US national security, such as military readiness and the economy. Indeed, by the mid-1980s, AIDS was not highly prevalent among military enlistees. In fact, during the first few years of the epidemic, President Reagan received briefings from Pentagon officials stating that there was no credible evidence showing that AIDS was quickly spreading among military personnel, or that a large percentage of enlistee applicants were HIV positive (Evans, 1988; Keller, 1985). Most of the success at containing AIDS within the military was attributed to the Department of Defense's aggressive awareness and prevention programs, such as educational materials, seminars, videos, and even the provision of condoms (Engal, 1985; Evans, 1988). While case prevalence rates were much higher in the navy than in other branches, which was mainly due to a higher enlistment of former drug addicts and alcoholics (Evan, 1988), prevalence rates in other military branches, such as the army, air force, and marines, was quite low (Gómez, 2007 Kellyer, 1985). By 1985, the Pentagon officially declared that AIDS was not a national security threat (Keller, 1985).

As a result, there was no sense of urgency to propose new bills and/or create agency divisions within the Department of Defense in order to enforce prevention and treatment policies onto the states. Moreover, no new state funding programs were suggested — if you recall from the previous chapter, these policies were common during the military's campaign to eradicate syphilis during the Second World War. Because of this, there was no interest on the part of the military to pursue a reform coalition between military officials and the president for a centralized response to AIDS.

During this period, AIDS was also not perceived as posing a threat to the economy. Because the epidemic was concentrated within the gay community and, gradually, intravenous drug users, the government did not believe that the virus would pervade the entire working population (Herek, 1990). Reagan was also a proponent of anti-worker discrimination. In fact, Reagan wanted the AIDS afflicted to contribute to the economy (Garrett, 1988). One must also keep in mind that the whole impetus under Reagan was to prune the federal budget and have the states finance most of the response to AIDS (Fox, 1992; Fox *et al.*, 1989). State economies were in disarray but this was not attributed to AIDS, but rather to a general fiscal recession. While federal funding for infectious diseases (including AIDS) was less than 5% of the total estimated costs for all diseases in the US (Fox, 1986), there was certainly a fear by the late 1980s that the states' financing of prevention and treatment programs was going to be expensive (Fox, 1986).

During this period, there was also an informal element that, perhaps more than anything else, affected the initial perceptions of the conservative Reagan administration. It was an element that is well documented and to a certain extent still exists to this day; namely, the moral, puritanical, and judgmental views of conservative politicians (Gusfield, 1986). As in the past with sexually transmitted diseases, such as alcoholism and prostitution, these moral beliefs shaped the initial perceptions of White House and congressional elites in ways that stymied their willingness to immediately respond to AIDS. Moral beliefs would be periodically used as a justification for legislative inaction and delay, especially within the White House.

In addition, during the first few years of the AIDS epidemic, conservative activists in society successfully influenced the White House's views on how it should respond to AIDS (Shilts, 2007). For the most part the conservative right convinced Reagan and his staff that AIDS was an immoral act, unworthy of immediate policy attention (Herek, 1990; Perrow and Guillén, 1990; Shilts, 2007). To a great extent, this had to do with the fact that there existed a conservative moral backlash against the sexual liberalism of the 1960s and 1970s. The moral conservatives were keen on strategically using this moral backlash for leverage when pressuring Reagan and his staff not to respond (Altman, 1986).

Moral conservatives in society were also successful at influencing Reagan's thoughts through national conventions, always arguing that AIDS was a divine judgment from God, cast upon the immoral sinners from high above (Morganthau *et al.*, 1983; *Christian Today*, 1985; *US News & World Report*, 1985a). Reporters at the time also noted that conservative Christian organizations were mailing hundreds of pamphlets proclaiming that: "homosexuals and the pro-homosexual politicians have joined together with the liberal, gay-influenced media to cover up the facts concerning AIDS" (Doan, 1987: p. 12).

Conservatives' influence was aided by the fact that the moral right was tightly aligned with the increasingly popularized "moral majority," led by a group of Christian evangelicals seeking to reinstill good Christian morals within government. Led by charismatic leaders such as Jerry Falwell, the growing popularity of televangelism, coupled with the unwavering support of conservative voters (especially in the southern part of the US), gave the moral majority greater leverage and influence when working with the White House (Berstein, 2004; Jonsen and Styker, 1993). Despite his track record as a Republican in support of gay rights when serving as governor of California, Reagan was very much influenced by the conservative right. Facing congressional elections in 1984, Reagan found himself in a difficult position and was essentially forced to support the moral majority's position on AIDS (Behrman, 2004; Bronski, 2004).

Civic Mobilization and Response

While the White House and Congress was not responding, civil society took the lead in mobilizing a response at the local level. Because the virus initially emerged among young gay men, the gay community was particularly concerned and immediately mobilized. The first community-based organization (CBO) to emerge was the San Francisco AIDS Association (SFAA) in 1982. Although SFAA was initially focused on research, it gradually started to provide prevention and treatment services, especially homecare (Ira and Elder, 1989). Soon thereafter the Gay Men's Health Crisis was formed in New York. In 1983, moreover, the National Association of People with AIDS (NAPWA), the National AIDS Network, and the Federation of AIDS Related Organizations were created.

These initiatives set the groundwork for the creation of a host of other AIDS NGOs throughout the 1980s and 1990s. Perhaps the most prominent among these was the American Foundation for AIDS Research (amfAR), which was created in 1985 by Dr. Mathilde Krim, Michael Gottleib, and Elizabeth Taylor. amfAR raised money for treatment and prevention, and soon became one of the largest not-for-profit organizations committed to domestic and international AIDS research and policy. Two years later, in response to escalating prices for the antiretroviral drug AZT (azidothymidine), ACT UP (AIDS Coalition to Unleash Power) was created in New York as a not-for-profit dedicated to pressuring the government to reduce drug prices. Thanks in part to their efforts, the price of AZT was eventually lowered. In addition to the rise of these two influential NGOs, several other grass roots organizations emerged during the 1980s and 1990s. It was a time of unprecedented growth and response by not only the gay community but also scientists, intellectuals, the church, and other organizations fighting for the rights of AIDS victims (Jonsen and Styker, 1993).

During this period, however, AIDS NGOs were rather fragmented and disorganized, failing to provide a unified front. Organizations in California and New York did not work together to create a unified response to federal inaction. NGOs in these cities were essentially working hard to overcome their own political battles with local health departments (Cohen and Elder, 1989; Shilts, 2007) — NGOs in New York apparently had the most difficult time achieving this (Perrow and Guillén, 1990).

While several AIDS NGOs emerged to provide crucial healthcare, prevention, and treatment services, during this period they did not help to build the CDC's AIDS programs. In large part this failure stemmed from the fact that members of the gay community and AIDS NGOs did not occupy positions within the CDC staff, especially in the highest tiers of leadership (Altman, 1988). Instead, NGOs and civic members remained in their communities, focusing on building programs and responses at the local level (Jonsen and Styker, 1993). Moreover, these NGOs were never part of a broader democratic movement for the right to universal healthcare (Hoffman, 2003). There was therefore a large disconnect between federal health officials and civil society when it came to strengthening the CDC and its national AIDS programs.

The Peril of Bureaucratic Fragmentation and Competition

When it came to the federal bureaucracy, while PHS efforts to work with the White House and Congress in strengthening the government's response to AIDS was impressive, the PHS itself was nevertheless hampered in its ability to respond. This was mainly due to a high level of inter-agency fragmentation and overlap in research and policy interests, as well as inter-agency competition, which was fueled by the lack of sufficient funding, insecurity, and the need for bureaucratic survival in a context of economic recession.

By the time AIDS emerged, there was a myriad of PHS agencies working on infectious diseases. These agencies included the CDC,

NIH and subdivisions of the NIH, which included the National Cancer Institute (NCI) and the National Institutes of Allergy and Infectious Disease (NIAD). There was also a considerable amount of policy overlap, as all of these agencies, with the exception of the HHS, were involved in conducting AIDS research (Panem, 1988). While the CDC was mainly focused on classifying, monitoring, and reporting the spread of AIDS, the NIH also monitored and reported the epidemic while conducting biomedical research (Chabner and Curt, 1984). Meanwhile the NCI viewed AIDS as being potentially a new form of cancer, thus prompting research into HIV's etiology and evolution (Currran, 2006).

By 1983, this overlap in policy interests instigated intensive inter-agency competition. Initially, the main issue was about which agency should be responsible for AIDS research and policy (Russel, 1984). As the challenge of defining and finding a cure intensified, the NIH insisted that it take the lead in conducting this work. However, the CDC resisted this idea. The CDC also wanted to be involved in research and discovery (Mason, 2006). The NIH was upset with the possibility of the CDC — and any other agency — staking claim over its research mission. In essence, there was a race between these agencies to discover and claim credit for a new and mysterious virus (Curran, 2006; *The New York Times*, 1984; Russell, 1984).

The struggle over financial resources also contributed to this high level of inter-bureaucratic competition. Bereft of sufficient funding, these agencies wanted to use the AIDS situation as an opportunity to obtain more financial support and to expand their programs. During the 1980s, the CDC faced severe budget cuts (Wilke, 1983; Meyer and Russell, 1981; Rich, 1982). The House's budgetary outlays for the CDC barely increased during the first few years of the epidemic. In this context, the CDC believed that creating an impressive research and policy response would impress the president and congresses, in turn capturing their attention and support for program expansion.

During this period, the NIH was also experiencing a sizable decrease in funding. Although it was not as extreme as the CDC's, projected budgetary outlays were not expected to increase. While funding for research remained steady, there were no immediate plans to increase funding for AIDS research (Mason, 2006). Staff size within the NIH also remained stable but did not decrease as suddenly and as markedly as it had within the CDC.

The intensive inter-bureaucratic competition that arose from these financial issues had serious consequences, especially when it came to research and policy. By 1983, the director of the CDC Task Force for AIDS, Dr. James Curran, and other officials complained that Dr. Robert Gallo of the NIH and his staff were not sharing important information. They were hoping to obtain from Gallo crucial blood tests and samplings that they could use to conduct research. However, Gallo resisted this idea. The conflict intensified to such an extent that HHS Undersecretary Edward Brandt, had to call Curran and Gallow into his office to help resolve the problem (Brandt, 2006). The purpose of the meeting was to help clarify matters and to make it clear to both Gallo and Curran that sharing information was important for creating effective policy (Brandt, 2006). Undersecretary Brandt believed that the main challenge concerned Gallo's pride and defense of his reputation; Gallo did not want to share information, and he just wanted all the credit and glory for discovering the HIV virus and proposing innovative policy recommendations (Brandt, 2006).

Initial Bureaucratic and Policy Outcomes

During the first few years of the AIDS epidemic, President Reagan was never fully committed to working with the HHS to overcome these bureaucratic challenges (Brandt, 2006; Engel, 1987). Reagan also never explored the possibility of creating a centralized agency within the HHS that could help coordinate all AIDS policy responsibilities as well as the HHS' work with the states. In fact, to senior HHS officials, Reagan appeared apathetic to their organizational and policy needs (Brandt, 2006; Curran, 2006; Mason, 2006).

Although the Reagan administration did eventually take the initiative to create an institution that incorporated the views of HHS officials and civil society, it was perceived as ineffective. In 1987, Reagan worked with White House staff to create the National AIDS Commission. The Commission's purpose was to serve as the president's main advisory group on AIDS. It comprised several health officials, including the secretary of HHS at the time, several agency heads, and representatives from the private sector and civil society. The Commission was mainly responsible for evaluating the government's current policies and proposals, while surveying the AIDS situation.

However, two problems emerged. First, there were no HIV positive individuals on the Commission. This upset the gay and HIV positive community. Reagan was criticized for lacking common sense and for being careless about his appointments to the commission (*The New York Times*, 1987). Second, after the Commission's first review, the White House received a very low mark across a host of policy and leadership measures (Johnson, 1988). The review's findings made it clear that the administration was divided and that HHS officials were not pleased with the government's performance.

Within HHS, however, there was a clear consensus that a more centralized, coordinated response to AIDS was needed. In an interview with former HHS Undersecretary Edward Brandt (1981–1983), he explained to me that within the US's decentralized public health system, a more centralized, coordinated bureaucratic response to AIDS was important for ensuring that prevention and treatment policies were implemented in an timely and effective manner (Brandt, 2006). Brandt went on to claim that the state and local governments did not have the resources needed to effectively respond on their own (Brandt, 2006).

Worse still, President Reagan also ignored a detailed presidential AIDS Commission report published in June 1988 informing him of the need to create an official AIDS position within the White House (Boodman, 1988). Some accused Reagan of ignoring essentially every policy recommendation from the 200-plus page report (Melillo, 1991). It quickly became apparent to Brandt and Mason that Reagan's disdain towards the AIDS situation was the main obstacle to creating a more centralized and coordinated response to AIDS (Brandt, 2006).

By 1987, Reagan was essentially forced to change his views on AIDS. But it is important to note that in addition to the overwhelming evidence that AIDS cases were increasing, as well as the infection of close personal friends (such as the actor Rock Hudson), the institutional landscape within which Reagan operated was also changing. It is important to keep in mind that in 1986, Reagan lost the Senate to the Democrats, a situation that could have arguably been just as important of a factor in changing Reagan's perception and interest in AIDS. The Senate was now controlled by Democrats pressuring the White House for a stronger response to AIDS; and with pressures from the House increasing as well, Reagan eventually had no choice but to strengthen his commitment to AIDS.

If creating a centralized AIDS agency was not a viable option, then perhaps increasing funding to those agencies' work on AIDS was. However, this was also problematic. Despite HHS Secretary Heckler consistently pressuring the White House for additional funding (Curran, 2006; Kurtz, 1983; *The New York Times*, 1983; *Frontline*, 2006; Russell, 1985; Wilke, 1983), the White House barely asked for any increase in congressional funding for her work at the CDC and NIH. This situation upset members of the congressional House. For example, Harry Waxman (Democrat — California), chairman of the House Energy and Commerce Subcommittee on Health, argued that "the administration's response to AIDS has been too little and all but too late. ... The administration has never asked Congress for money for AIDS and, in fact, has opposed congressional efforts to provide funds to the Centers for Disease Control and the National Institutes of Health," (Waxman quoted in Russell, 1983).

On the other hand, Congress' efforts to engage in a centralized response were just as unimpressive. Congress had essentially no interest in strengthening the PHS's initial response. This had serious implications for the CDC. From 1981 to 1986, the CDC was not obtaining sufficient funding to expand its AIDS staff (Gómez, 2008). In fact, the CDC saw a significant *decline* in the number of personnel working on AIDS (Gómez, 2008). From 1985 to 1986, the CDC lost nearly 500 employees (Gómez, 2008). The situation became so bad that by 1985, the director of the CDC, James Mason, had to impose a hiring freeze and obtain staff from other departments in order to save money (Mason, 2006). Furthermore, this occurred in spite of Mason's continued pressures on Congress and the White House for additional funding (Mason, 2006).

to securing funding for research. For example, in 1982 the House
earmarked $5.6 million for AIDS activities and $28.7 million in 1983
(Perrow and Guillén, 1990). Though modest in its contributions, this
was much more than what the White House initially requested
(Perrow and Guillén, 1990; Russell, 1985). By 1984, the House
increased its commitment and authorized $61.5 million for AIDS
research (54% more than Reagan's request) and $97.4 million the
following year (61% more) (Office of Technology Assessment, *Review
of the Public Health Service's Response*: p. 32; Perrow and Guillén,
1990). By the end of 1985, the House had passed an appropriations
bill that earmarked $190 million for AIDS research, $70 million more
than what Reagan requested (*US News & World Report*, 1985b).

The White House also provided financial assistance. In 1983, Reagan
asked for a total of $12.6 million in AIDS research, to be divvied up
among all of the PHS agencies working on AIDS (Gómez, 2008).
However, this funding request was quickly perceived as insufficient.
In response, the president's request for research funding increased to
$17.6 million the following year (Gómez, 2008). Funding for AIDS
initiatives increased after 1985, from $34 million in 1983, to $67 million in 1984, and $121 million in 1985 (Gómez, 2008). Beginning
in 1986, Reagan increased his funding request for AIDS research
from $86.6 million in 1986, to $351.1 million for 1987, and $790.9
million for 1988, followed by an approved increase in overall AIDS
funding from $457 million in 1986 to $872 million in 1987 and
$1.525 billion in 1989 (Gómez, 2008). Despite this increase in fund-
ing, HHS officials were still unsatisfied with the amount of provided
to them (Brandt, 2006).

There were two factors that contributed to Reagan's decision to
increase his funding requests. The first was an overwhelming amount
of empirical data showing that AIDS was clearly an epidemic threat.
From 1981 to 1984, the number of AIDS cases increased from 31 to
7,699 (Gómez, 2008). From 1985 to 1987, the number of AIDS
cases increased from 8, 224, to 13,197, increasing to 31,001 by 1988
(Gómez, 2008). Second, in 1986 Reagan's long-time friend and
Hollywood actor, Rock Hudson, was diagnosed and died from AIDS.

This underscored the dim realization that AIDS could affect anyone. Moreover, the fact that Hudson had to travel as far as France to obtain effective HIV treatment demonstrated the need for more national investment into AIDS medication.

And finally, during this period very little financial and technical assistance was provided to the states (Altman, 1986; Shilts, 2007). Despite the need for assistance in the cites most affected by HIV/ AIDS, such as San Francisco and New York, under Reagan no effort was made to provide grants and/or direct technical support to municipal health agencies (Altman, 1986; Shilts, 2007). Furthermore, no funding was provided to NGOs working on medical treatment and care (Altman, 1986; Shilts, 2007). It was a time when municipal health departments and civil society were left to work on their own. This situation, moreover, dovetailed nicely with the Reagan administration's commitment to federalism and decentralization in healthcare and other social services (Fox, 1992; Fox *et al.*, 1989).

However, do these findings suggest that the government would have never responded to AIDS in an aggressive, centralized manner? Let us consider for a moment that Walter Mondale, democratic presidential candidate in 1984, had won the presidential election that year. Would he have pursued a centralized response to AIDS? After all, he had a long and distinguished record as a senator of Minnesota (1966–1972) and vice president during the Jimmy Carter administration (1976–1980), proactively defending civil rights and, in particular, the rights of the poor and minorities. During his 1984 presidential campaign against Reagan, moreover, he stood firm on his commitment to Medicare and proposed national social welfare programs for the poor (Blumenthal and Morone, 2010). Additionally, Mondale also seemed very interested in foreign affairs, both as vice president — many claim he was responsible for creating the Camp David Accords — and later on in life as ambassador to Japan in 1993. In contrast to Presidents Reagan and George H.W. Bush, then, he could have been much more sensitive to international criticisms and pressures for a centralized response to AIDS.

Yet, it is not clear that if Mondale had been elected, that he would have pursued a different response to AIDS. First, consider the fact that Mondale did not campaign on the AIDS issue during the 1984 election (Ryan, 2004). This suggests that AIDS was not a major policy focus — which is puzzling, considering his endorsement for protecting the civic rights of AIDS victims and the LGBT (Lesbian, Gay, Bisexual & Transgender) community in 1984, as well as his realization that the gay community was rising in prominence (Easterbrook, 1983; National Gay and Lesbian Task Force, 2012).

Second, Mondale may have confronted staunch resistance from the PHS bureaucracy, which was, as we saw earlier, adamant in defending its ground, and securing its autonomy and power. The PHS would have vehemently resisted any efforts to take away its autonomy and influence. Furthermore, while Mondale would have had the support of the democratic Senate and Congress, justifying a large expense during an economic recession would have been challenging. Mondale's unwavering commitment to Medicare notwithstanding, even as vice president under Carter, Mondale often wondered how they would be able to afford an increase in Medicare spending (Blumenthal and Morone, 2010: p. 265). In addition, recall that during this period Congress was not entirely committed to increasing the CDC's budget for AIDS. Therefore, while Mondale certainly had an impressive track record in fighting for the rights and needs of minorities and the poor, it is not clear that he was highly committed to creating a stronger centralized bureaucratic and policy response to AIDS, nor would have the fiscal and political conditions been propitious for Mondale's policy ideas of creating such a centralized response, if indeed he had had them.

International Criticisms, Pressures, and Response (1987–present)

The year 1987 marked a turning point in the international community's attention to AIDS. Beginning with the creation of the World Health Organization's Global AIDS Program (GAP) that year, followed shortly thereafter by the emergence of new international organizations, NGOs, conferences, and media attention, by the late 1980s these movements began to reach common ground on the need to work in partnership with other nations for a more aggressive response to AIDS (Altman, 1999). By this point, key international donors, such as the World Bank, emphasized that eradicating AIDS and other diseases went hand in hand with poverty alleviation and economic development (Ruger, 2005). This signaled the beginning of what others refer to as the "Geneva Consensus" on how governments should respond to AIDS (Gauri and Lieberman, 2006; Lieberman, 2009).

By 1987, the US and other nations began to be criticized for their lackluster policy response to AIDS. WHO officials tried persuading the Reagan administration to make AIDS a priority. However, Reagan essentially ignored these requests (Behrman, 2004). In addition, that year, Jonathan Mann, the first GAP director and professor at the Harvard School of Public Health, also began to criticize President Reagan and Vice President Bush for their delayed response. By 1989, Mann warned the newly elected Bush administration and his AIDS Commission that they needed to overhaul their approach to prevention and treatment in order to curb the spread of AIDS (*The Boston Globe*, 1989). Mann went on to claim that the Bush administration's stance on prohibiting the entrance of HIV positive individuals into the country unmasked a high level of discrimination within government. Mann once commented: "This has put us in league with various discriminatory countries around the world and has really undermined US ability to portray an effective and active AIDS program and to exercise global leadership" (Mann quoted in NPR, 1993).

Mann's criticisms were followed up with a flurry of international AIDS activists and scientists discussing President Bush's failed policy response and his tenuous relationship with the international community (Altman, 1991; Bliss, 2012). In 1991, for example, scientists and activists at the 7th International AIDS Conference held in Milan, Italy, followed up with yet another criticism of the US's slow policy response (Bliss, 2012).

During this period, domestic and international activists also began to criticize the Bush administration for its harsh stances towards immigrants with AIDS, as well as its lack of participation in international conferences (Altman, 1991). In 1990, these tensions heightened when Bush failed to address the 6th International AIDS Conference in San Francisco. Not only did Bush fail to attend but he even refused to send in a videotape greeting to conference participants (*The San Francisco Chronicle*, 1990). Many were also upset with Bush's decision in 1987 to support Reagan's announcement at the 3rd International AIDS Conference in Washington DC that the government would not grant visas to foreign nationals testing HIV positive (Mesce, 1990; *St. Louis Post-Dispatch*, 1991). Bush essentially adopted Reagan's stance on mandatory HIV testing for any individual older than the age of 14; these policies were quickly perceived as a direct infringement on individual liberties.

Furthermore, in 1991 President Bush as well as Congress authorized a reduction in the number of research scientists sponsored by the government to attend international meetings (Bliss, 2012; *The Atlanta Journal-Constitution*, 1991a). It quickly became clear that Bush had no interest in working with the international community (Bliss, 2012). Yet, these actions also revealed that the White House was not interested in strategically using AIDS policy as a way to increase the US's reputation as a nation committed to eradicating AIDS (Behrman, 2004).

This apathy in increasing the government's international reputation reflected President Bush's view that he simply had no reason to do so. As the perceived leader of the international community, reinforced with similar beliefs and expectations from other nations, President Bush believed that there was no need to display the US's scientific, medical, and infrastructural capacity to build an effective response to AIDS. Moreover, given the government's ample resources and experience in eradicating disease, the international community essentially expected the US to develop its own effective response to AIDS, and that as in the past, the government would help other nations achieve the same (Behrman, 2004). Steeped in expertise, pride, and experience, the president and HHS leaders believed that they had their own policy solutions to AIDS and that they did not need any international assistance and recommendations.

Clinton's Reform Efforts

The international community's criticisms of the US gradually decreased with the arrival of President William Clinton in 1992. Clinton's poise for responding to AIDS stemmed from the epidemiological situation, the heightened death toll, and the media's increased coverage of the crisis. These factors motivated Clinton to campaign on the issue when pursuing presidential election in 1991. During the campaign train, Clinton envisioned a more centralized, coordinated bureaucratic and policy response, emphasizing the need for an "AIDS Czar," as well as an increase in funding for AIDS (Foreman, 1993). Because of these efforts, when combined with his commitment to international cooperation and support, international as well as domestic pressures began to subside shortly after his arrival into office (Behrman, 2004).

But these international criticisms also began to subside because Clinton, unlike his predecessors, attended several international AIDS conferences and constantly declared AIDS's threat to the world (McKinney and Pepper, 1990). While AIDS's global impact was certainly of interest, Clinton was nevertheless mainly concerned with domestic AIDS policy during his administration. He was not interested in how he could increase the US's international reputation in response to AIDS. Instead, he was more committed to spreading global awareness about the epidemic, and its prevention and treatment.

It was not until the end of his second term that Clinton began to escalate the government's commitment to global AIDS policy (Kaiser Family Foundation, 2009b). In 1999, Clinton established the Leadership and Investment in Fighting an Epidemic (LIFE) initiative. In cooperation with the USAID, HHS, and the Department of Defense, LIFE was dedicated to preventing the spread of AIDS in 14 African countries as well as India (Kaiser Family Foundation, 2009b). This program entailed four priority areas: (1) prevention policy, such as sex education; (2) improving community and home-based care treatment; (3) treating children affected by AIDS; and (4) ensuring effective healthcare infrastructure and capacity (United States Agency for International Development, 1999). Clinton succeeded in securing $100 million for fiscal year (FY) 2000 from the Congress for this initiative (United States Agency for International Development, 1999), essentially tripling US bilateral assistance for AIDS to $466 million by FY 2001 (William J. Clinton Presidential Center, 2012). Additionally, Clinton signed an Executive Decree order in May 2000 in order to ensure that medical technologies and drugs were more affordable throughout sub-Saharan Africa (William J. Clinton Presidential Center, 2012).

At the domestic level, Clinton also demonstrated strong leadership and commitment to AIDS policy reform. For example, he worked with Congress to increase the budget for Ryan White CARE, Medicare, and Medicaid (White House, 1999; William J. Clinton Presidential Center, 2012). Under his watch, funding for Ryan White CARE increased by 260% (White House, 1999), by 57% for AIDS research (William J. Clinton Presidential Center, 2012), while funding for HIV prevention increased by 36% (William J. Clinton Presidential Center, 2012). Moreover, even when the Republican-dominated Congress in 1995 sought to reform Medicaid by decentralizing most of the program's budgetary responsibilities to the states, Clinton opposed the effort because of his fear that this would lead to a decrease in funding for AIDS patients (Cimons, 1995); referring to this initiative, Clinton once commented: "If this Medicaid budget goes through, it is a stake in the heart of our effort to guarantee dignity to the people with AIDS in this country" (Clinton quoted in Cimons, 1995: p.1). The President's efforts smacked of an earnest commitment to keep all Medicaid funding centralized so as to ensure the equitable distribution of AIDS financing.

Clinton also took the lead in creating a more centralized bureaucratic response to AIDS. Interestingly, he was even accused by his own HHS director, Dr. Louis Sullivan, of trying to create more "bureaucracy" at a time when preexisting agencies and programs simply needed more funding (Neergaard, 1992). A good example of Clinton's state-building efforts came in 1993, when he created the ONAP. The ONAP was created in order to centralize coordination and policymaking processes between those PHS agencies working on AIDS. In 1995, Clinton also created the Presidential Advisory Council on HIV and AIDS in order to provide the administration with technical expertise on developing effective policies (*The Body*, 2010). The following year, he also crafted the White House National Leadership Forum, which was established in order to improve collaboration on preventative substance abuse and the spread of AIDS (*The Body*, 2010). Moreover, in 1998, Clinton also took the lead in working with NIH officials to create the NIH Office of AIDS Research (*The Body*, 2010).

These initiatives revealed that Clinton was aware of the bureaucratically fragmented, uncoordinated response to AIDS, as well as the need for presidential leadership and a coherent national plan. Clinton was also committed to working with the senior leadership at HHS, Congress, and civil society in order to ensure a more centralized, coordinated response. Nevertheless, the aforementioned accomplishments also suggested that Clinton was committed to introducing reforms on his own, as if to use his executive powers and leadership in order to circumvent the challenges of bureaucratic contestation. By the early 1990s, the media underscored the fact that an AIDS leader had finally emerged, one with a strong commitment to bureaucratic and policy reform (Duckett, 1993).

However, with the election of Republican President George W. Bush to the White House in 2000, one may have expected a quick reduction in presidential leadership and commitment to AIDS. Yet, this did not appear to be the case. Although Bush did not campaign on the AIDS issue, perhaps because of the Clinton administration's myriad of accomplishments, he did nevertheless realize the urgency of the situation and essentially had no recourse but to adopt Clinton's policy initiatives. It seems that Bush's actions were motivated by Clinton's policies, institutions, and international expectations that Bush would maintain the White House's response to AIDS (Dietrich, 2003). However, some claim that Bush was also a compassionate individual, filled with the loving principles of Christianity (Landers, 2012); and in these very principles, he could have contrived a "moral obligation" to help AIDS victims, both at home and abroad (Landers, 2012).

Bush's receptivity to Clinton's AIDS initiatives is somewhat puzzling, however, especially if one considers how political conservatism under the Reagan and H.W. Bush years hampered policy reform efforts. Shortly after entering office, Bush decided to inherit and even deepen several of Clinton's domestic and international policy initiatives. In 2001, for example, Bush worked with HHS Secretary

Tommy Thompson, to carry over Clinton's Presidential Advisory Council on HIV and AIDS (McQueen, 2001). Individuals serving under Clinton on this advisory council were allowed to finish their terms (McQueen, 2001). It also seemed that Bush was committed to maintaining Clinton's domestic agenda for AIDS spending, especially after working closely with Congress to reauthorize the Ryan White CARE budget in 1996 (Hopson, 2006). Nevertheless, there were doubts that Bush would sustain Clinton's commitment to ONAP and AIDS policy in general (Ross, 2001).

Many soon lost hope in Bush's commitment to AIDS, however. His decision to decrease funding for AIDS NGOs working on prevention among high at-risk groups, such as sex workers, upset AIDS activists (International Planned Parenthood Federation, 2012). Over time, Bush appeared increasingly apathetic to the need to increase HHS funding for AIDS, convincing many that he was not fully committed to policy reform (Bull, 2003).

Furthermore, Bush was not as committed to taking the lead in working with White House staff and the HHS to create a strong national bureaucratic and policy response to AIDS (Bull, 2003; Campbell, 2005). In fact, in April 2001, Bush proposed closing down the ONAP office (ACT UP, 2003). After vehement unrest and opposition from the AIDS community, Bush quickly reversed his decision (ACT UP, 2003). In an attempt to reaffirm his commitment to ONAP, Bush did a commendable job of selecting highly qualified, experienced ONAP directors. His first director was Scott Evertz, appointed in 2001, followed by Joseph O'Neill in 2002. Both were openly gay physicians with a long history of working with the AIDS community (*The Advocate*, 2004).

Interestingly, despite Bush's appointment of highly qualified ONAP directors, he was never committed to securing adequate funding for ONAP (Bull, 2003). The president was also criticized for failing to use ONAP as a "bully-pulpit" for advocating for more AIDS prevention and treatment funding (Bull, 2003). Some maintain that this occurred because Bush was seeking to appease the interests of conservative political and social forces, who emphasized abstinence above all else as an effective course of AIDS prevention (Bull, 2003).

Assembling an effective ONAP leadership team therefore seemed pointless.

However, President Bush also seemed apathetic to working closely with the HHS and CDC for increase bureaucratic coordination and policy effectiveness. Bush seemingly sustained the old republican tradition of completely delegating bureaucratic coordination and policy responsibility to the HHS.

In addition to the White House, by the early 1990s Congress also appeared to have changed its stance on AIDS. Partisan division was supplanted with a bipartisan consensus that AIDS prevention and treatment policy should be prioritized. The publication of scientific research illustrating the multiple ways in which HIV could be transmitted, both homo- and heterosexually, helped to subdue the historic stigma associated with the disease. The passing of the Ryan White Care Act in 1990 as well as the approval of continued support for the CDC and NIH essentially signaled the end of partisan differences over AIDS.

Bureaucratic Fragmentation and Competition

The absence of President Clinton's and especially President Bush's proactive effort to work with the HHS in overcoming the challenges of bureaucratic fragmentation and competition may also have do with the fact that this challenge subsided by the late 1990s. Since then, the CDC, NIH, and NCI appear to no longer compete among each other over funding. That the mysteriousness and mystique of HIV gradually declined by the late 1990s also contributed to a lack of competition between these PHS agencies, as a substantial amount of research and funding support, as well as knowledge of the viruses' etiological nature, had emerged. In recent years, moreover, HIV has been perceived as a manageable chronic disease, rather than a mysterious viral epidemic. There now seems to be a greater commitment to a collaborative effort between the CDC, NIH, NCI, and other PHS agencies (National HIV/AIDS Strategy for the United States, 2010). With time, HHS agencies have learned that more can be achieved through inter-agency cooperation in research and knowledge.

This does not mean that the PHS has been an agency completely devoid of inefficiency, however. Recently pundits have accused the HHS for being delayed in its handling of AIDS funding and the provision of grants to state health departments. Activist organizations, such as the AIDS Healthcare Foundation, have charged the HHS with being negligent and careless, at the expense of HIV and AIDS victims who are in need of funding (Yeghiayan, 2011). Especially in this climate of ongoing economic recession and unemployment, AIDS positive individuals are more than ever dependent on access to medications through Medicaid and ADAP (Aids Drug Assistance Program) (Yeghiayan, 2011).

Bureaucratic Reform

Notwithstanding the George H.W. Bush and William Clinton administrations' interest in increasing the government's response to AIDS, this never led to an effective centralized bureaucratic and policy response. Under President George H.W. Bush, no new centralized AIDS program or even White House initiative was created, nor was he committed to increasing funding for the CDC's AIDS programs and policies at the state level (*The Atlanta Journal-Constitution*, 1991b). During this period the CDC continued to find itself in need of financial assistance in order to expand its state and municipal AIDS programs (*The Atlanta Journal-Constitution*, 1991b). Furthermore, under Bush the CDC continued to see a decline in the number of personnel working on AIDS (*The Atlanta Journal-Constitution*, 1991b).

As an alternative to creating a federal agency and/or expanding the CDC's AIDS division, President George H.W. Bush eventually worked with Congress to provide financial assistance to the states. In 1990, he authorized Congress to pass the Ryan White CARE Act, which provided $4.5 billion in federal emergency relief to the states. He also worked with Congress to allocate more money for CDC, NIH, and NCI researchers. Pundits nevertheless argued that the states still needed more funding. In fact, some even accused Bush of ignoring new proposals to fund hospitals and infrastructure, such as beds and X-ray machines, as well as the provision of ARV medication (Hilts, 1990a; Perrow and Guillén, 1990).[3]

Despite the conservative political climate at the time and the Republican Party's interest in reducing the federal bureaucracy, the idea of creating a centralized bureaucratic and policy response was still considered. In fact, this idea was proposed by President George H.W. Bush's National AIDS Commission in 1990 (Gladwell, 1990; Hilts, 1991). Among a host of problems outlined in their report, the National AIDS Commission stated that the Bush administration failed to provide the leadership needed to increase coordination between health agencies for a more timely and effective response to the states, a problem which a centralized coordinating agency could easily resolve (Gladwell, 1990; Hilts, 1991). The AIDS Commission's report also called for more leadership in helping the HHS, the Veteran's Affairs administration, and the Department of Housing and Urban Development to coordinate more effectively.

In essence, the National AIDS Commission was calling for a centralized bureaucratic and even somewhat authoritarian approach to AIDS policy implementation. Indeed, the Commission's chairman, David E. Rogers, once commented: "What is all too evident to the Commission is a critical lack of any top-level federal group clearly accountable and capable of swift, authoritarian action to coordinate efforts ..." (Rogers quoted in Gladwell, 1990). Until that point, some were referring to the government's bureaucratic approach to AIDS as an "orchestra without a conductor ... a cacophony of musical parts without any kind of coordinative leadership" (Hilts, 1990b).

However, the National AIDS Commission's next proposal was even more striking. The AIDS Commission suggested that President George H.W. Bush create a "super-agency" for AIDS (Rudavsky, 1992; Knox, 1990). David Rogers claimed that this was needed because of an excessive amount of PHS fragmentation and a lack of leadership,

---

[3]It is important to recall that Bush never authorized a proposal put forth by Senator Edward Kennedy of Massachusetts and Senator Orrin Hatch of Utah requesting an additional $600 million a year in 1991 and 1992 to go to the cities and states for emergency help for hospitals and AIDS clinics, as well as paying for drugs and home treatment for patients (Hilts, 1990b).

which hampered the government's ability to organize medical care for people with AIDS, train healthcare workers at the state level, increase sex education, and coordinate drug addiction programs (Knox, 1990). The new proposal was viewed as a way to get Bush to "match the rhetoric of his first speech on the subject with his actions" (Knox, 1990). In fact, the chairman of the AIDS Commission, June E. Osborn, stated that the creation of an AIDS super-agency "would have been helpful several years ago ..." and that "it's the kind of thing that you would want to do if you saw a big emergency coming" (Osborn quoted in Knox, 1990).

Despite these recommendations, the Bush administration still did not respond. Furthermore, after two years of inaction, the National AIDS Commission once again approached the White House about the need to create a super-agency, or at least a new cabinet-level agency for AIDS (Rudavsky, 1992). June Osburn accused the White House of not taking the AIDS Commission's proposals seriously: "What disappointed me most profoundly was the sense that this was business as usual. This is not business as usual. This is a historic epidemic" (Hilts, 1992; Osburn quoted in Rudavsky, 1992, p. 2).

However, interest in creating a more centralized response to AIDS did seem to be on President Clinton's agenda. As I mentioned earlier, Clinton had campaigned on the issue, going so far as to propose the creation of an "AIDS Czar," promising administrative reform and a host of prevention and treatment policies if elected to office. Recognizing the excess bureaucracy that paralyzed the government's initial response, and realizing the need to assist the states in their endeavors, one of the first things Clinton did was to create the ONAP in 1993. Though not a formal agency within the CDC, ONAP was the first attempt to address the National AIDS Commission's repeated calls for a centralized bureaucratic response to AIDS. The ONAP's primary goal was to advise the president while working closely with the PHS and the states to implement policy.

Pundits nevertheless quickly accused Clinton of delaying the ONAP's construction while failing to provide adequate funding and support, and choosing ONAP directors that were inexperienced (Berke, 1993). ONAP's first director, Kristine Gibbie, was just 34 years old, a former health secretary for Washington state and PhD candidate at the University of Washington. She had no prior experience working with NGOs and the AIDS community. Several politicians, NGOs, and activists claimed that Clinton selected someone that was unqualified, mainly on the grounds that she was incapable of building coalitions in Congress, obtaining funding, and working closely with AIDS NGOs (Murray, 1993). After what appeared to be extensive criticism and lack of support, Gibbie resigned in October 1994. Gibbie defended her decision by claiming that her role as AIDS Czar was very unclear, and that she never felt like an "AIDS Czar" but rather a policy coordinator (Colburn, 1994). She claimed that from the beginning, the expectation that she would have authority and the ability to easily coordinate and change policy far surpassed her actual powers (Colburn, 1994).

In November 1994, Gibbie was replaced with Patsy Fleming, an African American woman with extensive HHS experience. Flemming had served as a special assistant to HHS Director Donna Shalala, as well as an assistant to the late Representative Ted Weiss (Democrat — New York) in the House, where she specialized in AIDS and other public health issues. However, Flemming was still perceived by AIDS activists as not having enough "on the ground" experience. Activists were also upset that neither Gibbie nor Flemming had received a cabinet-level position and lacked the authority needed to get things done quickly (Bedard, 1994). After three years in office, Flemming resigned.

In 1997, Flemming was replaced with Sandra Thurman. In contrast to the fist two ONAP directors, Thurman had spent several years as director of AIDS Atlanta, one of the largest and best-funded AIDS NGOs in the country. She had also served as the Director of Advocacy Programs at the Task Force for Child Survival and Development at the Carter Center in Atlanta, as well as being a member of the Presidential Advisory Council on HIV/AIDS and the Georgia State AIDS Task Force. Clinton was also reported as being very committed to working closely with her and maintained an "open door" attitude to her requests (Okie, 1989; Ross, 2001).

Despite this support and her extensive experience, AIDS activists and politicians still were not convinced that this would help get things done. The simple fact was that she and the ONAP office was still powerless, incapable of mustering a coalition for more funding within a Republican-dominated Congress. Mr. Steve Michael, co-director of the ACT UP office in Washington, DC, one of the largest AIDS NGOs in the US, declared that they wanted an ONAP director that was a politician and that could get more resources for AIDS (Bedard, 1997). Repeated recommendations for an ONAP office that was a cabinet-level position, with ample autonomy and resources was never acted upon. This failure, in addition to other problematic areas, such as the failure to pass legislation mandating federal funds for free needle exchange, led Clinton's very own Presidential Advisory Council in 1998 to mention that they had no confidence in Clinton's ability to respond to the ongoing AIDS problem (Egelko, 1998).

The absence of an effective ONAP program created several problems. First, it failed to help the PHS better coordinate for policy research and implementation. The ONAP was created with the expressed intent of increasing policy coordination between agencies that incessantly competed with one another over funding. Clinton's arrival into office provided a key opportunity to unify senior officials in the CDC, NIH, and NCI. While these agencies were, of course, working closer than before, coordination within the fragmented PHS system has always been needed. Both under Clinton and the subsequent George W. Bush administration, a lack of policy coordination delayed and complicated the government's ability to manage agency finances, and to devise and implement policy (Open Society Institute, 2006).

Second, the absence of a strong ONAP office also led to a decline in policy accountability and learning between agencies (Open Society Institute, 2006). A centralized coordinating agency was needed in order to closely monitor activities within the PHS and to hold administrators to account. Without such a system, avoiding fiscal profligacy and corruption could not be achieved (Open Society Institute, 2006).

Third, the ONAP was needed to help coordinate relations between the states and PHS agencies. Continued budgetary shortfalls at the state level, in addition to a dearth of healthcare infrastructural resources required the presence of an effective ONAP office possessing the funding needed to increase dialogue between the states and the PHS while pressing the latter to provide more direct assistance to the states. Furthermore, within a large, highly decentralized federal context, having a centralized agency that can monitor local government performance and hold the PHS accountable for failing to assist the states in meeting local needs could have facilitated policy implementation (Open Society Institute, 2006).

And finally, an ineffective ONAP contributed to the absence of a coherent national AIDS program. Despite Clinton's commitment to increasing funding for federal prevention and treatment policies, analysts note that policy guidelines and goals were never clearly articulated within the ONAP and other agencies. As one reporter put it, Clinton's publicized National AIDS Strategy in 1997 had prevention and treatment steps, yet "the action steps were vague, with no office identified to carry them out, and no timeliness set for completion of tasks" (Collins, 2007: p. 10). The same problem was found with President George W. Bush's HIV Prevention Strategic Plan, which was implemented in 2001 (Collins, 2007).

Even under the George W. Bush administration, there was no sense of a coherent plan and strategy for responding to AIDS. Soon after entering office, Bush displayed little interest in strengthening the ONAP, creating an alternative AIDS program or increasing funding to the states. Of course, one can see how the terrorist events of 9/11 took Bush's focus away from domestic social policy issues.

In addition to failing to construct an effective ONAP, the government also failed to increase the CDC's AIDS budget. Budget spending for the CDC's AIDS programs have essentially flat-lined since the late 1990s (Gómez, 2010b). In fact, the budget decreased from $976 million in 2003 to $838 million in 2006, rising slightly to $904 million in 2010 (Gómez, 2010b).

In addition, despite countless reports indicating that the states were in need of financial and technical assistance, the CDC never obtained the support needed to create new policies that would enhance its intervention at the state and municipal level. While one may view federal intervention as an effort to limit democratic decentralization processes, in a context of poorly funded municipal governments within a large geographic area, such an approach may be needed. Centralization for important health sectors can co-exist within a decentralized approach to healthcare (Gómez, 2012; Pritchett and Wolcock, 2004).

The CDC has also failed to introduce new initiatives increasing its centralized influence either through close partnerships with NGOs and/or through discretionary fiscal policies to the states. Although the CDC has encouraged local health departments to work with community leaders and the private sector for increased awareness (CDC, 2007), it has not contracted NGOs to monitor how effective health departments are in implementing AIDS policy. For example, in one of the highest HIV/AIDS at-risk groups, the African American community, the closest the CDC has come to working with community organizations is the CDC's creation of the African American HIV/AIDS Working Group, which, among other initiatives focused on prevention and awareness, merely tries to "explore opportunities to create new partnerships and strengthen existing partnerships" (CDC 2007: p. 4). Similarly, a 2005 report published by the National Alliance of State & Territorial AIDS Directors (NASTAD), a federal agency which brings together Governors and Mayors to address AIDS, stated that in the future the CDC and other agencies will need to work together in establishing partnerships with NGOs, CBOs, and community leaders while providing resources (NASTAD, 2005).

Congress has also failed to introduce new discretionary, performance-based fiscal programs motivating local governments to successfully implement policy. While discretionary funding through Ryan White, Medicare, and Medicaid continues, these transfers are not based on state and local governments' success in curtailing the spread of HIV through effective prevention and treatment policy. Plan B of Ryan White CARE is the closest Congress has come to imposing funding based on policy performance. However, it is important to note that it is not the quality and effectiveness of policy performance that is of concern but rather evidence of providing a list of important "medical services," such as outpatient and ambulatory healthcare services; ADAP; early intervention services; oral healthcare; hospice care; community-based organizational care; and medical case management and treatment adherence services (HRSA, 2008). To receive funding, local health departments must also demonstrate need, such as an increase in the number of individuals living with AIDS and funding shortfalls (Kaiser Family Foundation, 2013). However, merely showing that a local health department has implemented federally proscribed medical services says absolutely nothing about their quality and effectiveness.

The Absence of Civic Supporters

Why have the HHS and CDC been incapable of acquiring ongoing funding to expand their federal programs and create new policies? In essence, it was the absence of civic supporters that failed to provide CDC officials with the legitimacy and influence needed to achieve this outcome. As I discussed in Chapter 1, civic supporters emerge when well-organized NGOs and social health movements advocate policy ideas of a centralized bureaucratic and policy response to epidemics with a historically proven track record of success representing similar social health movements and organizations in the past. Bureaucrats partner with and use these civic supporters in order to increase their legitimacy and influence when seeking ongoing funding and political support for their centralization strategies. These civic supporters provide health officials with legitimacy because NGOs and social movements advocate policy ideas with a history of success, representing ideas that are well-known and supported by civil society as well as politicians. Moreover, politicians' recognition that these NGOs and social health movements represent a long, successful history of social health movements partnering with the bureaucracy further adds to contemporary bureaucrats' political credibility.

Yet, as we saw in Chapter 2, for the most part these civic supporters never emerged in the US. When it came to eradicating disease, civic organizations and social health movements in the past did not propose the creation of a central bureaucracy for increased federal policy intervention, nor did they continuously pressure Congress for federal financial and technical assistance (Hoffman, 2003). Civic organizations and social health movements often worked on their own (Hoffman, 2003), at times with the assistance of local government officials and PHS officials — officials that, as we saw in Chapter 2, were also advocating for a decentralized approach to public health (beginning in 1912). Furthermore, historically civic organizations and social health movements never established strong partnerships with the PHS based on the idea of immediately responding to epidemics in a timely manner. Scholars note that during the 19th century and early 20th century, public health officials in general repeatedly demonstrated little interest in establishing strong ties with social health movements for "big" policy ideas, such as universal healthcare reform (Hoffman, 2003). Therefore, by the time the AIDS epidemic emerged, there existed no rich tradition and expectation that AIDS officials would strategically use and work closely with AIDS NGOs in order to increase their legitimacy, influence, and ability to obtain ongoing support from Congress.

While HHS and CDC officials did respond early on by prioritizing the need to combat AIDS, and while they did work closely with the gay and intravenous drug community in order to learn more about their needs, they never engaged in a close partnership with AIDS NGOs and other community-based organizations in order to obtain ongoing congressional funding, expand programs, and introduce innovative policies (Gómez, 2010b). As I mentioned earlier, the CDC has only recently recognized the fact that it needs to engage in a stronger partnership with NGOs and CBOs working in the most at-risk communities, such as the African American and gay communities (CDC, 2007). CDC workshops were created in order to explore how the CDC can strengthen its partnerships with NGOs and CBOs (CDC, 2007), an issue which was vehemently supported by NASTAD (NASTAD, 2005). Nevertheless, no concrete effort was made to strengthen and maintain a close working partnership with NGOs and CBOs throughout the 1990s and early 2000s (NASTAD, 2005). In addition to failing to adequately meet the needs of at-risk groups, this has also appeared to decrease the CDC's justification for obtaining more funding from Congress. Without a clear partnership, support from civil society, and adequate information, in the future it may be difficult for the CDC to persuade the president and Congress to provide them with ongoing funding for their AIDS programs.

Global Policy Strategies

However, this kind of policy response is somewhat puzzling. As arguably the world's largest and leading economy, why has the US failed to continuously expand the congressional budget for AIDS? The answer to this question may be found by looking closely at the government's AIDS funding priorities. In recent years, especially under the George W. Bush administration, it seems that these priorities have not been focused on the domestic but rather the global level.

Indeed, the government's focus on global AIDS policy began to emerge under the Clinton administration. By the end of his second term, Clinton joined the international community in underscoring the importance of providing financial support to multilateral health agencies and developing nations in order to ensure an adequate supply of ARV medications, and technical and infrastructural assistance. As mentioned earlier, Clinton's LIFE program was created for that very reason. Clinton also realized that while he had done a lot at the domestic level, there was a pressing need to start focusing on global AIDS policy (Kates, 2012).

George W. Bush had the same interest. Under Bush, one could easily argue that there emerged a shift in the government's priority focus on AIDS from the domestic to the global AIDS policy level (Brodie *et al.*, 2004; Evertz, 2012; Kates, 2012; Platt and Platt, 2013). The global and domestic focus on AIDS exhibited completely different political logics (Tobias, 2012), with global AIDS receiving a stronger presidential interest and commitment (Kates, 2012).

It was under Bush, moreover, that we begin to see a White House leader claiming a "moral obligation" and "duty" to help other nations combat AIDS — mainly Africa, but also Latin America (Landers, 2012; McDonnell, 2007). Bush often emphasized his belief that he had a moral obligation to help those nations suffering from AIDS; that he was focused on "helping a neighbor in need" (Bush quoted in Bush, 2003). Bush once commented: "In the face of preventable death and suffering, we have a moral duty to act, and we are acting ... [to address] one of the most urgent needs in the modern world"

(Bush quoted in *Kaiser Health News*, 2003: p. 1). Bush further commented: "When I got into office, the devastation [of AIDS] was becoming so real that to have done nothing about it as president of the wealthiest nation would have been immoral" (Bush quoted in Landers, 2012; Hindman and Schroedel, 2010).

Bush's efforts also emerged at a critical juncture in international health politics, which may have further reinforced his focus on global policy (Garrett, 2012). 2001 was a key moment in the global fight against AIDS. As secretary general of the UN, Kofi Annan consistently reaffirmed and pressured government leaders to strengthen their focus on AIDS, while pressuring wealthier nations to contribute more funding to the global effort. In 2001, Annan also worked with the international community to create a new international funding initiative to help developing nations combat AIDS, tuberculosis, and malaria. Facilitated by a $50 million contribution from the Bill & Melinda Gates Foundation, what emerged from this endeavor was the Global Fund to Fight AIDS, Tuberculosis and Malaria. The Global Fund's emergence not only provided a new stream of funding for developing nations, but it also marked a shift in increased international attention and commitment from wealthier nations and philanthropists to help poorer nations combat these diseases (Brodie *et al.*, 2004; World Health Organization, 2008).

This turning point was further amplified with the creation of the 2000 Millennium Development Goals (MDG), endorsed by 189 country representatives, with the goal of reducing child mortality, improving maternal health, and combating AIDS, malaria, and other diseases by 2015 (World Health Organization, 2008). Shifts in international commitment to health were also prompted and facilitated by the 2001 Doha Declaration of access to essential medicines as a human right, where leaders from several developed and developing nations converged in Doha to declare a universal commitment to helping each other access medicines for AIDS (World Trade Organization, 2011). Thus, at a time when Bush was allowing his moral beliefs to shape his global AIDS agenda, the international community was also indirectly reinforcing Bush's commitment through its new global health campaigns. The timing and international climate could not have been more propitious for Bush and his focus on global AIDS policy (Garrett, 2012).

It is important to note, however, that civil society also approved of Bush's global policy endeavors. According to a nationwide survey conducted by the Kaiser Family Foundation in 2006, when asked if the US had the responsibility of leading the world in global health and providing bilateral assistance to combat AIDS, the percentage of individuals responding in the affirmative increased from 22% in June 2002, to 30% in May 2004, increasing again to 34% in April 2006 (Kaiser Family Foundation, 2009a). Those believing that the government should address AIDS problems at home before assisting other nations *decreased* from 71% in June 2002, to 62% in May 2004, and again to 55% in April 2006 (Kaiser Family Foundation, 2009a). Furthermore, when asked if the US is doing too much, too little, or about the right amount to help other countries combat AIDS, according to Kaiser Family survey, 34% believed in June 2002 that the US was doing too little, increasing to 56% in April 2006, while those believing that the US was providing the right amount of international support decreased from 34% in June 2002 to 13% in April 2006 (Kaiser Family Foundation, 2009a); on the other hand, those believing that the US did too much remained relatively stable, from 16% in June 2002 to 13% in April 2006 (Kaiser Family Foundation, 2009a).

Another condition facilitating President Bush's focus on global AIDS policy was the lack of bipartisan division over global versus domestic AIDS policy. It was politically easier to focus on spending for global AIDS versus increasing spending for the CDC's domestic AIDS programs (Garret, 2012; Kates, 2012), for several reasons. First, both Republican and Democratic senators and House members agreed with Bush that helping developing nations combat AIDS was the right thing to do (Garrett, 2012; Tobias, 2012); these bipartisan views, moreover, were heavily influenced by their constituents' beliefs that this was the proper, moral thing to do (Kaiser Family Foundation, 2012: p. 1).

Reaching this bipartisan agreement was a challenging process, however. As a politically important individual considered by many to be one of the biggest obstacles to shifting the congressional focus in favor of global AIDS policy, initially Senator Jessy Helms (Republican — North Carolina) needed convincing. In addition to pressures from AIDS activists to respond to international needs, Helms was also approached by the rock star Bono to address the AIDS epidemic in Africa (Evertz, 2012). Yet, even Bono's charm and popularity failed to convince Helms. Helms only became convinced after his close friends and colleagues approached him at a Republican dinner one evening in Washington. That night, one of Helms' closest colleagues, Janet Wasevany, asked Pastor Rick Warren of Saddleback Church in California to talk with Helms about AIDS in Africa. Warren explained how African woman and children were suffering from AIDS; that they needed their help; and that it was the proper, moral — better yet, Christian — thing to do. Apparently Helms welled up in tears and realized that from that moment on, he needed to work with the Democrats to strengthen their focus on global AIDS policy.[4] Soon thereafter, Helms commented:

> We have a higher calling, and in the end our conscience is answerable to God. Perhaps in my eighty-first year, I am too mindful of soon meeting Him, but I know that, like the Samaritan traveling from Jerusalem to Jericho, we cannot turn away when we see our fellow man in need. (Helms, 2002)

Other Republican senators agreed with Helm's views. Senator Bill Frist (Republican — Tennessee) and Richard Lugar (Republican — Indiana) (Lugar also served as chair of the Senate Foreign Relations committee), for example, placed bilateral assistance for AIDS top on their agenda. Frist's commitments were driven by his prior career as a physician as well as his previous work on global AIDS policy (Hindman and Schroedel, 2010). Moreover, even before Bush assumed office, Lugar had already been drafting bills to increase US bilateral assistance for AIDS in Africa (Hindman and Schroedel, 2010). Furthermore, House

---

[4] I would like to thank Laurie Garrett at the Council of Foreign Relations for sharing this story with me; interviewed by me on November 19, 2012.

Democratic Representatives Tom Lantos (Democrat — California) and Republican Henry Hyde (Republican — Illinois), advocates for Bush's PEPFAR bill, were already known for their commitment to human rights in access to healthcare (Hindman and Schroedel, 2010). All of these congressional members agreed with Bush that because of America's wealth, knowledge and expertise, the government should help Africa combat AIDS (Hindman and Schroedel, 2010).

Nevertheless, when it came to domestic AIDS policy, there was much more division and lack of consensus both within and between the House and Senate (Kaiser Family Foundation, 2012). This reflected the fact that domestically, AIDS in the US is still a highly contested bipartisan issue, conjuring up racial, poverty, and moral views within government and society (Avert, 2012; Lambda Legal, 2007; Tomaszewski, 2012).

It is also interesting to note that at the same time that Senator Helms was eventually advocating for a global response to AIDS, he was also blaming the domestic gay community for the epidemic, calling them "weak, morally sick wretches," and stating that "there is not one single case of AIDS in the country that cannot be traced in origin to sodomy" (Helms quoted in Tapper, 2008). Thus, even when Helms felt morally compelled to, as I quoted him stating earlier, help "a fellow man in need," interestingly it seems that he did not feel the same way towards AIDS victims in the US.

A large group of supportive evangelical religious groups also provided an encouraging environment for Bush to strengthen his focus on global AIDS (Evertz, 2012; Garrett, 2012; Kates, 2012; Tobias, 2012). As a self-proclaimed Christian, Bush maintained close ties with his evangelical support base, which comprised a host of Christian dominations — what is still commonly referred to as the "moral majority." Shortly after entering office, Christian leaders in the US and Africa pressured Bush to help Africa respond to AIDS (McGreal, 2008). As Bush drew plans to create his bilateral AIDS programs, such as PEPFAR, as well as other initiatives providing funding for faith-based groups adopting his abstinence-based approach to prevention (e.g., ABC, **A**bstinence first, **B**eing tested for HIV, **C**orrect and effective use of condoms), Bush received a lot of encouragement and support from his evangelical support base (Evertz, 2012; Garrett, 2012; Kates, 2012; Tobias, 2012). They viewed Bush's actions as a testament to the love and compassion of Christians (Evertz, 2010). Some have even claimed that this Christian connection inspired Bush to introduce and maintain PEPFAR (Hindman and Schroedel, 2010).

Several years after PEPFAR was introduced, Bush also received praise from popular Christian leaders, such as Pastor Rick Warren of Saddle Back Church in California — the very pastor that delivered the invocation for President Barack Obama's first inauguration (James, 2009). Warren praised PEPFAR and Bush's success in providing ARV medications to Africans with AIDS (*Time*, 2008). With the support and encouragement of his conservative friends, as well as liberal Democrats and Hollywood celebrities (for instance, in an interview with *The Atlantic*, Matt Damon recently commented that he would have kissed Bush on the lips for his work on global AIDS; Goldberg, 2012), this may have incentivized Bush to further deepen his commitment to global AIDS (Evertz, 2010).

However, Bush was so engrossed in the global AIDS effort that he appeared to overlook the importance of simultaneously investing in domestic AIDS policy (Garrett, 2012; Gómez, 2010b; Kates, 2012; Platt and Platt, 2013). Throughout his two terms in office, there never emerged any new policy initiatives and requests for increased congressional spending for domestic AIDS policy (Evertz, 2012; Gómez, 2010b; Kates, 2012); furthermore, this occurred even after the Bush administration received policy recommendations to apply its global policy innovations to the domestic level (Collins, 2007; Open Society Institute, 2006).

In fact, Bush's policy advisors recommended that Bush go so far as to create a "domestic PEPFAR." Bush initially liked this idea; however, it faced staunch opposition from HHS and PHS officials, many of whom felt threatened by such an endeavor. The fear was that a domestic PEPFAR would take away these officials' policy autonomy, powers that were cherished and safeguarded. Thus while the peril of bureaucrat fragmentation and competition had subsided, PHS officials were still territorial and opposed any effort to weaken their control and policy influence.

Complaints from the AIDS activist community also supported the notion that Bush was too focused on global AIDS policy. At the beginning of the Barack Obama administration, well known AIDS NGOs, such as amfAR, released documents stating that the Bush administration had been too complacent on domestic AIDS issues (amfAR, 2010); that the administration did not take the domestic AIDS situation seriously (amfAR, 2010); and that there was a need for an increased investment in innovative prevention programs targeting at-risk youth (amfAR, 2010). amfAR also criticized the administration for failing to ensure that the youth and other at-risk groups had sufficient access to healthcare infrastructure, testing, and treatment (amfAR, 2010). A host of other NGOs released policy statements stating that essentially nothing had been done to address domestic AIDS prevention and treatment (Kates, 2012).

Pundits soon joined these NGOs in their criticisms. For example, Rod McCullom, columnist for *The Advocate* newspaper, stated the following: "In the 2000s, during the Bush administration, a greater emphasis was placed on treating HIV/AIDS around the world as opposed to at home ... The Bush administration did a great thing as far as PEPFAR, the emergency plan for HIV/AIDS relief, which helped a lot of people in Africa and Asia. But on the other hand, HIV was neglected at home" (McCullom quoted in Pilecki, 2010).

Examining federal budgetary expenditures also suggested more of a commitment to global versus domestic AIDS policy. As Gómez (2010b) explains, from 2004 to 2009, while total federal spending for global bilateral and multilateral agencies was lower than total domestic spending for discretionary (Ryan White) and mandatory (Medicare and Medicaid) AIDS programs, US bilateral spending and contributions to the Global Fund seem to have increased at a higher yearly percentage growth rate during this same time period: from 1.9% to 5.5% for the Global Fund and 1.4% to 5% for US bilateral aid assistance — e.g., PEPFAR, versus 6.5% to 6.8% for domestic discretionary and 9.9% to 11.3% for domestic mandatory spending (Gómez, 2010b).

Alternatively, when measured in terms of yearly percentage changes in budgetary allocations for healthcare spending, the bias in favor of global AIDS policy seemed more apparent. As Gómez (2010b) maintains, bilateral and multilateral spending saw a higher annual percentage change increase from 2004 to 2009, from 121% in 2004 to 101% for the Global Fund and 135% in 2004 to 108% in 2009 for US bilateral assistance. In contrast, for this same time period annual percentage change increases for domestic discretionary and mandatory spending were significantly lower: 7.07% to 6.6% for mandatory versus 0% to 1.49% for discretionary spending (Gómez, 2010b). What these findings suggest is that each year Congress was increasing the budget for global AIDS at a consistently higher percentage change growth rate when compared to domestic AIDS programs.

President Barack Obama's AIDS Policy Strategy

Since entering office in January 2009, President Barack Obama has consistently argued that AIDS "remains an epidemic" in the US (*The Body*, 2010: p. 1) and that the government needs to increase its commitment to prevention and treatment policy — especially for high at-risk groups, such as the African American community. In response, Obama created the National Strategy on HIV/AIDS during his first year in office. Based out of the White House and managed by ONAP, this initiative had three primary goals: first, a reduction in HIV incidence; second, an increase in access to healthcare and optimizing health outcomes for those with HIV/AIDS; and third, a reduction in HIV-related health disparities (White House, 2010). The underlying goal of the National Strategy is to emphasize prevention and to address the root causes of AIDS, such as poverty and homelessness, issues which the Obama administration felt were neglected under the previous Bush administration (Barack Obama Presidential Campaign, 2008).

However, where did Obama's interest in reform come from? It seems that the president has been motivated by prior policy initiatives: that is, the Clinton and Bush's administration's recognition of the need to increase the government's commitment to domestic and, especially, bilateral assistance to developing nations. Especially under the Clinton administration, Obama inherited a domestic agenda that sought to strengthen the government's domestic policy response to

AIDS. Nevertheless, since efforts to fund prevention activities for at-risk groups were stalled under the prior Bush administration (Leff, 2003), Obama was particularly focused on addressing these issues when he entered office. Obama's commitment to AIDS therefore reflects both policy progress and policy retrenchment under prior presidential administrations.

When compared to the Bush administration, the Obama administration has not been as excessively focused on global AIDS policy, however (Evertz, 2012; Gayle, 2010). While Obama shared the George W. Bush administrations' view that it is the moral obligation and duty of the US to provide bilateral assistance for AIDS (*Council on Foreign Relations*, 2010), this has not distracted the White House from strengthening the government's domestic policy response (Gayle, 2010; Kates, 2012). Even before he was elected into office, appeared to be cognizant of the fact that prior administrations and the Congress were too focused on combating AIDS overseas and that not enough had been done domestically. Obama therefore entered office with a focus on simultaneously strengthening the government's domestic and international response to AIDS.

The Obama administration also seems to have taken centralized bureaucratic and policy reforms more seriously. In contrast to the Clinton and Bush administrations, Obama choose an ONAP director that was recommended by one of the highest at-risk groups in America: the gay community. On February 26, 2009, Mr. Jeffrey Crowley was appointed as the ONAP director. Crowley is an openly gay professional with extensive experience in connecting research with policy in increasing access to drugs and reducing health disparities. Prior to his appointment, he was deputy executive director for Programs at the National Association of People with AIDS, as well as a senior research scholar at Georgetown University (Stein, 2009). Crowley was also officially endorsed and recommended as the next ONAP director by the Gay & Lesbian Leadership Institute, an NGO focused on promoting the hiring and retention of gay professionals as presidential appointees. Unlike his predecessors, Crowley therefore had the civic support and legitimacy needed to do his job well.

In addition, since entering office, Obama has been committed to increasing HHS funding for AIDS. Unlike previous administrations, Obama's budget for the financial year of 2011 proposed an increase in federal funding for the NIH to conduct research on AIDS to $2.7 billion (Kaiser Family Foundation, 2010). Moreover, Obama's budget included an increase in spending from $6,312 billion in 2009 to $6,342 billion in 2010 for the CDC (OMB, 2010). Public health advocates and CDC officials consider this impressive, considering Obama's freeze on spending for other agencies due to the economic recession (Keefe, 2010). Obama's domestic budget for AIDS, which includes CDC programs, also increased from $26 billion in 2010 to $27.2 billion in 2011 (Kaiser Family Foundation, 2010). Domestic spending for healthcare for those living with HIV/AIDS, mainly through Medicare and Medicaid, has also increased by 7% since 2010, while Ryan White CARE has received a boost of $39.5 million more in funding for 2011 (Kaiser Family Foundation, 2010).

Furthermore, included in Obama's 2011 budget was a proposal to increase the CDC's staff by about 100 full-time employees, as well as funding new obesity projects and initiatives for reducing AIDS and other diseases within inner cities (Keefe, 2010). Other initiatives include $10 million to create a CDC Health Prevention Corps, which would recruit and train healthcare professionals and assign them to key inner city locations; $20 million for obesity prevention programs; and $23 million to strengthen the CDC's health statistics program (Kaiser Family Foundation, 2010).

The Obama administration has also increased its commitment to providing more assistance to the states. In addition to the aforementioned increase in federal spending for programs aiding the states, such as Ryan White CARE, Medicare, and Medicaid, Obama is working closely with the CDC to implement new initiatives targeting the highest at-risk groups for HIV in the US: the African American community (CNN, 2008).

For example, through an initiative called the Act Against AIDS program, the CDC is working closely with 14 African American organizations, ranging from newspapers to community-based organizations and churches to increase awareness about HIV, as well as treatment

(Sutton *et al.*, 2009). Those organizations selected to participate were chosen for their proven track record in reaching out to the black community (CDC, 2009a).[5] The overall goal is to harness the talent and commitment of community and media leaders in order to increase awareness and provide more effective HIV/AIDS treatment (CDC, 2009a). Those organizations involved receive funding from the CDC to hire an HIV coordinator who, in turn, uses their organization's membership network to disseminate awareness materials and other HIV prevention services (CDC, 2009a). Through this initiative, Obama seeks to harness the experience, talent, and proven commitment of community organizations in order to help prevent the spread of HIV and provide AIDS treatment to the black community.

However, the gay community, which is viewed as the second-largest at-risk group in the US, seems to have not received as much attention. While the CDC has known about the burgeoning rate of infection among gay men for several years (CDC 2010a, b), the Obama administration has not proposed any new programs for this group. The CDC has instead worked on its own, drawing attention to the issue while engaging in policy interventions focused on community building, awareness, and peer outreach (CDC 2010b). At the same time, the CDC provides funding for schools and CBOs implementing prevention programs (CDC, 2009b). However, the Obama administration has not proposed an initiative similar to the Act Against AIDS program mentioned earlier. Furthermore, the administration has not ensured that there is adequate funding for the CDC's programs focusing on the gay community, especially for schools and families for greater awareness and acceptance (amFAR, 2010; Melloy, 2010). This is somewhat surprising, considering that the new ONAP director is openly gay and has strong ties to the gay community.

---

[5] These organizations include: 100 Black Men of America; American Urban Radio Networks; Coalition of Black Trade Unionists; Congressional Black Caucus Foundation; National Action Network; National Association for the Advancement of Colored People; National Coalition of 100 Black Women; National Council of Negro Women; National Medical Association; National Newspaper Publishes Association; National Organization of Black County Officials; National Urban League; Phi Beta Sigma Fraternity; and the Southern Christian Leadership Conference.

Finally, when it comes to working with the state governments, there has still been no effort to create programs focused on increasing local government accountability and efficiency in rendering AIDS services. Yet again, efforts to increase the CDC's policy influence either through a strong partnership with AIDS NGOs or through the creation of performance-based fiscal transfers has not been pursued. While the Obama administration's ongoing financial support to the CDC and states certainly helps, until these innovative measures are implemented, state and especially municipal hospitals and community healthcare centers may not have the accountability and incentives needed to provide services in an effective manner.

At the international level, however, the Obama administration's effort to respond to AIDS is noteworthy. Obama shared the Bush administrations' view that it is the moral obligation and duty of the US to help other respond to AIDS (*Council on Foreign Relations*, 2010; Gayle, 2010; Kates, 2012). On May 5, 2009, the Obama administration unveiled its Global Health Initiative (GHI). GHI takes a holistic approach to bilateral aid in health. That is, GHI emphasizes not only AIDS but other neglected diseases as well, such as diarrhea, malaria, tuberculosis, women and children's health, and strengthening healthcare systems.

What is novel about GHI's approach is its emphasis on health systems strengthening, that is, increased government spending for human resources and infrastructure, such as beds and X-ray machines. This is an issue that the international development community has neglected for quite some time. While the reform of health systems has long been on the international agenda, the issue has mainly emphasized decentralization and privatization. GHI nevertheless realizes that this does not address the root cause of poor health policy outcomes. Just as important is investing in the training of doctors, nurses, and ensuring that hospitals and clinics have the beds, medical instruments, and scanners needed to provide healthcare services effectively (Gómez, 2010a).

The Obama administration also continues to support PEPFAR. While Obama is certainly committed to PEPFAR's focus on AIDS, he has nevertheless also requested PEPFAR officials to expand to other areas, such as addressing the HIV–TB co-infection problem, as well as the strengthening of health systems (PEPFAR, 2009; Gómez, 2010a). The goal is to expand PEPFAR to incorporate other related health issues, such as maternal and children's health. Furthermore, the USAID's new five-year plan for AIDS takes on a much more comprehensive approach bilateral aid assistance, seeking to invest in sustaining and strengthening healthcare systems, which requires more investment in human resources and infrastructure (PEPFAR, 2009).

However, Obama's GHI approach has also been criticized. AIDS activists and international NGOs, such as Médecins Sans Frontières (a French NGO focused on providing ARV treatment), claim that the US is failing to maintain its commitment to PEPFAR and in so doing, its moral obligation to helping other nations respond to AIDS (Council on Foreign Relations, 2010; Dickenson, 2010). Some are concerned that the AIDS epidemic is getting worse in Africa and that now is not the time to be experimenting with new approaches to global health (Dickenson, 2010; Tobias, 2012). This criticism reflects an ongoing debate in the public health community between those advocating for continued investments in vertical (centralized bureaucratic and policy) health systems approaches to AIDS versus those emphasizing a more horizontal, or holistic approach, which entails decentralization, healthcare infrastructure, human resources, and other neglected diseases.

In addition, perhaps more so than any other administration, Obama has been concerned with increasing the US's credibility as a government committed to working in close partnership with other nations. The president and Secretary of State Hillary Clinton have emphasized that part of GHI's mission is to strengthen the US's relationship with international organizations, such as the WHO and the Global Fund to Fight AIDS, Tuberculosis and Malaria, while working with other nations to eradicate AIDS; moreover, they view this as a way to bolster the US's credibility and diplomatic activities (Gómez, 2010a). For the first time, the US seems to be down-playing its leadership role in global health, realizing that it can achieve more by working in close partnership with the international community.

In yet another move to strengthen the US's credibility as a global partner in the fight against AIDS, in 2009 Obama issued an executive order officially repealing the ban on the entry of HIV positive individuals into the US. Since the denial of visas began under the George H.W. Bush administration in 1988, no foreign AIDS activists and researchers have been able to meet with the US policy community. Furthermore, since 1990 the annual International AIDS Conference had not been held in the US (Bliss, 2012; Preston, 2009), but was for the first time in Washington DC in July 2012. The repeal of this ban will help the government strengthen its ties with the international community. Moreover, this endeavor should help to increase the US's credibility for helping reduce the stigma surrounding AIDS (Bliss, 2012; Preston, 2009). This is an issue that the international community previously criticized the US government of and is an issue that continues to hamper policy responses in other nations, such as Russia and, to a certain extent, India and China.

Conclusion

When AIDS first emerged in the US, it was highly contested and did not elicit an immediate government response. During the first few years of the epidemic, the government's perception of the AIDS situation was negatively affected by the absence of credible epidemiological evidence; the absence of AIDS's threat to the national security; and the influence of well-organized moral-based interest groups. While the congressional House of Representatives was more interested in responding, due mainly to the presence of representatives from AIDS afflicted areas, there were no like-minded sympathizers in the Senate. In contrast, HHS and PHS officials were eager to respond, while seeking more political support and funding for their programs. While AIDS NGOs were forming at the local level, their fragmentation and reluctance to work closely with or within the CDC did not lay the groundwork for constructive partnerships with national AIDS officials. By the late 1980s, the government consequently did not engage in a strong centralized bureaucratic and policy response to AIDS.

Bureaucratic and policy reforms eventually emerged. Yet, this never led to the creation of effective national agencies and/or innovative federal programs assisting the states in their response to AIDS. At the same time, beginning in the late 1980s, heightened international criticisms and pressures had essentially no impact on presidential interests in pursuing these outcomes. President George H.W. Bush's perception that the US was a world leader, possessing the infrastructural capacity and knowledge needed to not only successfully respond to AIDS but also to lead the world in its response generated no interest in increasing the US's international reputation through a centralized bureaucratic and policy response. While President Clinton began to engage the international community by expressing concern and providing bilateral assistance towards the end of his administration, pursuing an aggressive centralized response as a means to strengthen the US's international reputation was never of interest.

The CDC's repeated inability to obtain financial and policy support from the White House and Congress also underscored a constraint that was derived from history. That is, the absence of civic supporters. In the absence of social health movements and AIDS NGOs collectively mobilizing and advocating for a centralized bureaucratic and policy response, and in the absence of CDC officials seeking out and establishing close partnerships with them, it seems that AIDS officials never garnered the legitimacy and influence needed to continuously obtain financial and policy support for their endeavors. While the CDC has recently sought to establish close partnerships with NGOs, especially in challenged African American communities, it is still not clear if and how CDC officials are harnessing their assistance to persuade Congress to provide additional funding. Until this is achieved, the CDC may not be able to consistently obtain the financial resources needed to expand their programs and implement innovative prevention, treatment, and fiscal transfer policies that, in turn, can help to ensure effective policy implementation.

These limitations notwithstanding, during the George W. Bush administration new bureaucratic and policy reforms were implemented. While the administration failed to strengthen the ONAP and prevention policy, it did nevertheless succeed in creating the largest federal bureaucracy ever created for helping other nations respond to AIDS: PEPFAR.

However, therein lays one of the biggest challenges to escalating the government's domestic response to AIDS. That is, particularly under the George W. Bush administration, the president and Congress appeared to be too focused on the global AIDS effort, while overlooking ongoing domestic policy needs. By the early 2000s, a critical juncture and combination of international and domestic political and social conditions, as well as Bush's moral beliefs, motivated him to place most of his interest and focus on global AIDS policy. It has only been under the Obama administration that efforts have been made to simultaneously increase support for global and domestic AIDS policies. Despite these efforts, the ongoing domestic economic recession has challenged Obama's ability to achieve these goals.

Let us now examine a nation that, in contrast to the US, did not lose its focus on domestic AIDS policy, one that placed this policy focus above and beyond any interest in helping other nations respond to AIDS: Brazil. For, as we will see in the next chapter, Brazil's international and domestic response to AIDS was rather different when compared to the US's, ultimately yielding a more successful, ongoing centralized bureaucratic and policy response to AIDS.

References

ACT UP (2003). *The Track Record on the Bush Administration on HIV/AIDS*, ACT UP Press, New York.

Aggleton, P. (2001). HIV/AIDS in Europe: The Challenge for Health Promotion Research, *Health Education Research*, **16**, 403–409.

Altman, D. (1986). *AIDS in the Mind of America*, Anchor Books Press/Doubleday Garden City, New York.

Altman, D. (1999). Globalization, Political Economy, and HIV/AIDs, *Theory and Society*, **28**, 559–584.

Altman, L. (1991). Amsterdam Picked for AIDS meeting, *The New York Times*, Section B, Column 1, September 12, p. 11.

amfAR (2010). amfAR for a Reassessment of HIV Prevention Efforts for Men who have Sex with Men (MSM) in the US. Available on-line: http://www.amfar.org/hill/article.aspx?id=8495. Accessed March 22, 2014.

Avert (2012). HIV & AIDS in the United States of America. Available on-line: http://www.avert.org/america.htm. Accessed March 22, 2014.

Baldwin, P. (2007). *Disease and Democracy: The Industrialized World Faces AIDS*, University of California Press, Berkeley.

Barack Obama Presidential Campaign (2008). *Barack Obama: Fighting HIV/ AIDS Worldwide*, Presidential Campaign Press release. Available on-line: http://change.gov/pages/the_obama_biden_plan_to_combat_global_ hiv_aids/. Accessed March 20, 2014.

Barringer, F. and Russel, C. (1983). CDC Chief Steps Down, Wins Plaudits, *The Washington Post*, page A21, April 7.

Behrman, G. (2004). *The Invisible People: How the U.S. Has Slept Through the Global AIDS Epidemic, the Greatest Humanitarian Catastrophe of our Time*, The Free Press, New York.

Bliss, K. (2012). *From Atlanta to Washington: History and Politics of the International AIDS Conferences, 1985–present*, Center for Strategic and International Studies, Washington, DC.

Blumenthal, D. and Morone, J. (2009). *The Heart of Power: Health and Politics in the Oval Office*, University of California Press, Berkeley.

Boodman, S. (1988). Commission's Chief Faults AIDS Response; Anti-bias Laws Urged; Mandatory Testing Hit, *The Washington Post*, First Section, June 3, p. A1.

Brandt, E. (2006). Personal interview. November 8.

Brodie, M., Hamel, E., Brady, L., Kates, J., and Altman, D. (2004). AIDS at 21: Media Coverage of the HIV Epidemic 1981–2002, *Columbia Journalism Review*, March/April, 1–8.

Bronski, M. (2004). Why Reagan Ignored AIDS, *The Advocate*, June 9. Available on-line: http://archive.is/5mCTV. Accessed March 20, 2014.

Bush, G. (2003). Remarks on Signing the United States Leadership Against HIV/AIDS, Tuberculosis and Malaria Act of 2003, *Public Papers of the President*, The White House Press, Washington, DC.

Bull, C. (2003). Bush on AIDS, *The Advocate*, November 11.

Campbell, D. (2005). *A Bird in the Bush: The Failed Policies of the George W. Bush Administration*, Algora Publishing, New York.

Carpenter, D. (2001). *The Forging of Bureaucratic Autonomy: Networks, Reputation, and Policy Innovation in Executive Agencies, 1862–1928*, Princeton University Press, Princeton.

CDC (Centers for Disease Control and Prevention). (2007). *A Heightened National Response to the HIV/AIDS Crisis among African Americans*, Centers for Disease Control, Atlanta.

CDC (Centers for Disease Control and Prevention) (2009a). *Act Against AIDS Leadership Initiative: Harnessing the Strength of African-American Organizations to Fight HIV and AIDS*, Centers for Disease Control and Prevention, Atlanta.

CDC (2009b). *HIV/AIDS and Young Men who have Sex with Men*, Centers for Disease Control and Prevention, Atlanta.

CDC (2010a). *HIV/AIDS and Men who have Sex with Men: What the CDC is Doing*, Centers for Disease Control and Prevention, Washington, DC.

CDC (2010b). *CDC Analysis Provides new look at Disproportionate Impact of HIV and Syphilis among US Gay and Bisexual Men*, Centers for Disease Control and Prevention, Atlanta.

Chabner, B. and Curt, G. (1984). War on AIDS: Prompt Entry by National Institutes of Health, *The New York Times*, Section A, May 1, p. 28.

Cimons, M. (1995). Clinton Says He'll Protect AIDS Funds, Care, *The San Francisco Chronicle*, December 7.

Cohen, I. and Elder, A. (1989). Major Cities and Disease Crisis: A Comparative Perspective, *Social Science History*, **13**, 25–63.

Cohen, J. (2001). *Shots in the Dark: The Wayward Search for an AIDS Vaccine*, W.W. Norton, London.

Collins, C. (2007). The Other Healthcare Debate, *The Huffington Post*, June 20.

CNN (2008). Report: Black U.S. AIDS rates rival some African Nations, *CNN*, July 29, p. 1.

Council on Foreign Relations (2010). Obama's NSS: Promise and Pitfalls, *Expert Roundup*, May 28, p. 1.

Curran, J. (2006). Personal interview. November 8.

Doan, M. (1987). Charges Media 'Cover-Up'; Jerry Falwell's Anti-AIDS Dollar Drive, *US News & World Report*, May 4, p. 12.

Duckett, R. (1993). 50 Brainstorm on AIDS Agenda/Advocates Develop National Plan, *Worcester Telegram & Gazette*, February 21.

Easterbrook, G. (1983). The Perpetual Campaign, *The Atlantic Monthly*, January.

Engel, M. (1987). AIDS and Prejudice: One Reporter's Account of the Nation's Response, *The Washington Post*, Health Section, December 1, p. Z4.

Evans, D. (1988). Military has its own Reasons for a War against AIDS, *The Chicago Tribune*, June 5, p. 1.

Evertz, S. (2010). *How Ideology Trumped Science: Why PEPFAR has Failed to Meet its Potential*, Center for American Progress and the Council for Global Equity, Washington, DC.

Evertz, S. (2012). Personal interview. November 20.

Foreman, C. (1993). AIDS and the Limits of Czardom, *Brookings Institution Review*, 11, 18–21.

Fox, D. (1986). AIDS and the American Health Policy: the History and Prospects of a Crisis of Authority, *The Milbank Quarterly*, 64, 8–12.

Fox, D. (1992). 'The Politics of HIV Infection: 1989–1990 as Years of Change', in Fee, E. and Fox, D. (eds), *AIDS: The Making of a Chronic Disease*, University of California Press, Berkeley, pp. 125–143.

Fox, D., Day, P., and Klein, R. (1989). The Power of Professionalism: Policies for AIDS in Britain, Sweden, and the United States, *Daedalus*, 118, 93–112.

Frontline (2006). Interview with former Secretary of Health and Human Services Margaret Heckler, May 30. Available on-line: http://www.pbs.org/wgbh/pages/frontline/aids/interviews/heckler.html. Accessed March 22, 2014.

Garrett, L. (1988). Reagan AIDS Agenda, *Newsday*, August 3.

Garrett, L. (2012). Personal interview. November 19.

Gauri, V. and Lieberman, E. (2006). Boundary Politics and HIV/AIDs Policy in Brazil and South Africa, *Studies in Comparative International Development*, 41, 47–73.

Gayle, H. (2010). Personal interview. July 12.

Gladwell, M. (1990). National Plan Urged for Battling AIDS, *The Washington Post*, April 25, p. A25.

Goldberg, J. (2012). Matt Damon: 'I Would Kiss George W. Bush on the Mouth' for His AIDS Work, *The Atlantic*, April 19. Available on-line: http://www.theatlantic.com/international/archive/2012/04/matt-damon-i-would-kiss-george-w-bush-on-the-mouth-for-his-aids-work/255992/. Accessed March 22, 2014.

Gómez, E. (2007). Bureaucratizing Epidemics: The Challenge of Institutional Bias in the United States and Brazil, *Global Health Governance*, 1, 1–24.

Gómez, E. (2010a). Stop Fighting Viruses, Stop Treating People: The Obama Administration's Broad Vision for Global Health, *Foreign Policy*. Available on-line: http://www.foreignpolicy.com/articles/2010/01/27/stop_fighting_viruses_start_treating_people. Accessed March 22, 2014.

Gómez, E. (2010b). What the US can learn from Brazil when it comes to combating HIV/AIDS: International Reputation and Strategic Centralization in a context of Health Policy Devolution, *Health Policy & Planning*, **25**, 529–541.

Gómez, E. (2012). Understanding Brazilian Global Health Diplomacy: Social Health Movements, Institutional Infiltration, and the Geopolitics of Accessing AIDS Medication, *Global Health Governance*, **5**, 1–29.

Gusfield, J. (1986). *Symbolic Crusade: Status Politics and the American Temperance Movement*, University of Illinois Press, Urbana Champaign.

Helms, J. (2002). We Cannot Turn Away, Speech given on March 24, in *The aWAKE Project: United Against the African AIDS Crisis*, W. Publishing Group, Nashville, p. 63.

Herek, G. (1990). 'Illness, Stigma, and AIDS', in Vandenbos, G.R. (ed.), *Psychological Aspects of Serious Illness*, American Psychological Association, Washington DC, pp. 203–150.

Hilts, P. (1981). 2 Mysterious Diseases Killing Homosexuals, *The Washington Post*, p. A15, August 30.

Hilts, P. (1990a). Bush, in First Address on AIDS, Backs a Bill to Protect its Victims, *The New York Times*, Section A, March 3, p. 1.

Hilts, P. (1990b). Panel Says Government is not Leading AIDS Fight, *The New York Times*, Section A, April 25, p. 1.

Hilts, P. (1991). Panel Faults Leaders on AIDS Epidemic, *The Washington Post*, September 26, p. 24.

Hilts, P. (1992). National AIDS Panel Says Administration Has Not Done Enough, *The New York Times*, Section A, June 26, p. 18.

Hilts, P. and Engel, M. (1985). Armed Forces to be Tested for AIDS, *The Washington Post*, p. A1, September 19.

Hindman, A. and Schroedel, J. (2010). *U.S. Response to HIV/AIDS in Africa: Bush as a Human Rights leader?* Unpublished manuscript, Claremont Graduate University.

Hoffman, B. (2003). Health Care Reform and Social Movements in the United States. *American Journal of Public Health*, **93**, 75–85.

Hopson, D. (2006). Testimony of Deborah Parham Hopson, Associate Administrator, HIV/AIDS Bureau, Health Resources and Services Administrator, U.S. Department of Health and Human Services. Washington, DC, April 26.

Hoye, S. (2012). Knocking on Doors to end HIV in Philadelphia, *CNN*. Available on-line: http://www.cnn.com/2012/09/06/health/philadel-phia-hiv-outreach/index.html. Accessed March 22, 2014.

HRSA (Health Resources and Services Administration) (2008). *The HIV/ AIDS Program: Ryan White Parts A–F*, Department of Health and Human Services, Washington DC.

International Planned Parenthood Federation (2012). Bush's War on Sexual Health and Defensive Strategies Against It. Available on-line: http://www.ippfwhr.org/en/node/595. Accessed March 22, 2014.

James, S. (2009). Pastor Warren Sets Inclusive Tone at Inaugural, *ABC News*, January 20. Available on-line: http://abcnews.go.com/Politics/Inauguration/rick-warren-invocation-president-obama-inauguration/story?id=6687731#.UJ0Hxo7LiEk. Accessed March 22, 2014.

Johnson, J. (1988). Bush is urged to be a Leader in the Fight on AIDS, *The New York Times*, Section B, December 2, p. 6.

Jonsen, A. and Styker, J. (eds) (1993). *The Social Impact of AIDS in the US*, National Academy Press, Washington DC.

Kaiser Family Foundation (2006). The Global HIV/AIDS Timeline. Available on-line: http://www.kff.org/hivaids/timeline/hivtimeline.cfm. Accessed March 22, 2014.

Kaiser Family Foundation (2013). The Ryan White Program, HIV/AIDS Policy Fact Sheet. Available on-line: http://kaiserfamilyfoundation.files.wordpress.com/2013/03/7582-07.pdf. Accessed March 21, 2014.

Kaiser Family Foundation (2009a). Survey of Americans on the U.S. Role in Global Health. Available on-line: http://www.kff.org/kaiserpolls/upload/7894.pdf. Accessed March 22, 2014.

Kaiser Family Foundation (2009b). U.S. Global Health Policy Fact Sheet. Available on-line: http://www.kff.org/hivaids/upload/3030-13.pdf. Accessed March 22, 2014.

Kaiser Family Foundation (2010). U.S. Federal Funding for HIV/AIDS: The President's FY 2001 Budget Request, HIV/AIDS Policy Fact Sheet. Available on-line: http://www.democraticunderground.com/discuss/duboard.php?az=view_all&address=389x9429077. Accessed March 21, 2014.

Kaiser Family Foundation (2012). 2012 Survey of Americans on the U.S. Role in Global Health. Available on-line: http://kff.org/global-health-policy/

report/2012-survey-of-americans-on-the-u-s-role-in-global-health/. Accessed March 21, 2014.

Kaiser Health News (2003). President Bush Signs into Law $15B International HIV/AIDS Bill; Some Democrats say White House Commitment 'Hollow', May 28. Available on-line: http://www.kaiserhealthnews.org/Daily-Reports/2003/May/28/dr00017940.aspx?p=1. Accessed March 21, 2014.

Kates, J. (2012). Personal interview. October 24.

Keefe, B. (2010). CDC Gets Boost under President's Budget Proposal, *The Atlanta Journal-Constitution*, February 1. Available on-line: http://www.ajc.com/news/cdc-gets-boost-under-288111.html. Accessed March 21, 2014.

Keller, B. (1985). AIDS Tests for Troops Assigned Abroad Asked, *The New York Times*, Section A, November 27, p. 17.

Knox, R. (1990). US Agency is Urged for AIDS: Commission Sees Need to Coordinate Effort, *The Boston Globe*, April 25, p. 3.

Kurtz, H. (1983). Address to Conference of Mayors; Heckler Discounts AIDS Disease Fear, *The Washington Post*, p. A1, June 14.

Landers, J. (2012). Bringing Africa Back to Life: The Legacy of George W. Bush, *Dallas News*. Available on-line: http://www.dallasnews.com/news/local-news/20120608-bringing-africa-back-to-life-the-legacy-of-george-w.-bush.ece. Accessed March 22, 2014.

Leff, L. (2003). CDC's New HIV Prevention Plan Facing Mounting Criticisms from AIDS Groups, *The Associated Press*, July 26, p. 1.

Lieberman, E. (2009). *Boundaries of Contagion: How Ethnic Politics have Shaped Government Responses to AIDS*, Princeton University Press, Princeton.

Mason, J. (2006). Personal interview. November 17.

McDonnell, M. (2007). *Case Study of the Campaigns Leading to The President's Emergency Plan for AIDS Relief*, US Coalition for Child Survival Press, Washington DC.

McGreal, C. (2008). George Bush: A Good Man in Africa, *The Guardian*, February 14. Available on-line: http://www.guardian.co.uk/world/2008/feb/15/georgebush.usa. Accessed March 22, 2014.

McQueen, A. (2001). Bush Administration to Keep Clinton — Era Panel on National AIDS Policy, *Associated Press*, July 20.

Melillo, W. (1991). Whatever Happened to AIDS? *The Washington Post*, p. Z10, September 24.

Melloy, K. (2010). CDC: MSMs hardest hit by HIV, Syphilis, *Edge Philadelphia News*, March 11, p. 1.

Mesce, D. (1990). WHO to Take Part in AIDS Conference, *The Associated Press*, April 20, p. 1.

Meyer, L. and Russell, C. (1981). Centers for Disease Control Facing Cuts That Could Cripple Programs, *The Washington Post*, p. A6, November 28.

Morganthau, T., Coppola, V., Carey, J., and Cooper, N. (1983). Gay America in Transition, *Newsweek*, August 8, p. 30.

Nathanson, C. (1996). Disease Prevention as Social Change: Towards a Theory of Public Health, *Population and Development Review*, 22, 609–637.

National Gay and Lesbian Task Force (2012). *History of Nondiscrimination Bills in Congress*. Available on-line: http://www.thetaskforce.org/issues/nondiscrimination/timeline. Accessed March 22, 2014.

National HIV/AIDS Strategy for the United States (2010). The White House Press, Washington DC.

Neergaard, L. (1992). More Bureaucracy Won't Cure AIDS, Sullivan Says, *Associated Press*, December.

NPR (National Public Radio) (1993). Clinton to Lift Ban on HIV-Positive Immigrants, February 9, p. 1.

Okie, S. (1989). AIDS Shifting to Drug-Plagued Inner Cities, *The Washington Post*, August 27, p. A3.

OMB (Office of Management and Budget) (2010). *Budget of the United States Government, Fiscal Year 2011*, The White House Press, Washington DC.

Padgug, R. and Oppenheimer, G. (1992). 'Riding the Tiger: AIDS and the Gay Community', in Fee, E. and Fox, D. (eds), *AIDS: The Making of a Chronic Disease*, University of California Press, Berkeley, pp. 245–278.

Panem, S. (1988). *The AIDS Bureaucracy*, Harvard University Press, Cambridge.

Parker, R. (2003). Building the Foundations for the Response to HIV/AIDS in Brazil: The Development of HIV/AIDS Policy, 1982–1996, *Divulgação em Saúde para Debate*, 27, 143–183.

PEPFAR (2009). *The US President's emergency plan for AIDS relief: 5 year strategy*, United States Agency for International Development, Washington DC.

Perrow, C. and Guillen, M. (1990). *The AIDS Disaster: The Failure of Organizations in New York and the Nation*, Yale University Press, New Haven.

Pilecki, M. (2010). The New Epidemic: Assigning Blame & Searching for Solutions for Skyrocketing Youth HIV Infections, *EDGE News*, November 8. Available on-line: http://www.edgepalmsprings.com/index.php?ch=news&sc=culture&sc3=&id=112579&pg=1. Accessed March 22, 2014.

Platt, M. and Platt, M. (2013). *From GRID to Gridlock: The Relationship between Scientific Biomedical Breakthroughs and HIV/AIDS Policy in the US Congress.* Unpublished manuscript, Harvard University, Department of Government.

Preston, J. (2009). Obama lifts Ban on Entry into US by HIV Positive People, *The New York Times*, October 30.

Price-Smith, A. (2002). *The Health of Nations: Infectious Disease, Environmental Change, and their Effects on National Security and Development*, MIT Press, Cambridge.

Price-Smith, A., Tauber, S., and Bhat, A. (2004). State Capacity and HIV Incidence Reduction in the Developing World: Preliminary Empirical Evidence, *Seton Hall Journal of Diplomacy*, Summer/Fall, 149–160.

Pritchett, L. and Woolcock, M. (2004). Solutions when the Solution is the Problem: Arraying the Disarray in Development, *World Development*, **32**, 191–212.

Rich, S. (1982). Budget Director Seeking Deep Cuts in Health Agencies, *The Washington Post*, p. A1, December 1.

Rich, S. (1985). HHS is Skirting Law, Weicker Says, by Curbing NIH Research Grants, *The Washington Post*, Federal Report, p. A19, March 6.

Rosenbrock, R. and Wright, M. (eds) (2000). *Partnership and Pragmatism: Germany's Response to AIDS Prevention and Care*, Routledge Press, London.

Ross, S. (2001). White House Reverses Course on AIDS, *Associated Press*, February 8.

Rudavsky, S. (1992). AIDS Panel Faults Bush Administration Leadership, *The Washington Post*, June 26, p. A3.

Ruger, J. (2005). Democracy and Health. *Quarterly Journal of Medicine*, **98**, 229–304.

Russell, C. (1983). Deadly AIDS is Called 'No. 1 Priority' of Public Health Service, *The Washington Post*, p. A5, May 25.

Russell, C. (1984). AIDS Probes Cast as Rivals for Recognition, *The Washington Post*, p. A1, April 23.

Russel, C. (1985). Inside the Public Health Service: Agency Chief Pushes for 55% Rise in AIDS Budget, *The Washington Post*, p. A23, September 27.

Ryan, B. (2004). Among the Top Candidates for the Democratic Nomination, is there a Clear Choice for AIDS Advocates? *HIV Plus: Research and Treatment*, February, 24–29.

Sen, A. (1999). *Development as Freedom*, Knopf Press, New York.

Shilts, R. (2011). *And the Band Played On: Politics, People, and the AIDS Epidemic*, St. Martin's Press, New York.

Stein, R. (2009). Crowely to Direct Office of National AIDS Policy, *The Washington Post*, February 26. Available on-line: http://voices.washingtonpost.com/44/2009/02/26/crowley_to_direct_office_of_na.html. Accessed March 22, 2014.

Sutton, M., Jones, R., Wolitski, R., Cleveland, J., Dean, H., and Fento, K. (2009). A Review of the Centers for Disease Control and Prevention's response to the HIV/AIDS Crisis Among Blacks in the United States, 1981–2009, *American Journal of Public Health*, **99**, 351–359.

Talbot, D. and Bush, L. (1985). At Risk, *Mother Jones*, **10**, 28–37.

Tapper, J. (2008). Elizabeth Dole Tries to Rename the AIDS Bill After Jesse Helms, *ABC News Political Punch*, July 16, p. 1.

The Advertiser (1987). No AIDS 'Witch-Hunt' in Forces, October 31.

The Advocate (2004). Bush Names New ONAP Director, May 15, p. 1.

The Atlanta Journal-Constitution (1991a). Washington in Brief; Another 100 Scientists cut from AIDS Conference Roster, June 14.

The Atlanta Journal-Constitution (1991b). CDC Suffering Setbacks from Budgetary Ailment, April 26, p. 1.

The Body (2010). Obama, Municipalities Honor AIDS Testing Day, June 28. Available on-line: http://www.thebody.com/content/prev/art57216.html. Accessed March 22, 2014.

The Boston Globe (1989). The AIDS Momentum, November 6, p. 16.

The New York Times (1983). Mrs. Heckler Asks for More AIDS Funds, August 18, p. 19.

The New York Times (1984). A Viral Competition over AIDS, April 26, p. 22.

The New York Times (1987). The Reagan AIDS Strategy in Ruins, October 11, p. 26.

The San Francisco Chronicle (1990). Bush Decides Not to Address AIDS Meeting, February 12, p. A7.

St. Louis Post-Dispatch (1991). Nations Seek Help with AIDS Experts Lash U.S. at World Conference, June 17, p. 1A.

TIME (2008). Is Obama Scaling Back Bush's AIDS Initiative? December 2. Available on-line: http://www.time.com/time/politics/article/0,8599, 1944554,00.html. Accessed March 22, 2014.

Tobias, R. (2012). Personal interview. November 26.

Tomaszewski, E. (2012). *Understanding HIV/AIDS Stigma and Discrimination*, National Association of Social Workers, Washington DC.

Trafford, A., Witkin, G., Dobbin, M. and Thorton, J. (1985). The Politics of AIDS — A Tale of Two States, *US News & World Report*, November 18, p. 70.

UNAIDS (2004). *Three Ones Key Principles*. UNAIDS Press, Geneva.

United States Agency for International Development (1999). *Leadership and Investment in Fighting an Epidemic*, USAID Press, Washington DC.

US News & World Report (1983). Fear of AIDS Affects the Nation, June 27, p. 13.

US News & World Report (1985a). The Backlash Builds Against AIDS, November 4, p. 9.

US News & World Report (1985b). New AIDS Forecast: A Long, Long Siege, October 14, p. 14.

Vallgarda, S. (2007). Problematizations and Path Dependency: HIV/AIDS Policies in Denmark and Sweden, *Medical History*, **51**, 99–112.

Washington Post (1983). Heckler Visits AIDS Victim in the Hospital, *The Federal Triangle*, p. A27, August 18.

White House (1999). *The Clinton/Gore Administration: A Record of Progress on HIV and AIDS*, The White House Press, Washington, DC.

White House (2010). National HIV/AIDS Strategy, Office of National AIDS Policy, Washington DC.

Whitman, D. (1987). C. Everett Koop Takes on Intractable Issues as Surgeon General — But He's also Made Enemies; A Fall from Grace on the Right, *US News & World Report*, May 25, p. 27.

Wilke, J. (1983). AIDS Mystery U.S. Priority, Officials Say, *The Washington Post*, p. A3, August 3.

William J. Clinton Presidential Center (2012). Record of Accomplishment. Available on-line: http://www.clintonfoundation.org/clinton-presidential-center. Accessed March 22, 2014.

World Health Organization (1994). World Health Organization Urges Sex in Schools to Prevent AIDS, *Sozial — und Praventivemedizin*, **39**, 325.

World Health Organization (2008). *Maximizing Positive Synergies between Health Systems and Global Health Initiatives*, World Health Organization Press, Geneva.

World Health Organization (2009). *Injecting Drug Use (IDU) and Prisons*, World Health Organization Press, Geneva.

World Trade Organization (2011). 10-Year Old WTO Declaration has Reinforced Health Policy Choices, Lamy tells Symposium, *WTO News*, November 23. Available on-line: http://www.wto.org/english/news_e/news11_e/trip_23nov11_e.htm. Accessed March 22, 2014.

Yeghiayan, L. (2011). HHS Funding Delays & Mistakes Hurting AIDS Programs nationwide, says AHF, *Enhanced Online News*, August 22. Available on-line: http://eon.businesswire.com/news/eon/20110822006551/en/HHS/Ryan-White-CARE-Act/HIV%2FAIDS. Accessed March 22, 2014.

Chapter 4

Contesting AIDS in Brazil

In the early 1980s, Brazil joined the US in its confrontation of the AIDS epidemic. In line with what others have argued, considering Brazil's lack of experience of long-lasting democracy, elections, political accountability, the representation and inclusion of civil society's interests in policymaking, as well as lower levels of healthcare funding, and technological and infrastructural resources (Lieberman, 2009; Parker, 2003), one would expect Brazil to have responded poorly to AIDS. The US and other advanced industrialized nations, on the other hand, possessed these democratic, financial, and infrastructural preconditions (Aggleton, 2001; Altman, 1986; Baldwin, 2007; Nathanson, 1996; Price-Smith, 2002; Price-Smith *et al.*, 2004; Rosenbrock and Wright, 2000; Ruger, 2005; Sen, 1999; Vallgarda, 2007), thus prompting one to expect a more aggressive policy response when compared to Brazil. Yet, despite these advantages, and as we saw in the previous chapter, the US did not engage in an aggressive centralized bureaucratic and policy response. Furthermore, in contrast to what we would expect, this chapter maintains that Brazil eventually surpassed the US in its centralized response.

Indeed, for several years, international health organizations, the media, and scholars have praised Brazil's response to the epidemic. In addition to receiving the 2003 Bill & Melinda Gates Foundation award for having the best governmental response to AIDS (*Agnencia Estado*, 2003; *US News Wire*, 2003), in 2009, CNN's Dr. Sanjay Gupta went as far as to call Brazil's AIDS program the "envy of the world" (Gupta, 2009).

However, many may be unaware of the fact that before the early 1990s, Brazil's response to AIDS was just as delayed and lackluster as the US's; that is, a national government that was essentially apathetic about the AIDS situation as well as ineffective in its centralized bureaucratic and policy response. Created in 1986, the Ministry of Health's (MOH) national AIDS program was poorly organized, having little financial and political support. It did nothing to help at-risk groups and insolvent state governments respond to the epidemic. These outcomes were the result of intensive inter-elite contestation, which derived from disputes over the threat that AIDS posed to civil society, the lack of credible epidemiological evidence, the presence of multiple diseases and healthcare needs, and the absence of international criticisms and pressures.

Considering this kind of response, how did Brazil's national AIDS program eventually become the "envy of the world"? Why did the program gradually transform into a massive federal agency with ample financial and political support, continuously implementing a host of innovative prevention and treatment programs? Was it a purely domestic response to the burgeoning number of AIDS cases and deaths? Or were there new international circumstances that generated incentives for policymakers to engage in a strong centralized bureaucratic and policy response?

This chapter argues that the reason for Brazil's eventual success could be found in where policymakers positioned themselves in the geopolitical sphere. Presidents and senior MOH bureaucrats, as elites perceiving themselves as leaders of an influential emerging nation, capable of swiftly eradicating disease, developing the economy and prospering, wanted to demonstrate to the international community that they could join the advanced industrialized nations in curbing the spread of AIDS. In this context, it was the rise of international criticisms and pressures, not domestic pressures from civil society, which led to a stronger national government response. By the early 1990s, President Cardoso and his policymakers believed that strengthening the national AIDS program would help to achieve their goal of increasing Brazil's international reputation. Furthermore, in a context of fiscal instability and exorbitant debt, the acquisition of a World Bank loan in 1993 provided the financial means with which to achieve this goal. Policymakers were therefore receptive to working in close partnership with the international donor community, not only to obtain resources but also new policy insights on how they could strengthen their response to AIDS.

Interest in international reputation building not only generated new incentives to confront AIDS, but it also provided support for previously ignored — and even criticized — AIDS bureaucrats. Equipped with presidential blessings, these bureaucrats gradually emerged to strengthen their position within government and to finally start working closely with civil society. They did so by engaging in a strategy that found its roots in the early 20th century: that is, and as we saw in Chapter 2, finding and using civic supporters through social health movements and NGOs sharing similar centralization ideas and policy beliefs, while resembling similar social movements and ideas in the past. By partnering with the *sanitaristas* and AIDS NGOs, AIDS officials' legitimacy and influence increased, in turn facilitating their ability to obtain ongoing political and financial support. Given their ideas' historically proven track record, as well as the fact that the *sanitaristas* and AIDS NGOs represented a long, successful tradition of state–civil society partnerships to eradicate disease, politicians assigned great credibility to these ideas and to those bureaucrats partnering with civil society.

This chapter begins with a discussion of the government's initial response to AIDS. I then discuss why and how the national government eventually responded, highlighting the pivotal role of the international community. I close with a discussion of the lessons learned and how Brazil's response to AIDS compared to that of the US.

The First Few Years of the AIDS Epidemic

The first cases of AIDS emerged in the city São Paulo in 1982, followed shortly thereafter in Rio de Janeiro and some cities in the northeast, such as Salvador and Fortaleza. As in the US, the virus created a great deal of fear and uncertainty. Initially, the virus was found among individuals in the gay community as well as famous artists and celebrities (*Veja*, 1985; *Visão*, 1985). In a context where the gay community was constantly discriminated against (Mott, 2003), essentially all of the culpa was put on them. This further magnified the already high level of preexisting stigma and discrimination towards the gay community (Gómez, 2010; Laserda, *Jornal do Brasil*, 1985b; *Veja*, 1985).

Similar to what we saw in the US, the Brazilian government did not immediately respond (Da Costa Marques, 2003; Parker *et al.*, 1999). In fact, it took the government approximately eight years before the president would publically address AIDS (Da Costa Marques, 2003; *Folhão de São Paulo*, 1991; Galvão, 2000: p. 125) — substantially longer than it took the US government.

Several antecedent conditions explain the government's initial perceptions and delayed response. First and foremost was the president and senior MOH officials' belief that AIDS did not pose a serious national health threat (Parker, 2003). In part this was influenced by the fact that the government was confronting a host of diseases when the HIV virus emerged. For, as some scholars point out, "early in the epidemic, within the Ministry of Health in Brasília, some officials argued that AIDS did not satisfy the epidemiological criteria of 'transcendence,' 'magnitude,' and 'vulnerability,' necessary to warrant a response from public institutions" (Gauri and Lieberman, 2006: p. 59). Throughout the 1980s the MOH was trying to respond to a myriad of diseases, such as tuberculosis, hanseniase, samparo, and malaria. The fact that prevalence rates for these diseases were much higher than AIDS, save for samparo, further contributed to the president and MOH's belief that AIDS was not a serious public health threat. In fact, in 1985, the minister of health, Carlos Santa'Anna, claimed that AIDS was not a priority and that the government needed to tend to other more pressing health matters (*Folhão de São Paulo*, 1985; *Jornal do Brasil*, 1985a).

Second, during this period the government was fully committed to decentralizing healthcare services. In addition to the belief that decentralization would render healthcare services more efficiently, decentralization also dovetailed with the government's preexisting commitment to democratization (Souza, 1997). Even before the 1988 constitution, political and bureaucratic elites started to invest heavily in healthcare decentralization processes (Heirmann, 2002;

Nascimento, 1999), approving programs and granting administrative authority to the states (Gómez, 2008). These efforts contributed to the president and MOH's belief that they should not pursue a centralized response for AIDS, and that any movement in that direction could stall the democratization process.

Third, international criticisms and pressures were absent during this period. International organizations, such as the World Health Organization (WHO), the World Bank, the Inter-American Development Bank, and the Pan American Health Organization (PAHO) were not yet criticizing Brazil for its delayed and ineffective response (Fontes, 1999; Galvão, 2000). Furthermore, the international movement in response to AIDS, through the creation of UN organizations, conferences, and international AIDS NGO-networks (what others have referred to as the "Geneva Consensus") had yet to emerge (Fontes, 1999; Lieberman, 2009). In the absence of these international criticisms and pressures, Brazil's leadership had little reason to respond.

During this period the response to AIDS mainly occurred at the state level. In 1983, the governor of São Paulo, André Montoro, created the first AIDS program in the nation. Sympathetic to the gay community and seeking to deepen the democratization process, in response to growing pressures from the gay community the governor and his state health secretary worked closely with the gay community to assemble an AIDS program focused on prevention and social awareness (Parker, 2003; Parker, 2009). The gay community's efforts also benefited from the presence of a vibrant democratization movement, namely the *sanitarista* movement, which, as I discuss in more detail shortly, not only contributed to a sense of social solidarity but also pressured the military government for human rights and equal access to healthcare (Berkman *et al.*, 2005). The São Paulo program quickly emerged as a model for how other cities should respond to AIDS.

Amidst burgeoning AIDS cases and deaths, governors and mayors were repeatedly pressuring the MOH to provide them with the financial resources needed to regulate the blood supply, increase the number of hospital beds, equipment, and prevention services (*Visão*, 1985). For example, while São Paulo's AIDS program was in operation by 1983, it was still very much in need of federal assistance

(Teixeira, 1997). São Paulo and other municipal health departments turned to the MOH for help; nevertheless, the MOH had essentially no interest in providing this help (Da Costa Marques, 2003; Teixeira, 1997).

Further complicating the MOH's initial response to the states' needs was the presence of conflicting policy views and contestation within the bureaucracy. On one hand, political appointees in the MOH sided with the president and Congress' view that the government should not immediately respond to AIDS (Gómez, 2008; Gómez, 2010). Loyalty to the president's interests was reinforced by his centralized control and distribution of benefits, remnants of the outgoing military regime (Gómez, 2008). These officials' perceptions of the AIDS epidemic were therefore influenced by the president's interests and concerns, not by epidemiological evidence, pressures from civil society, and the states' needs. At the same time, senior MOH and planning officials were relying on a decentralized response to AIDS, expecting the states to bear the brunt of the policy response (Da Costa Marques, 2003: p. 124). The idea of the MOH financing the response to AIDS was resisted, considering that there was not yet a universal healthcare system in place and that INAMPS, the healthcare provider at the time, should take full responsibility in doing so.[1]

Conversely, there were those officials within the MOH and the national AIDS program that emphasized providing immediate assistance to the states, for the creation of an effective national AIDS program, and for the universal provision of prevention and treatment policy. Their motivation stemmed from the belief that, as in the past,

---

[1]In fact, prior to the new constitution in 1988, which consolidated all policy responsibilities under the MOH, MOH Secretary Santa'Anna did not want to be responsible for financing AIDS policy — keep in mind that this was two years after the national AIDS program was created (Teixeira, 2007). Because the INAMPS (national health insurance system) was still in existence, and because it had more money than the MOH, Santa'Anna wanted INAMPS to finance all AIDS policies. However, INAMPS officials believed that AIDS was a public health issue, which meant that the MOH should be responsible for funding AIDS policies. INAMPS believed that it was only responsible for providing health insurance for workers (Brazil by this point still did not have universal healthcare). These disputes went on for months (Teixeira, 2007). Eventually, the MOH decided that it should be responsible for funding and implementing AIDS policy.

and as we saw in Chapter 2, the central government should immediately intervene in order to curb the spread of disease, regardless of their etiology and the population they affected (Gómez, 2011; Hochman, 1998; Teixeira, 2007). Influenced by this tradition, AIDS officials believed that it was the government's responsibility to guarantee universal access to healthcare. This was a view that comported with the *sanitarista* community's beliefs and a policy principle that was included in the 1988 democratic constitution (Berkman et al., 2005; Galvão, 2000). However, in the absence of presidential, congressional, and MOH support, these officials were often marginalized, ignored, and ridiculed. In fact, Teixeira (1997) writes that during this period, AIDS bureaucrats seeking reforms were criticized by senior MOH officials, mocking them for trying to centralize control over AIDS policy in a context of increased healthcare decentralization (Teixeira, 1997: p. 55).

Despite these conflicting viewpoints within the MOH, things began to change when the president started to take the AIDS situation more seriously. By 1985, the José Sarney administration became more concerned and interested in AIDS. The emergence of several effective state AIDS programs, especially in São Paulo, but also by this point throughout several states, such as Alagoas, Bahia, Ceará, Minas Gerais, Paraná, Pernambuco, Santa Catarina, Rio Grande do Norte, Rio Grande do Sul, and Rio, when combined with increased pressures from the gay and NGO community, gradually increased the national government's interest in AIDS. Moreover, by 1982 most of the political opposition had won state elections, and anti-AIDS programs were implemented as one of several means to democratic deepening. One must also keep in mind that the federal government was on the verge of transitioning from an authoritarian government to a democracy, which was, at least in theory, fully committed to universal rights and access to social services. In fact, the architects of the 1988 constitution were wholeheartedly committed to universal healthcare as a key aspect of the new constitution. Therefore by 1984, a culmination of factors led to a gradual shift in presidential and MOH beliefs that the AIDS situation was important and that the government should respond.

By 1986, the government began to respond through the MOH's creation of the national AIDS program, namely the Departamento de DST, AIDS, e Hepatites Virais (henceforth, national AIDS program). The program fell under the MOH's purview. Led by Dr. Lair Guerra Macedo Rodrigues (henceforth, Lair Guerra) and a staff of about 20, the national program's mission was to monitor HIV, disseminate prevention programs, finance medical treatment, and establish technical norms for how policy should be implemented (Teixeira, 1997). Furthermore, and in contrast to what was seen in the US, the government realized early on that one centralized AIDS agency, not several, should be in charge of research, evaluation, and policy.

Civic Mobilization and Bureaucratic Infiltration

During this period, civil society also began to mobilize rather quickly and effectively. Mobilization efforts first emerged in the city of São Paulo. The gay community came together to pressure the city's secretary of health, João Yunes, to enact prevention and treatment services (Parker, 2003). The timing of the gay movement's efforts was propitious, as it emerged alongside the influential *sanitarista* movement. Emerging in the 1960s, this movement had a long history of advocating for democratization, decentralization, and health as a human right (Berkman *et al.*, 2005; Parker, 2003, 2009).

In part because of the gay movement's efforts and success, several AIDS NGOs soon emerged. In São Paulo, GAPA (Grupo de Apoio á Prevenção á AIDS, Support Group for the prevention of AIDS) was created in 1985, while ABIA (Associação Brasileira Interdisciplinar de AIDS, Interdisciplinary Association for AIDS) was created in the city of Rio de Janeiro in 1986. A host of AIDS NGOs soon began to emerge throughout the nation. By 1985, approximately 11 NGOs had emerged (Parker, 2003). They helped state health departments to construct AIDS prevention and treatment programs (Parker, 2003). The *sanitarista* movement also helped to build local AIDS policies while working within the MOH to help construct the national AIDs program (Teixeira, 1997). The religious and business community also began to help the AIDS NGO movement (Parker, 2003). By the early 1990s, the Catholic Church helped to increase prevention through its controversial advocacy of condom use, while the business community pressured the national AIDS program to fund awareness and prevention programs for businesses (Parker, 2003).

Despite these proactive civic efforts, the national AIDS program was not initially committed to taking NGO policy views and recommendations seriously. What's more, this lack of government attention to civil society even occurred after the MOH created the National AIDS Commission in 1987. This commission was explicitly designed to incorporate the views of civil society, government officials, as well as the private sector (Da Costa Marques, 2003; Darah, 2006). Those NGO members on the commission were not instrumental in guiding the creation of policy; rather, they were seen as opinionated advisers (Da Costa Marques, 2003). Further, during this period scholars note that the national AIDS program's relationship with NGOs was very weak and unsupportive (Parker, 2003). At the time national program directors also failed to meet international organizations (Parker, 2003). During this period those invited to participate on the National AIDS Commission were select members of the national AIDS program, international officials, such as WHO and PAHO officials, academics, and a handful of human rights activists (Do Nascimento, 2005). The failure to take civil society's suggestions seriously was one of several problems with the national AIDS program at the time.

Initial Government Response

Despite the creation of a national AIDS program in 1986, the president and Congress was not fully committed to strengthening the program. It was as if the entire program was created mainly to encourage civil society that something was being done, when in reality, very little was. During the program's first few years, funding appeared to be the biggest concern. No matter how often and how much money the director of the program, Lair Guerra, asked for, she never got what she requested (Da Costa Marques, 2003: pp. 127–28). Seeking to expand the program's policies, hire the best staff, and fund the provision of antiretroviral (ARV) medication (De Costa Marques, 2003: p. 125), Lair was criticized for incessantly pressuring Congress for more funding (Do Nascimento, 2005: p. 100). But, because the president and Congress still had not viewed AIDS as posing a major health threat, there was no interest in meeting her needs (Terto, 2008).

In addition, the national AIDS program was poorly organized and managed (Filho, 2006; Teixeira, 1997; Terto, 2008; *Visão*, 1985). There was essentially no interest in reorganizing the program for greater efficiency and responsiveness to the needs of civil society (Galvão, 2000; Teixeira, 1997). Lair also received little guidance from the president and Congress on how to strengthen her management skills (Da Costa Margues, 2003).

It soon became clear that the national AIDS program had very little substance to it. Activists claimed that the government did not have a coherent national AIDS strategy and that it was not committed to helping the gay and intravenous drug community (Daniel, 1991; Miguez, 1989). Famous gay activists, such as Herbert Daniel, traveled throughout the nation, giving speeches and book tours claiming that the national AIDS program was nothing but a scam (Daniel, 1991; Miguez, 1989).

Furthermore, the president and Congress had no interest in helping the national AIDS program provide assistance to the states, such as medical supplies, test kits for blood examinations, and hospital beds (*O Globo*, 1987b; *Folhão de São Paulo*, 1985; *Jornal do Brasil*, 1985a). The Presidential Palace and Congress did virtually nothing when it found out that most of the public hospitals in São Paulo, Rio, and other major cities were going bankrupt (*O Globo*, 1988). As in the US, at the time President Fernando Collor de Mello believed that the states should be the first responders and that the epidemic provided a good opportunity to test the efficacy of Brazil's newly decentralized healthcare system — namely, SUS (Sistema Único de Saúde).

During this period the AIDS program was also viewed as having a poorly designed and ineffective information awareness and prevention campaign (Parker, 2003; Rochel de Camargo Jr., 1999). A consensus had emerged in society suggesting that the national AIDS program was providing inadequate information on how to have safe sex. For instance, in 1991 a random survey conducted by the media in the nation's capital, Brasilia, stated that approximately 95% of those individuals randomly selected for a poll claimed that they were unsatisfied and had no confidence in the information being provided by the national AIDS program (*Jornal do Commercio*, 1992). While the national program encouraged the usage of condoms as well as clean needles in order to prevent the further spread of HIV, and while the program repeatedly televised info commercials about AIDS, its causes and how to avoid it, pundits claimed that the information was not very detailed, understandable, and thus informative (Daniel, 1991; *Jornal do Brasil*, 1985b; Silva, 1991). This prompted prominent figures in society, such as Betinho, a famous hemophiliac and the creator of the ABIA (an AIDS NGO based in Rio), to argue that the poor quality of information was contributing to a sense of fear and uncertainty in society (*O Globo*, 1987a).

To make matters worse, the national AIDS program was criticized for providing offensive information. For example, Dr. Eduardo Cortes, who succeeded Lair Guerra as director of the national AIDS program in 1990, was chastised for approving prevention campaign slogans such as "*Se voçe não se cuidar, a AIDS vai te pegar,*" (if you don't take care of yourself, AIDS will take you) and "*Eu tenho AIDS e vou morrer*" (I have AIDS, and I'm going to die) (Silva, 1991). These slogans were viewed as offensive, providing little hope for those living with AIDS (Galvão, 2000: p. 23; Silva, 1991). What AIDS activists and patients wanted to hear was a slogan that not only educated them, but more importantly, one that also gave them hope and a purpose to live (Miguez, 1989; Reis, 1989).

Criticisms reached an apogee when in 1992 Cortes decided not to attend the opening of the yearly carnival festivities in Rio. Worse still, he did not ask his staff to go. It was embarrassing. He was immediately made the culprit. The pressure was so intense that Cortes quickly tendered his resignation. In his defense, he blamed the overly bureaucratized, burdensome AIDS program for giving him too much work to do and not enough time to do it (*Diario Popular*, 1992; *Folhão de Tarde*, 1992).

And finally, during this period the national AIDS program had no interest in working closely with the AIDS community in order to quell discrimination and to make it feel socially accepted (Rochel de Camargo Jr., 1999). In a context of heightened fear and insecurity, this response was needed in order to ease tensions on the part of civil society and protests against the state. However, the minister of health and the national AIDS program director never went out of their way to meet with the gay and intravenous drug community (Filho, 2006). Despite the fact that the gay community decreased in size and almost collapsed by 1984 (the year before the democratic transition), failing to meet with the few gay organizations that remained smacked of apathy and discrimination, especially in a context of redemocratization and proclaimed government commitment to human rights.

In response, by the late 1980s, several gay NGOs asked for national AIDS program director Lair Guerra's resignation (*Boletim pela Vidda*, 1990). Gay activists often relished in referring to her as "the bitch," mainly because of her arrogant attitude and apathy towards working with them (Filho, 2006). This added to the wider belief in society that the national AIDS program was operating on its own, as a distant federal agency that was not interested in creating an effective program.

International Criticisms, Pressures, and the Incentives for Reforms

Scholars claim that the mid-1980s signaled a major turning point in the international community's fight against AIDS (Lieberman, 2009). Shortly thereafter, an outpouring of international conferences and heightened media attention started to address the epidemic (Lieberman, 2009). International criticisms of Brazil's response to AIDS emerged during this period. Dr. Anthony Fauci, at the time director of the National Institute of Allergy and Infectious Diseases in the US, criticized Brazil for its delayed response to AIDS; he emphasized that the government needed to heighten its policy response (*O Estado de São Paulo*, 1987: p. 26). In 1987, the same year Fauci made his remarks, at a conference on the epidemiology and surveillance of AIDS in

Latin America held in Puerto Rico, Brazil was singled out as having the worst AIDS situation in the region (*O Estado de São Paulo*, 1987: p. 26). And by 1990, the World Bank would claim that if the government did not quickly escalate its policy response, it would see approximately 1,200,000 cases of AIDS by 2000 (Brazil, Ministry of Health, 2005: p. 7); add to this comments made by the Bank in 1993 that Brazil was failing to adequately invest in strengthening of its public health system (De Souza, 1993; *O Estado de São Paulo*, 1993).

While the government implemented prevention and treatment policies by the late 1980s, most of these criticisms emerged because of President Fernando Collor de Mello's (1990–1992) poorly designed AIDS policies, as well as his decision to stop cooperating with the international community (Parker, 2003). After resigning due to charges of corruption, Collor's predecessor, Itamar Franco, also failed to aggressively respond to AIDS (Lieberman, 2009). Franco seemed apathetic to the issue. He was mainly focused on revitalizing the integrity of the office of the presidency. Although the World Bank engaged in negotiations with Brazil in 1991 for a series of loans to help fund the national AIDS program, it took until March 1994 for an agreement to be reached. This delay revealed the World Bank's reluctance to work with Brazil because of its climate of corruption and instability (Parker, 2003).

This new international context provided a reason and opportunity for Brazil to respond and to increase its reputation as an effective democratic state committed to eradicating AIDS. As we saw in Chapter 2, beginning with the Gutelio Vargas administration (1930–1945), policymakers in Brazil were always committed to showing the world that they could effectively respond to health epidemics. Also recall in Chapter 2 that under Vargas, Brazil became internationally recognized for its fight against syphilis, malaria, and yellow fever, in turn establishing a rich tradition of responding to the emergence of pandemics in order to prove muster with the international community. International criticisms of Brazil's lackluster response to AIDS therefore instigated an immediate effort to rejuvenate Brazil's international reputation as a nation committed to eradicating disease and developing.

The office of the presidency in Brasília showed the most interest in achieving this objective (Fontes, 1999; Gómez, 2008, 2013). In an interview conducted with me, former two-term president of Brazil, Fernando H. Cardoso (1994–2002), stated that, when confronted with international criticisms and pressures, he was concerned about Brazil's international reputation, and that building this reputation was a factor motivating him, as well as his staff, to escalate their policy response to AIDS (Cardoso, 2007). President Cardoso's statements were corroborated by health officials that knew him and worked with him at the time (Chequer, 2008; D'Avila, 2008). Yet, Cardoso also believed that it was important to show the world that his government would work with other nations in achieving the global consensus of providing universal access to healthcare and medical treatment as a human right, while at the same time demonstrating that he was unwaveringly committed to eradicating AIDS (Cardoso, 2007). Helping further fuel Cardoso's endeavors was his awareness of Brazil's long history of being a world leader in the fight against disease, sharing knowledge and resources while building international institutions, such as the WHO. This history contributed to his yearning to build — and indeed, sustain — Brazil's strong international reputation in health (Cardoso, 2007).

Could it be that Cardoso was only interested in establishing his international reputation in health? Or were there other factors motivating his decision to expand the national AIDS program?

As a presidential candidate in 1993, it could be that Cardoso was interested in using the AIDS situation for electoral reasons. However, this cannot be accurate, as recent research documents the fact that Cardoso at no point campaigned on the issue (Gauri and Lieberman, 2006; Lieberman, 2009). But perhaps Cardoso was trying to bolster his general popularity and support in society? This also cannot be true because he was already very well known for having rejuvenated the economy and tamed inflation through his role as minister of finance, when he introduced the successful Real stabilization program of 1993 (Resende Santos, 1997). But perhaps it was the widespread fear and panic that the AIDS situation created by the early 1990s — especially as it began to touch the lives of popular social figures, such as artists and actors, in turn making it nearly impossible to ignore; this dire situation could have essentially forced Cardoso and his health ministers to increase their financial and political commitment to AIDS. Yet again, this argument cannot hold, as the dire AIDS situation was already well known by the mid-1980s and the government had, as mentioned earlier, acknowledged the virus' spread (Parker, 2009). Moreover, many famous individuals were already afflicted by AIDS during the late 1980s (Parker, 2009). Thus, it was neither political self-interest nor heightened media attention, fear, and escalating epidemiological case rates which instigated Cardoso's interest in increasing his response to AIDS. Instead, the main motivating factor seemed to be his interest in building Brazil's international reputation in health.

In order to begin strengthening the government's international reputation, President Cardoso and the MOH began to attend several international AIDS conferences while inviting international organizations to visit Brazil and examine their policies (Da Costa Marques, 2003; Galvão, 2000). By engaging in these activities, it was hoped that the government could convince international organizations, such as the WHO, that Cardoso's administration could effectively respond and that it was committed to eradicating AIDS (Da Costa Marques, 2003). Galvão (2000: 116–117) writes that it was a time when the government was trying to establish itself as a world pioneer in the fight against AIDS.

Despite the government's new interest and commitment to AIDS policy, having the fiscal capacity to achieve its goals was an entirely different issue. By the late 1980s, fiscal instability and hyperinflation burgeoned, leading to a phalanx of fiscal stabilization policies.[2] By 1988, economists predicted that the MOH and the AIDS program would lose approximately 30% of its budget (*Jornal do Brasil*, 1988).

---

[2] They were the Cruzado Plan (1986–1990), the Collor Plan (1990–1992), and the Real Plan (1993–present); all three were introduced to tame hyperinflation through privatization and tax reform. The Real Plan, created and implemented by then Finance Minister Fernando Cardoso, finally succeeded in stabilizing the economy. And in 2000, the Chamber of Deputies (Congress) and the Senate passed the Fiscal Responsibility Law, which imposed several hard budget constraints on state and municipal governments in order to avoid fiscal deficits and debts.

In response, the national AIDS program requested approximately CZ600 (Cruzeiro) million in federal assistance to continue supporting their prevention and treatment activities (Da Costa Marques, 2003).

By the early 1990s, the national AIDS program found itself in a dire fiscal situation. The World Bank noticed these challenges and how it was delaying the government's response to AIDS (Araújo de Mattos *et al.*, 2003). Bank officials believed that the MOH would not have the resources needed to escalate prevention activities and purchase ARV medications.

In need of financial resources and technical support, the prospect of obtaining a loan from the World Bank helped to increase the government's attention and commitment to AIDS (Barbosa, 2008; D'Avila, 2008). With the World Bank's assistance, President Cardoso could now achieve his goal of increasing the government's international reputation by creating a more effective national AIDS program.

After several rounds of negotiation, in 1994 the World Bank offered a loan of $120 million dollars, with the possibility of being renewed every five years. Amidst escalating fiscal deficits and government downsizing, World Bank funding helped the government finance its programs, such as funding to NGOs for AIDS awareness and prevention (Galvão, 2000; Lewis, 2006). Establishing a safe blood supply system was also a priority (Gauri, 2004). More important for our interests, the World Bank loan clearly stipulated that part of the money be used for strengthening AIDS administration, such as centralizing policy control, expanding staff size, increasing salaries, and providing technical assistance (Galvão, 2000; Lewis, 2006; Mattos *et al.*, 2003). Despite the growing need for ARV medications, such as azidothymidine (AZT), World Bank officials nevertheless emphasized that none of their funding was to be used for purchasing or producing ARV medicine (Mattos *et al.*, 2003).

But was the provision of international funding the key catalyst for reform? Or was it the government's reputation-building interests? It seems that the latter was more important, as external funding without reputation building would not have provided the incentives needed to increase and more importantly sustain the government's commitment to reform. Alternatively, reputation-building interests in the absence of funding would not have led to ongoing reforms, as the state would not have been capable of affording ongoing program and policy expansion. Thus, World Bank funding provided the *means* through which Brazil could establish its international reputation and deepen its centralized response.

Shortly after the loan paperwork was signed, World Bank officials and the NGO community began to notice changes within the national AIDS program. Dr. Maureen Lewis, the World Bank economist in charge of the first loan to Brazil, noticed that the AIDS program director, Lair Guerra, who came back to the national program after Eduardo Cortes' resignation in 1992, became very enthused and excited about the loan package and her ability to introduce new policies (Lewis, 2006). Shortly after the first loan installment, Lair began to increase her attention to the AIDS situation and became more committed to working with the World Bank (Lewis, 2006). In an interview with me, Lewis commented that before the first World Bank loan, the AIDS program was poorly organized and had very little support from the president (Lewis, 2006). From what she could see, Lair was the only person fully committed to restructuring the program. Lewis also explained that with the loan money, Lair began to hire the best technical and managerial staff that she could find (Lewis, 2006). Others note that this was a period of rapid technocratic recruitment and specialization within the national AIDS program (Gālvao, 2000; Nunn, 2009; Teixeira, 1997).

The president's new interest in responding to AIDS and the arrival of World Bank support also helped to ameliorate tensions within the MOH. For the first time, AIDS and senior MOH officials started working together to expand the national AIDS program (Chequer, 2008; Teixeira, 2007). MOH officials who had previously sided with the president, who favored the idea of decentralizing the government's response to AIDS, started to find an interest in AIDS officials' efforts to seek a more centralized bureaucratic and policy response (Chequer, 2008; Teixeira, 2007; Terto, 2008). In addition, the fact that the World Bank shared similar interests with AIDS officials helped to provide them with even more credibility and influence (Barbosa, 2008; Gālvao, 2000; Terto, 2008).

Centralized Bureaucratic and Policy Outcomes

By the mid-1990s, new efforts were made to centralize the national AIDS program and its policies. Bureaucratic centralization increased with the president and MOH's delegation of increased policymaking autonomy to the national AIDS program. The minister of health, José Serra, and President Cardoso gave the AIDS program authority to create and implement policy without getting approval from other agencies (Cardoso, 2007; Galvão, 2000; Teixeira, 1997). Sera and Cardoso believed that AIDS officials had the technical knowledge and experience needed to work on their own and that they would be most effective that way.

In addition, and in sharp contrast to the other health and social welfare agencies at the time, because of this high level of autonomy the national AIDS program did not have to follow standard procedures when applying for congressional funding. Since the early 1990s, the AIDS program does not have to fill out the required paperwork that other agencies have to complete in order to obtain congressional funding (Moherdai, 2006). With the continued assistance of the World Bank and an easier way of obtaining congressional funding, the AIDS program has had the resources needed to centralize, specialize, and grow.

AIDS bureaucrats believed that they needed to increase their policymaking authority over the states (De Costa Marques, 2003). Furthermore the AIDS program believed that all states and municipalities had to implement their policy prescriptions (Teixeira, 1997). To help solidify the national program's centralized control, it also created the Comissões Municipais de AIDS (Municipal AIDS Commissions) (Teixeira, 1997). These institutions monitor sub-national policy performance, reported findings to the national program office, while providing financial and technical assistance to the states (Teixeira, 1997). Yet the governors resisted this interference, mainly because of the national governments commitment to decentralization.

But this does not mean that the national AIDS program became a completely isolated, despotic agency. Although it strengthened its centralized policy approach, since the early 1990s it has been simultaneously committed to consulting and representing the interests of civil society through NGOs while working in cooperation with other federal agencies. While the program started to work with other agencies before the first World Bank loan, after the loan it started working closely with other federal ministries, such as education and law. In addition, and as I discuss later, although the AIDS program was initially reluctant to work with the national TB Program (out of fear of losing its political influence), eventually it did start to work closely with TB officials in order to ensure that the World Bank's prevention and treatment policies were effectively implemented.

And finally, under the Cardoso administration several new prevention and treatment programs were implemented. For example, beginning in the mid-1990s, a series of awareness campaigns in the media targeting the most at-risk groups, such as gay men and women, were introduced (Levi and Vitoria, 2002). Moreover, in 2002 a media campaign was created focusing on helping young gay men learn more about AIDS (Levi and Vitoria, 2002). By 2007 the national program also began to focus on AIDS's spread among woman, creating the Plano Integrado de Enfrentamento da Feminização da Epidemia de Aids e otras DST. Through this program, NGOs work with AIDS officials to provide HIV testing, female condoms, as well as educational materials (Brazil, National AIDS Program, 2007). Finally the national program created several sex education curriculum programs in 2009 (Arnquist *et al.*, 2011).

With respect to general preventative efforts, the national program also stepped up its commitment to distributing condoms, going so far as to promise the distribution of 3 billion condoms yearly to the states in 1994 (Lieberman, 2009). A universal HIV testing program was also introduced (Lieberman, 2009). By 1996, moreover, based on President Cardoso's policy recommendation, Congress passed Decree Act No. 9313, which constitutionally guaranteed the universal provision of free ARV medication (Mattos *et al.*, 2003; Nunn *et al.*, 2009). Brazil became the first nation in the world to legally guarantee the universal distribution of AIDS drugs. Finally Congress also passed legislation in 2000 ensuring that clean needles be distributed to the states (Paiva *et al.*, 2006).

Thus, by the late 1990s, the national AIDS program reversed its course, introducing new prevention and treatment policies while starting to work more closely with civil society. But why did AIDS officials finally start to work closely with civil society? As the next section explains, for those AIDS bureaucrats seeking a stronger centralized bureaucratic and policy response, working closely with civil society was eventually perceived as a strategic way to obtain the legitimacy and influence needed to continuously obtain financial and political support for their endeavors. To that end, AIDS bureaucrats began to view and use the *sanitaristas* and AIDS NGOs as helpful civic supporters.

Connecting with Civic Supporters

Understanding the national AIDS program's successful transformation requires that we briefly rehash our discussion from Chapter 2 of the historical genesis of social health movements working in partnership with public health officials. As I discussed in that chapter, beginning in the early 20th century, public health officials established strong partnerships with social health movements in order to construct effective, centralized public health institutions (Carrara, 1996; Hochman, 1998).

Despite the emergence of TB and syphilis as the 20th century progressed, because there was a myriad of other diseases present in Brazil, TB and syphilis were highly contested between politicians and bureaucrats over their threat to society. Consequently the government did not immediately respond (Nasciemento, 1991; Nascimento, 2005). Nevertheless, in 1899 and 1915, the Liga contra a Tuberculose (henceforth, Liga) and the Sifilógrafo social health movements (focused on syphilis) arose to instigate domestic and international awareness about these epidemics, while advocating for a centralized response (Carrara, 1996, 1997; Do Nascimento, 2005; Filho, 2001; Nascimento, 1991).

Health scientists, academics, doctors, and activists came together to form the Liga and Sifilógrafo movements. Because famous medical scientists were involved in both movements, and because they traveled the world sharing their scientific findings and winning awards, both movements garnered considerable attention, respect, and legitimacy (Carrara, 1996; Gómez, 2008; Nascimento, 1991). As proud scientists and public intellectuals, members of these movements were also committed to bolstering Brazil's world recognition for cutting-edge research, as well as its reputation in successfully combating disease (Carrara, 1997; Filho, 2001; Nascimento, 1991; Peard, 1999).

Aside from world fame, the Liga and Sifilógrafo also found themselves in agreement with the international community's policy preferences, such as the creation of a centralized bureaucratic and policy response to diseases while guaranteeing the universal provision of essential medicines; these ideas were popularly espoused in western Europe and inspired members of both social movements (Carrara, 1996; Nascimento, 1991). These movements also pressed the government to follow western Europe's lead in creating universal prevention campaigns as well as the free distribution of medication and treatment (Araujo, 1939; Carrara, 1996; Filho, 2001; Nascimento, 1991). But the Liga and Sifilógrafo also did not believe in working alone. They believed in strength in numbers and thus sought to establish a close partnership with national health officials in order to achieve their policy goals (Gómez, 2008, 2010).

For health officials, partnering with these social movements was perceived as potentially helping them convince presidents to strengthen existing public health institutions, such as the Departmento Geral de Saúde Público (DSP) (1900–1930) and the Ministerio da Educação e Saúde Público (MESP) (1930–1945) (Gómez, 2008). In order to persuade the president that there was a need to create a similarly centralized institutional response to TB and syphilis, DSP and MESP officials worked with Liga and Sifilógrafo members, seeing them as highly regarded, influential allies in their cause for reform (Carrara, 1996; Nascimento, 1997, 1991).

A good example is the work of Dr. Oswaldo Cruz, director of Public Health. So as to help convince presidents and congressional policymakers that they should build a centralized agency focused exclusively on TB, and in order to build his credibility and influence, Cruz engaged in a close partnership with Liga and Sifilógrafo members (Carrara, 1996; Nascimento, 1997, 1991); subsequent DGHSP and MESP health officials would do the same (Carrara, 1996).

Seeking to build centralized institutions together, the fact that DGHSP and MESP officials sought to work with the Liga and Sifilógrafo movement underscored their similar types of policy ideas and beliefs: that is, establishing a centralized bureaucratic and policy response to health epidemics. This helped to establish a sense of cohesion as well as a unified policy mission. Aiding this process was the fact that several DGHSP and MESP officials emerged from these and other social health movements (Carrara, 1999). But, more importantly, working with these social health movements helped to increase the legitimacy and policymaking influence of DGHSP and MESP officials (Nascimento, 1991, 1997).

Working Closely with Civic Supporters in Response to AIDS

When the AIDS epidemic first emerged in Brazil, there was a preexisting commitment to healthcare decentralization. Healthcare decentralization was viewed as an effort to deepen the democratization process, as it helped to increase civic accountability and participation in policymaking.

Nevertheless, it is important to emphasize that the government's first interest in healthcare decentralization emerged under the military governments (1964–1985) (Falleti, 2010). In 1971, for example, the government created the Assistance Fund for Rural Workers, FUNRURAL; this fund provided healthcare services to the poor, especially in hard to reach rural areas (Fundo de Assistencia ao Trabalhador Rural) (Falleti, 2010). Yet the military's biggest commitment to decentralization emerged with the Program of Internalization of Health and Sanitary Actions, PIASS (Programa de Interiorização das Ações de Saúde e Saneamento), which was established in 1976. Through the PIASS the MOH instructed sub-national health departments to construct public health outposts, while providing better sanitation services and clean water (Falleti, 2010). Further efforts to decentralize came in 1982, when the MOH created the Integrated Health System, AIS (Ações Integradas de Saúde) (Harmeling, 1999).

Through the AIS the government imposed greater healthcare policy responsibilities onto the state governments (Harmeling, 1999). The goal was to establish a strong primary care system (Harmeling, 1999).

By the early 1980s, the military was politically and ideologically committed to healthcare decentralization (Falleti, 2010; Gómez, 2011; Merhy, 1977). In addition to decentralization's political benefits (Falleti, 2010; Lobato, 2000), this processes was also aided by the *sanitarista* movement's belief in healthcare decentralization (especially civic participation and control) and their successful attempt to assume key leadership positions within the MOH and the Ministry of Planning (Weyland, 1995; Falleti, 2010).

Despite the return to democracy in 1985 and the adoption of decentralization as the primary policy instrument for ensuring universal healthcare in the 1988 constitution, by the early 1990s MOH and national AIDS program officials began to question decentralization's effectiveness. There emerged little confidence in decentralization's ability to quickly respond to AIDS patients, and to provide prevention and treatment services (Gómez, 2011; Rich, 2010). For example, there was an ongoing shortage of beds in public hospitals (Buss and Gadelha, 1996) as well as inadequate funding for biomedical tests and X-ray image tests (Portela and Lotrowska, 2006). There were also several administrative challenges, such as effective healthcare service management, and limited operational hours and staff meetings (Portela and Lotrowska, 2006). State and municipal health departments were also becoming notorious for mishandling healthcare budgets (Rich, 2009), and they were also accused of neglecting to ensure that their AIDS prevention and treatment programs were working effectively (Gómez, 2011; Rich, 2009). On top of all this, by the early 1990s President Cardoso was also expressing his dissatisfaction with healthcare decentralization processes, emphasizing the dearth of funding, poor administration, and lack of accountability (Pasche *et al.*, 2006).

Civil society was quick to respond to this context. Much like what had occurred during the early 20th century, in response to a highly contested epidemic (AIDS), the *sanitarista* movement arose to pressure the government for effective policy action (Barreira, 2012; Brito,

2012; Galvão, 2000; Massé, 2009; Rich, 2009). Shortly after the World Bank loan was provided, the *sanitaristas* reemerged as a globally integrated, well-organized movement dedicated to strengthening the national AIDS program (Brito, 2012; Galvão, 2000; Gómez, 2011; Massé, 2009; Rich, 2009; Villela, 1999). The *sanitaristas* believed that the government should strengthen public health agencies, and emphasize disease prevention while universally distributing medications (Barreira, 2012; Brito, 2012; Falleti, 2010; Galvão, 2000). This is similar to what the Liga and Sifilógrafo had advocated for in the past. Moreover, the *sanitaristas* emphasized that patients and activists should be more involved in the policymaking process (Barreira, 2012; Brito, 2012; Merhy, 1977); and furthermore, that the state and civil society once again establish a partnership to advocating a similar, state-centered, universal policy commitment to AIDS and other diseases (Barreira, 2012; Brito, 2012; Rich, 2009). The end result was a social health movement that turned quickly from advocating decentralization to joining concerned AIDS officials in pursuing a centralized bureaucratic and policy response to AIDS (Gómez, 2011; Nunn, 2009).

Furthermore, by the early 1990s the *sanitaristas* were so concerned about the AIDS situation that many of them changed their policy preferences, from decentralization to a centralized approach to administration and policy (Barreira, 2012; Campos, 2012; Filho, 2012; Gómez, 2011; Grangeiro, 2012; Nunn, 2009; Varas, 2012). Those preferring a decentralized approach to AIDS policy soon outnumbered those sanitaristas in civil society that preferred a decentralized approach (Gómez, 2011; Nunn, 2009). Keen on enhancing their credibility, influence, and justification for building their national program, AIDS officials strategically used and advocated the *sanitaristas'* ideas of administrative and policy centralization.

The *sanitarista* movement also helped the national AIDS program strengthen its commitment to centralization (Barreira, 2012; Berkman *et al.*, 2005; Biehl, 2004; Campos, 2012; Filho, 2012; Gómez, 2011; Grangeiro, 2012; Nunn, 2009; Solano, 2000; Varas, 2012). With a large influx of policy consultants, many of whom were funded by the aforementioned World Bank loan, there were now many new people within the AIDS program dedicated to a centralized bureaucratic and policy response, believing in and advocating AIDS officials' centrist ideas (Barreira, 2012; Biehl, 2004; Campos, 2012; Filho, 2012; Gómez, 2010; Grangeiro, 2012; Varas, 2012); this infiltration bolstered the number of AIDS officials committed to a centrist response (Biehl, 2004; Berkman et *al.*, 2005; Galvão, 2000; Gómez, 2010; Nunn, 2009). Since many of these consultants had extensive experience implementing universal prevention and treatment policies in their state governments (Camara, 2002; Nunn, 2009), they were in full agreement with AIDS officials' centrist views (Gómez, 2011).

The fact that many of these new World Bank consultants, as well as those hired through the MOH, were *sanitarista* members also facilitated the national AIDS program's ability to work with and through the *sanitarista* community at the local level, many of whom were influential politicians and bureaucrats (Barreira, 2012; Berkman *et al.*, 2005; Brito, 2012; Darrah, 2006; Nunn, 2009; Parker, 2003). As Gómez (2011) notes, these *sanitarista* infiltrators maintained their relationship with the fellow *sanitarista* members throughout the country, as well as NGOs, repeatedly going back and forth to their states, following up on projects, and making sure that they were being implemented effectively. When called to work at the national level, former *sanitarista* state AIDS officials, who had established strong networks of support and partnerships with NGOs and the *sanitarista* community in their cities, took these experiences and networks back with them to the national program. These *sanitarista* networks within the national program helped AIDS officials to achieve their policy objectives (Abadia, 2003; Brito, 2012; Barreira, 2012; Darrah, 2006).

AIDS NGOs also helped to provide support to the *sanitaristas* working within the national AIDS program. On their own, however, these NGOs were also very influential. Much like the Liga and Sifilógrafo movements before them, AIDS NGOs were highly involved at the international level, attending a myriad of AIDS conferences, while working with NGOs in other nations (Bastos, 1999). AIDS NGOs in Brazil also had strong connections with international organizations, such as the WHO and the UNAIDS (the Joint United Nations Programme on HIV/AIDS), and frequently met with officials there

to help increase awareness about AIDS and to provide advice to other
nations (Bastos, 1999). Yet, many of Brazil's NGOs were also passionate about working with international financial institutions, such as
the World Bank and the UK's DFID (Department for International
Development), in order to provide funding to other community-
based organizations and NGOs (Bastos, 1999). Through these activities, Brazil's NGOs also encouraged governments in other nations to
include civil society into the AIDS policymaking process (Bastos,
1999). Through these activities, AIDS NGOs in Brazil were able to
increase their popularity, making them influential — and thus attractive — partners in the quest to engender an effective centralized
bureaucratic and policy response to AIDS (Barreira, 2012; Camara,
2002; Gómez, 2011).

It is important to note, however, that the policy ideas that the
NGO community was espousing comported with the Liga, Sifilógrafo,
and *sanitarista* social movements' ideas. More specifically, these
NGOs' ideas were centered on the establishment of a strong national
AIDS program, fully capable of creating universal medical treatment
policies, progressive prevention campaigns, while continuously providing technical and financial assistance to state and municipal governments (Barreira, 2012; Brito, 2012; Gómez, 2010; Teixeira, 1997;
Varas, 2012). Another key emphasis for NGOs was combating discrimination (Parker, 2003; Teixeira, 1997). Finally, NGOs also believed
that national AIDS officials should join them in participating in
domestic and international conferences and meetings, sharing information and policy recommendations (Bastos, 1999; Rich, 2009).

Adding to the NGOs' influence was their exponential growth in
number (Camara, 2002; Villela, 1999). For example, by 1994, at the
6th annual National AIDS NGO Conference, approximately 400
NGOs had signed up to work with AIDS NGOs (Villela, 1999; *VI
Encontro Nacional de ONGs/AIDS*). The popularity of working with
AIDS NGOs burgeoned, especially as these organizations obtained
ongoing financial support from the World Bank — which translated
to jobs for many unemployed activists (Massé, 2009).

NGOs and the *sanitarista* movement were therefore complemen-
tary groups of dedicated activists, incessantly working to engender a

more effective national AIDS response. However, it is interesting to note that in addition to sharing similar policy ideas, these two groups also closely resembled the Liga and Sifilógrafo movements (Barreira, 2012; Brito, 2012; Campos, 2012; Dhalia, 2012; Filho, 2012; Grangeiro, 2012; Schaffer, 2012; Varas, 2012).

As Gómez (2011) maintains, AIDS NGOs and the *sanitaristas* therefore represented social movement legacies that were dedicated to centralized government intervention and universal healthcare policy (Barreira, 2012; Brito, 2012; Campos, 2012; Dhalia, 2012; Filho, 2012; Grangeiro, 2012; Schaffer, 2012). What's more, AIDS NGOs and *sanitaristas* also represented a rich tradition of social health movements working in strong partnership with national health officials to achieve these policy goals.

Civil society as well as government officials recognized these partnership efforts and supported them (Barreira, 2012; Campos, 2012; Dhalia, 2012; Filho, 2012; Gómez, 2011; Grangeiro, 2012; Nunn, 2009; Schaffer, 2012). Yet politicians also came to recognize the connection that the *sanitaristas* and AIDS NGOs had with these historic social health movements; this led politicians to respect the *sanitaristas* and NGOs' efforts, their ideas, as well as those AIDS officials working with them (Barreira, 2012; Campos, 2012; Dhalia, 2012; Galvão, 2000; Gómez, 2010; Grangeiro, 2012; Maherdai, 2012; Nunn, 2009; Schaffer, 2012).

The social and, hence, political legitimacy and ability of AIDS NGO officials to implement policy nevertheless rested on the support that they obtained from the *sanitarista* and AIDS NGOs (Barreira, 2012; Brito, 2012; Campos, 2012; Dhalia, 2012; Gómez, 2010; Grangeiro, 2012; Schaffer, 2012; Varas, 2012). Congress' heightened interest and sensitivity to support from society for this partnership was further reinforced by the transition to democracy and the consolidation of electoral institutions (Ciconello, 2008).

Motivating AIDS officials' interest in seeking out and working with the *sanitaristas* and AIDS NGOs was officials' knowledge of the similarities between these civic groups and the historic Liga and Sifilógrafo movements (Barreira, 2012; Brito, 2012; Grangeiro, 2012; Teixeira, 2007). Paulo Teixeira, former director of the national AIDS Program, commented to me in an interview that he was often reminded of the Liga and Sifilógrafos movements, as well as the strong partnership that they had with health officials, when working on the AIDS situation (Teixeira, 2007). Teixeira further commented how this historic knowledge motivated him to seek out and work with the *sanitaristas* and AIDS NGOs (Teixeira, 2007); moreover, he believed that doing so would help to increase the national program's political legitimacy and influence (Teixeira, 2007).

Teixeira's comments to me were corroborated with the interview testimony of other AIDS officials working with him at the time (Barreira, 2012, 2009; Brito, 2012; Campos, 2012; Dhalia, 2012; Grangeiro, 2012; Schaffer, 2012). Interviews with former national AIDS officials also revealed that during the 1990s, these officials were inspired by the long history of state–civil society ties in combating health epidemics (Barreira, 2012, 2009; Brito, 2012; Campos, 2012; Dhalia, 2012; Grangeiro, 2012; Schaffer, 2012). Like Teixeira, this knowledge also motivated these officials to seek out *sanitarista* and AIDS NGOs that not only resembled the Liga and Sifilógrafos, but that were also advocating similar historical policy ideas of centralized government intervention (Barreira, 2012, 2009; Brito, 2012; Campos, 2012; Dhalia, 2012; Grangeiro, 2012; Schaffer, 2012). According to interview testimonies from these officials as well as *sanitarista* members, they were also aware of the historically proven track record of this type of policy intervention (Barreira, 2012; Campos, 2012; Filho, 2012; Grangeiro, 2012; Schaffer, 2012).

Further aiding officials in their ability to recall these successful historical partnerships were the efforts of AIDS NGOs to periodically remind officials of them. NGOs also reminded officials of the long history of civil society working closely with federal health officials to eradicate disease, and how they shared and were unified by common policy ideals and strategies (Terto, 2008; Teixeira, 2007; Gómez, 2008).

AIDS officials' ability to work with civil society was also aided by the presence of several venues and opportunities for meetings. For example, the National AIDS Commission (Comissão Nacional de Aids, CNAIDS), which was created in 1986, provided a place where AIDS officials and civil society could meet. CNAIDS was created by the national AIDS program in order to bring together key stakeholders in the policymaking process — with actors from civil society being key members of this process. At these meetings, AIDS officials and representatives from civil society exchanged policy ideas and strategies for implementing policy (Barreira, 2012; Brito, 2012; Campos, 2012; Crespo and Spink, 2003). But meetings were also held at the local level. Rich and Gómez (2012) maintain that periodic, informal meetings, often organized by the NGOs, were held between AIDS officials and NGOs, and that the purpose of these meetings was to learn from each other; furthermore, they maintain that at these meetings they shared similar policy ideas and interests in policy centralization (Barreira, 2012).

The legitimacy and political influence of AIDS officials was strengthened because of their partnership with the *sanitaristas* and AIDS NGOs (Barbosa, 2008; Barreira, 2009, 2012; Brito, 2012; Campos, 2012; Dhalia, 2012; Filho, 2012; Grangeiro, 2012; Schaffer, 2012; Varas, 2012). AIDS officials' legitimacy and influence increased because many politicians were cognizant of this relationship, as well as the MOH's long history of having a successful centralized approach to disease eradication (Barreira, 2012; Brito, 2012; Carrara, 1996; Campos, 2012; Filho, 2012; Grangeiro, 2012; Hochman, 1998; Schaffer, 2012). Through information gathered from MOH publications and the media, moreover, politicians assigned great credibility to AIDS officials' policy ideas (Barbosa, 2008; Barreira, 2009, 2012; Brito, 2012; Campos, 2012; Filho, 2012; Grangeiro, 2012; Schaffer, 2012). The product of this attention and support was AIDS officials' ability to secure ongoing political support for their centralized policy interventions (Barbosa, 2008; Barreira, 2009, 2012; Brito, 2012; Campos, 2012; Dhalia, 2012; Filho, 2012; Grangeiro, 2012; Varas, 2012; Schaffer, 2012).

Civic Supporters and Centralization Strategies

There were administrative benefits to partnering with civic supporters. By the mid-1990s, for example, this partnership contributed to a substantial increase in congressional spending for the national AIDS program. More specifically, spending for hiring more administrative staff, consultants, and the provision of universal prevention and treatment burgeoned (Barbosa, 2008; Barreira, 2009, 2012; Brito, 2012; Campos, 2012; Dhalia, 2012; Filho, 2012; Gómez, 2010; Grangeiro, 2012; Schaffer, 2012; Varas, 2012). And because many international donors, such as the World Bank, encouraged governments to establish a strong partnership with NGOs, AIDS officials were able to obtain the support of the international community repeatedly; this, in turn, further added to their domestic credibility and ability to obtain support from Congress (Gómez, 2010).

Even more telling about the government's commitment to spending was the fact that the national AIDS program did not fall into the traditional trap of donor aid dependence. Domestic spending for AIDS far surpassed the amount of money provided by the World Bank (Gómez, 2010). What's more, spending occurred amidst the economic recession of 1998, which adds even further credence to the notion that the government was fully committed to combating AIDS.

The government's ongoing support for AIDS officials' centralized bureaucratic and policy efforts also led to policy initiatives contributing to the national AIDS program's ongoing centralized influence. Despite the national program's decision in 2002 to gradually decentralize more financial and policy responsibilities to municipal health departments, in 2003 AIDS officials obtained congressional and MOH approval for the creation of a new discretionary — performance-based — fiscal transfer policy that assists municipal AIDS officials complying with the national program's conditionalities and policy recommendations (Barboza, 2006; Brazil, Ministry of Health, 2010; Pires 2006).

Called the Ministerial Ordinance No. 2313, Política de Incentivos Fundo-a-Fundo program (henceforth, Política de Incentivos), as long as municipal health agencies adhere to the conditionalities imposed by the national AIDS program, they are eligible for grant assistance (Barboza, 2006; Brazil, Ministry of Health 2010;). To qualify for a grant, the following conditionalities must be met: (1) a high incidence of AIDS cases, at a minimum of 50,000, as well as evidence of quickly escalating case rates; (2) a municipal AIDS program's participation in the first two World Bank loans (1994–1998; 1999–2003) — which signifies need for financial and infrastructural resources; and (3) budgetary evidence that municipal health agencies are already committed to acquiring technical equipment and managerial capacity (Barboza, 2006; Gómez, 2011).

Furthermore, the national AIDS program put forth several policy conditionalities. They include the following:

1. A commitment to building the institutional, infrastructural, and managerial capacity needed to effectively implement prevention and treatment policy (Barbosa, 2006; Pires, 2006).
2. Commitment to ensuring a high quality of prevention and medical treatment services for AIDS victims (Barbosa, 2006; Pires, 2006).
3. An agreement that those municipalities receiving grant assistance would provide, when needed, financial assistance to other municipalities that did not participate in the Política de Incentivos program (Barbosa, 2006; Pires, 2006).
4. A commitment to strengthening civil society's participation in policymaking as well as monitoring the implementation of policy (Barbosa, 2006; Pires, 2006).
5. And finally, a promise to ensure that municipal health departments purchase and distribute ARV medication (Barboza, 2006; Brazil, Ministry of Health, 2010; Pires, 2006).

Yet, it was *how* the Política de Incentivos was introduced that further underscored the national AIDS program's strategies to sustain its centralized influence after decentralization. In 2003, for example, the national program sent thousands of technical consultants to municipal health agencies to monitor whether these agencies were adhering to the national program's policy recommendations (Barboza, 2006). Furthermore, all technical publications and manuals were published and distributed by the national program (Barboza, 2006). These strategies implied that the national program wanted to reduce municipal health agencies' policymaking autonomy, while also revealing that the national program had essentially no confidence in the municipal officials' ability to create and implement policy (Gómez, 2011). Since the Política de Incentivos was created, most of the funding has gone to the areas hardest hit by AIDS, such as the southern states. The city of São Paulo, for example, has by far received most of the money, with an estimated receipt of 33.4% from 2002–2010 (Gómez, 2011). By 2010, approximately 26 states and 489 municipalities received Política de Incentivos assistance (Brazil, Ministry of Health, 2010; Gómez, 2011).

The Congress has also been committed to consistently providing funding for the Política de Incentivos. Furthermore, funding has increased despite the provision of a World Bank loan in December 2008 providing state governments with funding for SUS as well as AIDS programs (Godinho, 2009; World Bank, 2008).

At the same time, since the early 2000s the national AIDS program was engaged in formal spent money in order to bolster its centralized bureaucratic and policy influence, while at the same time engaging in informal policy strategies to achieve the same outcome. It did this mainly by contracting NGOS to carefully monitor state and especially municipal health department commitments to implementing AIDS policies, thus providing much needed information to the center about the performance of municipal agencies. Therefore this informal policy strategy had the added benefit of increasing municipal health departments' accountability to the national program (Rich and Gómez, 2012). Moreover, this informal partnership encouraged NGOs to consistently pressure municipal governments to ensure that policies were being implemented effectively (Rich and Gómez, 2012). National AIDS officials realized that they did not have a large enough staff at the national level that could do this kind of monitoring work. The national program therefore relied on NGOs to be their local eyes and ears, taking advantage of the rich abundance of NGOs presence at the municipal level (Rich and Gómez, 2012). Many of these NGOs were lacking in funding and thus eager to be hired and work for the national government (Gómez, 2011; Massé, 2009).

But how did the national program establish this informal partnership with NGOs? AIDS officials achieved this by incessantly meeting with NGOs at the municipal level, such as through the Commissions for Articulation with Social Movements (CAMS) (Rich, 2010; Rich and Gómez, 2012). Organized by municipal health officials and civil society, CAMS is a participatory municipal AIDS policy committee that invites policymakers, activists, and HIV positive individuals to formulate policy recommendations together (Rich, 2010; Rich and Gómez, 2012). It is at this venue where national AIDS officials have frequently meet with AIDS NGOs in order to share information, and to learn about municipal needs and local AIDS officials' commitment to sound policy implementation. But it is also at CAMS that NGOs provide AIDS officials with their information and experience in working with municipal officials (Rich, 2010; Rich and Gómez, 2012). In fact, extensive field work conducted by Rich (2010) found that after interviewing national AIDS officials at approximately 21 CAMS meetings, these officials acquired information from NGOs about municipal health agencies' often poor commitment to prevention and treatment policy as well as the limitations to decentralization processes. At these meetings Rich (2010) additionally found that AIDS officials also strategize with NGOs about how they can more effectively monitor municipal officials, as well as the different types of pressure tactics that they can use in order to help make municipal officials more accountable and committed to sound policy implementation.

Conclusion

While Brazil's response to AIDS may certainly be viewed as the "envy of the world," it took a long time for the government to achieve this reputation. Similar to what we saw in the US, Brazil's government did not immediately respond to AIDS. While a national AIDS program was created by 1986, it was poorly funded, organized, and supported. At the same time, there was no legislative and MOH assistance to state and municipal health departments, which were hampered in their response due to fiscal imbalances and debt. Worse still, during this period the national AIDS program did not respond to the needs of civil society.

By the late 1980s, however, international health agencies, such as the UN's Global Program on AIDS, as well as leading scientists and the World Bank, began to criticize Brazil for its delayed response. But as President Fernando Cardoso positioned Brazil as an emerging nation striving to increase its international reputation, these criticisms and pressures had a positive impact on his reform interests. Cardoso wanted to show the world that Brazil could join other advanced industrialized nations in having the policies and the political commitment needed to eradicate AIDS, while working closely with the international donor community to obtain the financial and technical assistance needed to achieve this goal. By responding in this manner, Cardoso and his MOH officials could help to increase Brazil's international reputation as a modern state capable of overcoming any obstacle to development.

With this goal in mind, by the mid-1990s Cardoso and the MOH increased their commitment to constructing a more effective national AIDS program. While a generous loan from the World Bank certainly facilitated this process, it was Cardoso's international reputation-building interests that motivated him to support previously ignored AIDS officials. Cardoso delegated a high level of policymaking autonomy to the national program while facilitating AIDS officials' ability to obtain funding from Congress. Armed with strong political and financial backing, AIDS officials implemented a host of prevention and treatment policies while assisting the states in their endeavors.

However, noticing that healthcare decentralization through SUS was not helping achieve an effective response, national AIDS officials soon realized that effective policy implementation would depend on their ability to maintain their centralized policy influence while nevertheless operating within the confines of SUS. AIDS officials achieved this by not only hiring AIDS NGOs to monitor municipal government performance and reporting their findings back to the national program, thus increasing municipal accountability to the center, but also by introducing new discretionary fiscal transfer policies, such as the Política de Incentivos. Since its inception in 2003, Política de Incentivos has not only provided financial assistance to municipal health departments in consistent need of funding AIDS services, but it has also helped to hold the mayors more accountable for their policy actions.

Despite policymakers' renewed interest and commitment to reform, achieving these and other policy objectives ultimately depended on AIDS officials' ability to find and strategically use civil society, that is, civic supporters. Beginning in the early 1990s, these officials strategically sought out and used the *sanitarista* and AIDS NGO community in order to increase officials' legitimacy and influence when seeking ongoing support for their policies.

AIDS officials pursued this partnership for a good reason. As we saw in Chapter 2, like their predecessors during the early 20th century, i.e., the Liga Contra a Tuberculose and the Sifilógrafo, the *sanitaristas* and AIDS NGOs advocated policy ideas that had a historically proven track record of success — that is, an immediate, centralized bureaucratic and policy response to epidemics. Partnering with these supporters and using their ideas increased AIDS officials' legitimacy and influence, especially when compared to more contemporary policy ideas, such as decentralization. With the rise of hundreds of AIDS NGOs by the mid-1990s as well as a more proactive *sanitarista* movement, AIDS officials strategically and successfully tapped into and used these civic supporters for their strategic advantage.

Thus by the late 1990s, Brazil gradually overcame what Prod'homme (1996) referred to as the "dangers of decentralization" by creating a highly centralized AIDS program capable of consistently implementing innovative prevention and treatment policies. Because of its success, newly reported cases of HIV and AIDS have dramatically declined, while awareness and prevention within at-risk-groups has increased.

These outcomes are particularly striking when we compare Brazil to the US. As we saw in the previous chapter, AIDS officials in the CDC never obtained the political support needed to engage in these centralization strategies; nor did they have access to civic supporters.

But what about the US's and Brazil's responses to other contested epidemics? In recent years, obesity in the US has emerged as a visceral point of contention between politicians and public health officials. In the next chapter, we will look at how the US responded to obesity, followed by Brazil's response to its most recently contested epidemic, tuberculosis.

References

Aggleton, P. (2001). HIV/AIDS in Europe: The Challenge for Health Promotion Research, *Health Education Research*, **16**, 403–409.

Altman, D. (1986). *AIDS in the Mind of America*, Doubleday Press, New York.

Araújo de Mattos, R., Terto, V., and Parker, R. (2003). World Bank Strategies and the Response to AIDS in Brazil, *Divulgação em Saúde para Debate*, **27**, 215–27.

Arnquist, S., Ellner, A., and Weintraub, R. (2011). *HIV/AIDS in Brazil: Delivering Prevention in a Decentralized Healthcare System*, Harvard Business School, The President and Fellow of Harvard College, Cambridge.

Baldwin, P. (2007). *Disease and Democracy: The Industrialized World Faces AIDS*, University of California Press, Berkeley.

Barbosa, E. (2008). Personal interview. August 10.

Barboza, Renato. (2012). *Gestão do Programa Estadual DST/Aids de São Paulo: Uma Análise do Processo de Descentralizacão das Acões no Perído de 1994 a 2003*, Masters Thesis, Post Graduate Program in the Sciences, University of São Paulo, São Paulo.

Barreira, D. (2009). Personal interview. October 10.

Barreira, D. (2012). Personal interview. August 6.

Berkman, A., Garcia, J., Muñoz-Laboy, M., Paiva, V., and Parker, R. (2005). A Crucial Analysis of the Brazilian Response to HIV/AIDS: Lessons Learned for Controlling and Mitigating the Epidemic in Developing Nations, *American Journal of Public Health*, **95**, 1162–1172.

Boletim pela Vidda (1990). N.3, March edition.

Brazil, Ministry of Health, National AIDS Program (2005). *Portaria 2313*, Ministry of Health, Brasília.

Brazil, National AIDS Program. (2007). *Plano Integrado de Enfrentamento da Feminização da Epidemia da Aids*, Ministry of Health, Brasília.

Brazil, Ministry of Health. (2010). *O que é Transferencia Fundo-a-Fundo?* Ministry of Health, Brasília.

Brito, A. (2012). Personal interview. September 19.

Campos, R. (2012). Personal interview. September 3.

Cardoso, F. (2007). Personal interview. November 1.

Carara, S. (1996). *O Tributo a Vênus: A Luta Anti-Vanérea no Brasil no fins do Século XIX até os anos 40*, Casa Oswaldo Cruz Press, Rio de Janeiro.

Carrara, S. (1997). A Geopolítica Simbólica da Sífilis: Um Ensaio de Antropologia Histórica, *Historia, Ciencias, Saúde*, 3, 391–408.

Carrara, S. (1999). 'A AIDS e a História das Doencas Venéreas no Brasil', in Parker, R., Bastos, C., Galvão, J., and Pedrosa, J. (eds), *A AIDS no Brasil*, ABIA press, Rio de Janeiro, 273–306.

Chequer, P. (2008). Personal interview. August 5.

Crespo, M. and Spink, J. (2003). *A Comissão Nacional de Aids: A Presença do Passado na Construção do Futuro*, Ministry of Health, Brasília.

D'Avila, S. (2008). Personal interview. August 14.

Da Costa Marques, M. (2003). *A História de Uma Epidemia Moderna: A Emergencia Política da AIDS/HIV No Brasil*, RiMa/Eduem Press, São Paulo.

Daniel, H. (1991). A Doenca Burocracia, *Jornal do Brasil*, June 10.

Dhalia, C. (2012). Personal interview. August 31.

Diario Popular, São Paulo (1992). Coordenador da AIDS se demite, March 6.

Falleti, T. (2010). 'Infiltrating the State: The Evolution of Health Care Reforms in Brazil, 1964–1988', in Mahoney, J. and Thelen, K. (eds), *Explaining institutional Change: Ambiguity, Agency, and Power*, Cambridge University Press, New York, pp. 38–62.

Filho, E. (2006). Personal interview. June 30.

Filho, C. (2012). Personal interview. September 3.

Folhão de São Paulo (1985). Hospitais Recusam Casos de AIDS, duz Teixeira, August 7.

Folhão de São Paulo (1991). Leia o Discurso do Presidente.

Folhão de Tarde (1992). Governo Demite Coordenador de Combate á AIDS.

Fontes, M. (1999). 'Interface entre as Políticas Internacionais e Nacionais de AIDS', in Parker, R., Galvão, J., and Bessa, M. (eds), *Saúde, Desenvoliento e Política: Respostas Frente á AIDS no Brasil*, ABIA Press, Rio de Janeiro, pp. 91–122.

Gazeta Mercantil (1994). O Ministério da Doença, January 14.

Galvão, J. (2000). *AIDS no Brasil: A Agenda de Construção de uma Epidemia*, ABIA Publishers, São Paulo.

Gauri, V. (2004). 'Brazil Country Case Study', in Ainsworth, M. (ed.), *The Effectiveness of the World Bank's HIV/AID Assistance: Preliminary Findings from an Independent Evaluation*, The World Bank Press, Washington DC, pp. 7–13.

Gauri, V. and Lieberman, E. (2006). Boundary Politics and HIV/AIDS Policy in Brazil and South Africa, *Studies in Comparative International Development*, **41**, 47–73.

Gazeta do Povo (2010). April 29.

Godinho, J. (2009). Personal interview. October 15.

Gómez, E. (2008). A Temporal Analytical Approach to Decentralization Processes: Lessons from Brazil's Health Sector, *Journal of Health Politics, Policy and Law*, **33**, 53–91.

Gómez, E. (2010). What the United States can learn from Brazil's response to HIV/AIDS: International Reputation and Strategic Centralization in a context of Health Policy Devolution, *Health Policy & Planning*, **25**, 529–541.

Gómez, E. (2011). Overcoming Decentralization's Defects: Discovering Alternative Routes to Centralization in a Context of Path Dependency Health Policy Devolution: Lessons from Brazil's Response to HIV/AIDS, *Global Health Governance*, **5**, 1–35.

Gómez, E. (2013). An Inter-Dependent Analytical Approach to Explaining the Evolution of NGOs, Social Movements, and Government Response to HIV/AIDS and Tuberculosis in Brazil, *Journal of Health Politics, Policy & Law*, **38**, 123–159.

Grangeiro, A. (2012). Personal interview. September 6.

Gupta, S. (2009). Why the Brazilian Response to AIDS is the Envy of the World, *CNN*, August 27. Available on-line: http://edition.cnn.com/video/#/video/international/2009/08/27/vital.signs.gupta.brazil.bk.a.cnn?iref=allsearch. Accessed March 22, 2014.

Heirmann, L. (2002). *Decentralização do Sistema de Saúde no Brasil*, Nucleo de Investigação em Servicos e Sistemas de Saúde, São Paulo.

Hochman, G. (1998). *A Era do Saneamento: As Bases da Política de Saúde Pública no Brasil*, Editora Hucitec-Anpocs, São Paulo.

Jornal do Brasil (1985a). AIDS Contamina 32,4% da População Homosexual do Rio, August 25.

Jornal do Brasil (1985b). Gabeira pede Informacões Sobre a AIDS, August 21.

Jornal do Brasil (1988). Programa da Aids perde Cz$ 900 milhões, September 9.

Jornal do Commercio (1992). Burocracia Prejudica Campanha sobre AIDS, February 26.

Lacerda, F. (1985). Brasil é o Terceiro País em Incidencia de Aids, *Jornal do Brasil*, July 21.

Levi, C. and Vitoria, M. (2002). Fighting against AIDS: The Brazilian experience, *AIDS*, **16**, 2373–2383.

Lewis, M. (2006). Personal interview. December 7.

Lieberman, E. (2009). *Boundaries of Contagion: How Ethnic Politics have Shaped Government Responses to AIDS*, Princeton University Press, Princeton.

Maherdai, F. (2012). Personal interview. August 6.

Massé, M. (2009). *From Cycles of Protest to Equilibrium: Explaining the Evolution of AIDS-Related Non-Governmental Organizations in Brazil*, MPhil Thesis, Oxford University.

Mattos, R., Terto, V., and Parker, R. (2003). World Bank Strategies and the Response to AIDS in Brazil, *Divulgação em Saúde para Debate*, **27**, 215–227.

Miguez, A. (1989). Aidéticos Vão á Rua contra Discriminacão, *Jornal do Brasil*, June 18.

Mott, L. (2003). *Homossexualidade: Mitos e Verdades*, Editora Grupo Gay de Bahia, Salvador.

Nascimento, E. (ed.) (1999). *Decentralização de Saúde no Brasil*, Nucleo de Investagação em Servicos e Sistemas de Saude, São Paulo.

Nathanson, C. (1996). Disease Prevention as Social Change: Towards a Theory of Public Health, *Population and Development Review*, **22**, 609–637.

Netto, G. (1985). AIDS: O Mal do Fim do Século, *Folhão de São Paulo*, August 7.

Nunn, A. (2009). *The Politics and History of AIDS Treatment in Brazil*, Springer Press, New York.

Nunn, A., Massard da Fonseca, E., Bastos, F., and Gruskin, S. (2009). AIDS Treatment in Brazil: Impacts and Challenges, *Health Affairs*, **28**, 1103–1113.

O Globo (1987a). Para Presidente de Associacao, Aids Assusta por Desinfomacão, September 24.

O Globo (1987b). Kits estão Acabando e Deixarão de ser Feitos 40 mil Testes contra AIDS, September 27.

O Globo (1988). Política do Governo no Combate á AIDS é Criticada, July 13.

O Globo (1994). Tuberculose Ameaca Elevar Número de Mortes port Aids, August 11.

Paiva, V., Pupo, L., and Barbosa, R. (2006). The Right to Prevention and the Challenges of Reducing Vulnerability to HIV in Brazil, *Revista de Saúde Pública*, **40**, 1–10.

Parker, R. (1997). *Políticas, Instituições e AIDS: Enfrentando a AIDS no Brasil*, ABIA Publications, Rio de Janeiro.

Parker, R. (2003). Building the Foundations for the Response to HIV/AIDS in Brazil: The Development of HIV/AIDS Policy, 1982–1996, *Divulgação em Saúde para Debate*, **27**, 143–183.

Parker, R., Galvão, J., and Bessa, M. (eds) (1999). *Saúde, Desenvolvimento, e Política: Respostas frente á AIDS no Brasil*, ABIA publications, Rio de Janeiro.

Pasche, D., Righi, L., Thome, H., and Stolz, E. (2006). Paradoxos das Políticas de Descentralização de Saúde no Brasil, *Revista Panamericana de Salud Pública*, **20**, 416–422.

Price-Smith, A. (2002). *The Health of Nations: Infectious Disease, Environmental Change, and their Effects on National Security and Development*, MIT Press, Cambridge.

Price-Smith, A., Tauber, S., and Bhat, A. (2004). State Capacity and HIV Incidence Reduction in the Developing World: Preliminary Empirical Evidence, *Seton Hall Journal of Diplomacy*, Summer/Fall, 149–160.

Reis, C. (1989). Entrevista: Tenho Aids, mas Continuo Vivo: Herbert Daniel Fala do Choque e do Otimismo que a Luta Pede, *Revista Afonse*, August 1.

Resende-Santos, J. (1997). 'Fernando Henrique Cardoso: Social and Institutional Rebuilding in Brazil', in Dominguez, J. (ed.), *Technopols: Freeing Politics and Markets in Latin America in the 1990s*, Pennsylvania State University Press, University Park, pp. 145–94.

Rich, J. (2010). *Grassroots Bureaucracy: Mobilizing the AIDS Movement in Brazil, 1983–2010*. PhD Dissertation, Department of Political Science, University of California at Berkeley.

Rich, J. and Gómez, E. (2012). Centralizing Decentralized Governance in Brazil, *Publius: Journal of Federalism*, **10**, 1–26.

Rochel de Camargo Jr., K. (1999). 'Políticas Públicas e Prevencão em HIV/AIDS', in Parker, R., Galvão, J., and Bessa, M. (eds), *Saúde, Desenvolvimento, e Política: Reespostas frente á AIDS no Brasil*, ABIA Publications, Rio de Janeiro, pp. 227–262.

Rosenbrock, R. and Wright, M. (eds) (2000). *Partnership and Pragmatism: Germany's Response to AIDS Prevention and Care*, Routledge Press, London.

Ruger, J. (2005). The Changing Role of the World Bank in Global Health, *American Journal of Public Health*, **95**, 60–70.

Schaffer, M. (2012). Personal interview. September 13.

Sen, A. (1999). *Development as Freedom*, Knopf Press, New York.

Silva, P. (1991). O governo não cumpre seu papel: Herbert Daniel denuncia o estado de preconceito contra aidéticos, *Nacional*, July 8.

Souza, C. (1997). *Constitutional Engineering in Brazil: The Politics of Federalism and Decentralization*, St. Martin's Press, New York.

Teixeira, P. (1997). 'Políticas Públicas em Aids', in Parker, R (ed.), *Políticas, Instituicões e Aids: Enfrentando a Epidemia no Brasil*, ABIA Publications, Rio de Janeiro, pp. 43–68.

Teixeira, P. (2007). Personal interview. February 22.

Terto, V. (2008). Personal interview. June 22.

US New Wire Inc. (2003). Brazilian National AIDS Program Receives 2003 Gates Award for Global Health, May 28.

Vallgarda, S. (2007). Problematizations and Path Dependency: HIV/AIDS Policies in Denmark and Sweden, *Medical History*, **51**, 99–112.

Varas, M. (2012). Personal interview. September 12.

Veja (1985). AIDS, August 14.

Villela, V. (1999). 'Das Interfaces Entre os Níveis Governamentais e a Sociedade Civil', in Parker, R. (ed.), *Saúde, Desenvoliemento e Política: Respostas frente á AIDS no Brasil*, ABIA Publications, Rio de Janeiro, pp. 177–226.

Visão: Revista semanal de informacção (1985). A Verdade onde Estara? October 16.

World Bank (2008). *Implementation and Completion and Results of a Loan in the Amount of US$100 million to the Federal Republic of Brazil for a Third AIDS and STD Control Project*, Report No. ICR0000783, The World Bank Group, Washington, DC.

Chapter 5

Contesting Obesity in the United States

In recent years, the US government has confronted yet another highly contested epidemic, one that is a byproduct of heightened economic growth, international trade, technological advancements, and increased sedentary lifestyles: obesity. According to most scholars, one would assume that because of the presence of the US's long-lasting democratic electoral institutions, the incorporation of the interests of civil society into legislative committees, increased legislative accountability to civil society, and a high level of per capita healthcare spending as well as advanced medical infrastructure that the government would immediately and aggressively respond to obesity (Aggleton, 2001; Altman, 1986; Baldwin, 2007; Nathanson, 1996; Price-Smith, 2002; Price-Smith *et al.*, 2004; Rosenbrock and Wright, 2000; Ruger, 2005; Sen, 1999; Vallgarda, 2007). Nevertheless, this chapter suggests that this kind of response never emerged.

For years the US government's response has in fact been delayed because of conflicting political, bureaucratic, and civil society views over obesity's overall threat to the nation. After several years of ongoing debate, the US government still has not constructed an effective centralized response. In essence, it is the same problem as usual: as we saw with the government's historic response to syphilis, malnutrition, and AIDS, when it came to obesity, the president and Congress' failure to be convinced of obesity's threat to US national security, coupled with the absence of the president and other government leader's personal experiences and interests in obesity, failed to instigate an immediate centralized response.

However, since the gradual rise of obesity's threat, Pubic Health Service (PHS) officials had different views and responded in a different manner. As early as the 1970s, they immediately pressured the president and Congress for greater attention to obesity and recommended a centralized response, while incessantly warning and publically declaring obesity's threat to the nation. Moreover, these proactive efforts occurred well before the surgeon general's Call to Action in 2001. In contrast to what we saw with AIDS in Chapter 3, however, the response of social health movements and NGOs was minimal and divided at best. There never emerged a proactive network of social health movements and/or NGOs focused on obesity, constantly pressuring the government for policy reform while seeking to establish cooperative partnerships with PHS officials. Because of this, no civic supporters ever emerged for obesity, which, in turn, further hampered the government's centralized bureaucratic and policy response.

The more recent phase of obesity politics (2001–present), demarcated by the rise of international criticisms, pressures, and policy recommendations for a more aggressive centralized response, ushered in new hope and opportunity. As we saw in the past, however, the White House once again ignored these international criticisms and pressures. President George W. Bush was far from interested in working closely with the international community, such as the World Health Organization (WHO), and increasing the government's international reputation through innovative bureaucratic and policy reforms. In addition, under Bush, the CDC (Centers for Disease Control and Prevention) was forbidden to work with the WHO on obesity issues. With Congress heavily influenced by private sector interests, during this period there was no support for expanding the CDC and its work with the states.

The only positive to emerge during this period was the president, bureaucrats, and other political leaders' personal experiences and fears and how this, in turn, prompted them to eventually place obesity on the national agenda. President Bush's unwavering passion for exercise and fears of weight gain, when combined with likeminded leaders in the PHS and sub-national governments, helped to increase attention to the obesity problem within government. Despite the creation of new exercise programs for the White House and the Department of Health and Human Services (HHS), and despite Bush and the HHS's call on civil society to get in shape, ironically Bush never focused his energy on strengthening the HHS's and PHS's obesity programs and assistance to the states.

Nevertheless, Bush set the stage for a more aggressive response under the Barack Obama administration. In contrast to Bush, Obama has pursued a closer relationship with the WHO over the obesity issue, encouraging the CDC to establish stronger ties with the WHO, as well as civil society. This certainly increases the prospects of building a constructive partnership between the international community, the bureaucracy, and civil society.

Similar to the Bush administration, the personal interests, fears, and empathy of political and bureaucratic leaders has also helped to place obesity on the national agenda. In 2010, for example, First Lady Michelle Obama's concern about her children's weight gain prompted the creation of a new federal campaign to address childhood obesity (ABC, 2010a; Obama, 2010). Moreover, Surgeon General Regina Benjamin, as well as the Secretary of Agriculture, Tom Vilsack, have expressed their personal struggles with weight gain, displaying empathy towards others and an unrelenting commitment to addressing obesity (ABC, 2010b; Obama, 2010). When combined with First Lady Michelle Obama and the military's recent declaration that obesity now poses a national security, which is mainly due to the challenges of passing physical fitness tests and recruitment (Park, 2010), it seems that a coherent national strategy for combating obesity may soon emerge.

The First Few Years of the Obesity Epidemic

The obesity epidemic did not arise as mysteriously and as suddenly as AIDS. Instead, the number of obese individuals started to gradually increase throughout the 1980s and 1990s, burgeoning in case notification rates by the mid to late 1990s. From 1960 to 1980, CDC researchers using NHANES survey estimates (National Health and Nutrition Examination Surveys) noted that the number of obese Americans, measured in terms of BMI (body mass index), increased by 8%. This percentage increase jumped to 22% from 1988 to 1994

(Flegal, *et al*, 2002). By 2002, the CDC reported that approximately 30% of the US population was obese.

There was also a rising trend in obesity cases among children. The number of overweight cases (again measured in terms of BMI) for children increased from 15.1% between 1971–1974 to 50.1% from 2003–2004. Cases of childhood obesity continued to grow. These trends convinced PHS officials that childhood obesity was indeed a national epidemic.

Although scholars claim that it was not until recently that presidents paid sufficient attention to the epidemic (Kersh and Morone, 2005), a closer look at the evidence suggests otherwise. Presidential concern with overweight and obesity began with the Johnson and Carter administrations (Nestle and Jacobson, 2000). While Johnson indirectly addressed the issue through the formation of his Presidential Commissions for Exercise, Carter would go further by making weight loss one of 17 new national health initiatives, others including the consumption of less salt, alcohol, and more exercise (Booth, 1991). Carter was passionate about diet and exercise. For him, taking preventative action against disease was the most important thing; this was a belief, moreover, that stemmed from Carter's childhood upbringing in the southern part of the US, where local community doctors stressed preventative medicine (Blumenthal and Morone, 2009). Carter made it a goal to reduce the percentage of overweight individuals to 10% for men and 17% for women by 1990.

Carter's interest, however, was just that, an interest, and no substantive effort was made to place obesity on the national policy agenda (Nestle and Jacobson, 2000). More than anything, Carter's concerns reflected growing interest in civil society about better fitness and health. While the PHS was warning about America's burgeoning weight problem since the 1970s, these warnings also comported with the general mood in society that people should be taking better care of themselves. But these bureaucratic warnings were not enough to convince Carter that he should respond. While Carter may have been aware of the growing obesity epidemic, the PHS was not yet stating that an epidemic crisis was at hand.

However, it was the William J. Clinton administration that seemed to receive most of the criticism and blame for policy inaction. While the CDC was, by the mid-1990s, frequently testifying before Congress and asking it and the HHS for additional funding (Koplan, 2007), and while the CDC was publishing reports about the epidemic in 1994, special interest groups were arguing that the Clinton administration was being unresponsive to their needs. These groups also accused Clinton of failing to secure their individual rights. The National Association for Fat Acceptance (NAFA) in particular was upset that Clinton was not passing legislation for anti-discrimination in the labor force while failing to propose legislation requiring that health insurance companies cover obesity-related medical costs (Rosin, 1994). While the CDC was limited in its ability to meet directly with the White House (it always has to work up the chain of command by first meeting with HHS directors and then Congress, unless there is a public health emergency), it did nevertheless indirectly inform the Clinton administration of the problem. By 1994, the media began to publish stories about a president that was ignoring America's new obesity epidemic (Price, 1994; Rosin, 1994).

Several factors contributed to Clinton's policy perceptions and lack of response. First, and again similar to what we saw with AIDS, the absence of obesity's threat to US national security meant the issue failed to obtain the government's attention and to prompt a response. Obesity was not perceived as posing an immediate threat to military readiness and soldiers' ability to fight in war. Notwithstanding the fact that Presidents George H.W. Bush and Clinton were at war when overweight and obesity trends were increasing (1980–2001), i.e., the first Gulf War (Desserts Storm and Shield) and Somalia, respectively, obesity never affected the military's fighting capabilities. For example, the number of military personnel having to separate from active duty because of their failure to meet weight and body composition standards declined from 1999 to 2002 (Institutes of Medicine of the National Academy, 2003).

Furthermore, during this period the economic consequence of obesity was not of concern. While the CDC and researchers noted that the costs for businesses and state-level health programs were gradually increasing due to obesity-related diseases, such as high blood pressure, diabetes, and heart disease, during the 1980s and 1990s they were not yet considered as serious threats to the economy (Finkelstein *et al.*, 2005; Runge, 2007). Most studies during this period emphasized the burden for businesses, especially with regards to escalating health insurance premiums for obesity-related conditions, a decline in worker productivity and absenteeism, as well as a lack of career opportunities and prospects of promotion (Finkelstein *et al.*, 2005; Runge, 2007). The grander economic burden of obesity had not yet emerged.

Yet another factor contributing to Clinton's lack of interest in obesity seemed to be associated with the fact that he had no personal interest in the matter. During his time in the White House, despite being overweight, Clinton refrained from taking his weight problem seriously (Shut, 2011). It essentially seemed that he had no fear and no concern about being overweight. Clinton never believed that his condition warranted a heightened commitment to exercise and better nutrition. In an interview with CNN's Sanjay Gupta in 2011, looking back at his health during his time in the White House, Clinton stated that he felt as if he had been "playing Russian roulette," freely eating and taking risks, regardless of the potential health consequences (Shut, 2011: p. 1). This is supported by the fact that Clinton very rarely, if ever, spoke about the challenges of obesity in the press — let alone, his personal health issues.

Perhaps the biggest problem with Clinton's apathy towards his own health was that it did not motivate him to put obesity on the national agenda. In addition to not addressing the issue in public, Clinton never proposed any legislation, nor did he encourage the HHS to do more work on the obesity issue (Burros, 1994). In addition, Clinton did not encourage and remind his staff and other government officials about the need to lose weight and to stay in shape.

A similar lack of interest was found in the House and Senate. Legislative views were first influenced by the fact that throughout the 1980s and 1990s, obesity was not perceived as a major health threat. While more cases were being reported, obesity was perceived as a slowly moving chronic condition that most people believed could be easily avoided through self-discipline and willpower. Consequently, obesity did not prompt the emergence of well-organized social health movements or non-governmental organizations (NGOs) pressuring the government for a centralized response. The only obesity-related NGO that existed during this period was the NAFA, which was very small and ineffective in mustering sufficient pressures for policy reform.

In this climate, political parties, especially within a Republican-dominated House and Senate, were not eager to respond. This was reflected by the fact that there were no bills or proposed legislation to address obesity (Nestle and Jacobson, 2000). While there were periodic hearings about the issue (led by concerned congressional members), they were few and parcel, never leading to concrete policy initiatives (Nestle and Jacobson, 2000).

Additionally, and again similar to what we saw with the issue of malnutrition in Chapter 2, the ongoing influence of the private food industry and their interest in opposing any type of regulatory policy hampered a legislative response (Brownell, 2007; Jacobson, 2007). Major private corporations consistently and successfully lobbied the House and Senate at even the mere hint of an interest in federal regulation. Because of the fact that major food companies, such as Kraft, General Mills, Coca-Cola, and Pepsi are amongst the biggest contributors to political campaigns, Republicans in both legislatures repeatedly refrained from imposing regulatory measures on the fast food industry (Brownell, 2007).

If the private sector influenced the interests and motivations of Republican political party members, the agricultural sector did the same for the Democrats. Democrats linked to major agricultural industries (in the mid-west, especially) were committed to protecting the latter's interests. Fearful of imposing regulations on a weakening yet critical constituency base contributed to the lack of interest in tackling obesity (Tillotson, 2004; Jacobson, 2007). It is important to keep in mind that from 1900 to 2000, the House passed more than 70 acts protecting the agricultural food industry (Tillotson, 2004).

The same conditions shaping bureaucratic elite perceptions of the AIDS epidemic also emerged for obesity. That is, the HHS's and PHS's views were in large part influenced by the ongoing tradition of viewing epidemics from a purely scientific perspective. As we saw in Chapter 2, moral and judgmental political and policy views were never found within the public health bureaucracy. For although the case could be made that obesity was a moral issue, based on puritanical principles of sloth and gluttony, these beliefs never affected the views of public health officials (Dietz, 2007).

Finally, the need to survive within a competitive fiscal environment also contributed to an increase in the CDC's interest in obesity. However, in contrast to what we saw with the PHS's response to AIDS, these conditions did not kindle increased inter-bureaucratic competition and lack of cooperation between PHS agencies. What is in fact surprising about this period is that there was an interest on the part of the PHS to work closely with other agencies in response to obesity. Intra-PHS (CDC/NIH (National Institutes of Health)) and inter-agency (USDA (US Department of Agriculture)/CDC/NIH) collaboration was focused mainly on research and reporting obesity cases. Over time, inter-agency collaboration would focus on prevention and new policy initiatives, generated primarily through the creation of new inter-agency initiatives. During the first few years of the obesity epidemic, however, because the PHS was still learning about the problem, these inter-agency initiatives were few and parcel.

The impetus for engaging in inter-agency cooperation stemmed primarily from the fact that there was no race to find a biological cure for obesity. There was no mysterious, unknown virus that, as we saw with AIDS, kindled inter-agency competition to find a cure first. At the same time, presidential apathy towards the issue failed to put obesity on the national agenda, while there were few incentives for agency heads to compete with each other for congressional attention and funding.

Always in search of additional funding, the CDC was committed to collecting and publishing data alluding to the presence of an obesity epidemic. CDC officials repeatedly used this data to justify an increase in budgetary spending (Oliver, 2006a, 2006b). Nevertheless, it seems that the CDC was not socially constructing an epidemic in order to garner more resources, as some scholars maintain (Oliver, 2006a, 2006b). Instead, the CDC was simply reporting escalating obesity case rates, trends that they had been writing about since the mid-1990s.

The PHS and the HHS were the first to label obesity as an "epidemic." By 1997, the director of the CDC, Dr. David Satcher, started to publicly address obesity as such, followed by his successor, Dr. Jeffrey Koplan, and yet again by Satcher as surgeon general in 1998. But it is important to note that until 1997, the PHS was simply warning the government of an impending obesity epidemic. Because of this, I have divvied up the PHS's initial response into two time periods: *warnings* and *declarations*.

Warnings

By 1974, well before the general public became aware of America's obesity problem, the NIH started holding meetings and writing reports warning the government that rates of overweight and obesity were increasing at an accelerated pace. As Table 5.1 illustrates, since 1974, several reports were published by the NIH and the HHS providing strict policy guidelines for the prevention of obesity through diet and exercise (Nestle and Jacobson, 2000). On February 13, 1985, the NIH even held a public symposium in which it described obesity as a "killer disease" and stated that people who are even five pounds overweight should have cause for concern (Rovner, 1985). The panel of experts provided evidence showing that about 34 million Americans weighed 20% or more above their desirable body weight, the point at which physicians should be treating the problem. The report also argued that obesity should get the same amount of

Table 5.1 Examples of policy guidelines for obesity and general nutrition published by the HHS and NIH in the 1970s and 1980s

1974	National Institutes of Health: *Obesity in Perspective*
1977	National Institutes of Health: *Obesity in America*
1977	US Senate Select Committee on Nutrition and Human Needs: *Dietary Goals for the United States, 2nd Edition*
1979	US Department of Health, Education and Welfare: *Healthy People: The Surgeon General's Report on Health Promotion and Disease*
1980	US Department of Health and US Department of Agriculture: *Dietary Guidelines for Americans, 2nd Edition*
1988	US Department of Health and Human Services: *The Surgeon General's Report on Nutrition and Health*

Source: Nestle and Jacobson, 2000

attention as smoking, high blood pressure, and other health risks (Gustaitis, 2005).

One must of course keep in mind that all the hype about obesity boded well with the times. The 1980s was an era of increased public consciousness and interest in being in shape, eating low calorie foods, and feeling good. People frequently watched Richard Simmons and Jane Fonda engage in exercise activity on TV. Weight loss programs and low calorie snacks were in high demand. In this sense, these PHS reports therefore boded well with the times. However, it is important to understand that these reports were to a large extent reflecting a general health craze; they were not yet emblematic of what the PHS believed to be a genuine obesity epidemic.[1]

By the early 1990s, the CDC started becoming a bit more concerned about obesity. By 1991, the CDC published reports discussing how Americans were getting heavier and failing to see its health consequences (Booth, 1991). By 1994, the CDC warned that if the government did not address the issue, especially for children, a national epidemic would most certainly arise (Elder, 1999; Russell, 1994). According to Dr. William Dietz, Director of the CDC's Division on Nutrition and Physical Activity, the CDC spent a considerable amount of time warning the George H.W. Bush and Clinton administrations that obesity was going to be the next big epidemic if the government did not respond (Dietz, 2007). Even before coming to the CDC, Dietz was warning Clinton about the problem in his position as Director of Clinical Nutrition at the New England Medical Center in Boston (*Capital Times*, 1994; McMurrie, 1994).

It is important to understand, however, that all of this was occurring in a different social context. Heightened social interest in getting in shape had essentially come to an end by the 1990s. By 1991, CDC researchers showed that data on self-reported leisure time for physical activity indicated that 58.1% of adults reported irregular or no leisure time for physical activity (Kuczmarksi *et al.*, 1994). The NIHS (National Institutes of Health Survey) also found that the percentage of adults who exercised on a regular basis declined from 1985 to

---

[1] I would like to thank James Morone of Brown University for pointing this out to me.

1990, especially among Blacks, Hispanics, low income individuals, and unemployed individuals (Kuczmarksi *et al.*, 1994; Piani and Schoenborn, 1990). More and more children were failing presidential fitness exams (McCall, 1991). The broad fitness craze that had swept across America in the 1980s had gradually declined by the mid-1990s (Ahmad, 1997). The arrival of home computers, video games, and, by the late 1990s, the internet, incentivized people to stay home. The sedentary, lazy, and comfortable American lifestyle that is today well known in the media had finally emerged (Schnurr, 1992). From then on, PHS reports would take on a different tone, addressing a different audience. These reports were no longer writing to appease a health-conscious society. They were now trying to seriously warn the government that it had to respond to obesity.

In addition to this change in social climate, two additional factors contributed to the PHS's heightened interest in obesity. First, AIDS was no longer usurping most of the resources and attention within the PHS. By the early-to-mid-1990s, it was being perceived as a controllable (yet still chronic) disease, far from a crisis. At the same time, obesity among children was quickly growing. These two conditions provided a new opportunity for the HHS and CDC to start focusing more on obesity — as well as a host of other ailments, such as tobacco and alcohol (McGinnis, 2007). In essence, these two conditions provided the PHS with more time to focus on obesity and to warn the government and the public about it (McGinnis, 2007).

This is precisely what happened. "We are going to reap what we sow!" argued CDC health officials at the time (Russell, 1994). Researchers at the CDC revealed that obesity cases, especially among children, were quickly escalating (Russell, 1994). Conferences organized by the CDC, such as the one held in Miami in fall of 1995, immediately garnered a lot of media attention. Findings at the Miami conference revealed that the number of obese children and teens (ages 6–17) increased from 6 to 11% nationwide (Somerson, 1995). Moreover, the report revealed the growing racial disparity in obesity among children, highlighting the fact that black females were, for example, the most obese and the least active, with 60% reporting that they watched at least three hours of TV a day.

Declarations

Amidst this backdrop, government officials in other agencies started to become more critical of the government, opening declaring that nothing was being done and the government was facing a serious epidemic threat. In 1994, Dr. Philip Lee, then undersecretary for HHS, argued that the Clinton administration had no national campaign or plan to address the issue (Burros, 1994). In a *The New York Times* article published on July 7, 1994, Lee was quoted as stating: "the Government is not doing enough. It is not focused. We don't have a coherent across-the-board policy" (Burros, 1994). He went on record to criticize the White House for only giving $50,000 on average to the states, mainly for programs focused on nutritional education (Burros, 1994). While Dr. Lee was not claiming that there was an obesity epidemic, he was nevertheless committed to creating a more aggressive national campaign (Lee, 2007).

HHS director Donna Shalala also began to express concern. By January 1995, she proposed a campaigned called "10 Health Resolutions," of which losing weight (through diet and exercise) was one of them (*The Washington Post*, 1995). The second New Year's resolution she proposed was called "Get off of the couch!" (*The Washington Post*, 1995). Shalala established a clear connection between poor diet and exercise. Poor diet, she argued, was associated with 300,000 deaths a year (*The Washington Post*, 1995). Shalala also worked closely with Surgeon General David Satcher to educate Americans about physical fitness and nutrition. She was also the mastermind behind Healthy Vision 2010, which encouraged Americas to eat better, exercise, and to have more proactive lifestyles (Strumpf, 2004).

By 1997, Surgeon General David Satcher was quoted in several newspapers declaring that "childhood obesity is at epidemic levels in the U.S." (Squires, 1998; Associated Press, 1998). He went on to argue that: "We have been remiss in shedding light on this problem, which leads to so many other health problems, particularly when we consider the threats that this disease imposes on our children. Today, we see a nation of young people seriously at risk of starting out obese and dooming themselves to the difficult tasks of overcoming a couch illness" (Satcher quoted in Squires, 1998). That same year, Satcher took his message to several televised news stations. In several interviews he again referred to obesity as an "epidemic," emphasizing the need to address the issue and respond (KING-TV, "King Five News at Five," October 27, 1998, at 5pm; WAGM-TV, "Age Day," November 12, 1998, 5:30pm; WCBS-AM, "Newsradio 88"; WCNC-TV, "6 News at 6," October 27, 1998).[2] Satcher's public declarations continued throughout 1999 (Lasalandra, 1999), setting the stage for his "Healthy People 2000" report and eventually the surgeon general's Call to Action in 2001.

By the fall of 1999, Satcher felt compelled to begin criticizing President Clinton for his lack of response to obesity (*The Hill*, 1999). Satcher wanted Clinton to pressure Congress for the creation of more obesity prevention polices, especially those focused on healthy lifestyles (*The Hill*, 1999). Satcher also wanted the administration to provide more funds for nutrition education and exercise, especially in schools (Krucoff, 1997). Nevertheless, Satcher's requests were not being taken seriously (Ahmad, 1997; McFeatters, 1999; McMurtrie, 1994).

Satcher's rhetoric and recommendations comported with the views of CDC Director Jeffrey Koplan (1988–2002). Koplan was equally as vocal about the epidemic and pressured the administration for a more centralized response (Koplan, 2007). Like HHS Undersecretary Philip Lee before him, Koplan realized that no administration up to that point had devised a coherent national plan. Koplan once commented: "It's time to create a national obesity-control policy ..." and that a new "national effort is needed to control it" (Rubinowitz, 1999). Unfortunately, Koplan's views and requests for funding were also ignored by the Clinton administration and Congress (Koplan, 2007). With the exception of a few supportive congressional representatives, neither the White House, Congress, nor the HHS was ever willing to provide him with the additional resources needed to finance his prevention programs (Koplan, 2007).

---

[2] In all of the transcripts to these televised news interviews, Satcher was quoted as referring to childhood obesity as an "epidemic."

Civil Society Responds

Social concern about the rise of overweight and obesity slowly began to emerge during the 1950s and 1960s. Civil society's response was essentially divided between those groups seeking to increase awareness and prevention versus those that fought for social acceptance and civil rights. With regards to the former, since 1952 the American Heart Association (AHA) and the National Cancer Institute (NCI) advocated for improved dietary lifestyles and nutrition. The AHA was focused on highlighting obesity's risk for heart disease while advocating for better diet and exercise (Kersh and Morone, 2002). During this period, several federal agencies as well as NGOs, such as the American Diabetes Association, the American Cancer Society, and the AHA emerged to promote healthy eating and to monitor diseases commonly associated with being overweight, such as heart disease, cancer, stroke, and diabetes (Nestle and Jacobson, 2000).

Instead of trying to influence federal legislation, however, the focus of these NGOs was on what individuals should do to avoid excess weight and its associated ailments (Nestle and Jacobson, 2000). It was also believed that the government should not attempt to remedy these health issues through proactive preventative policy (Nestle and Jacobson, 2000). Consequently, NGOs began to mobilize and promote better health awareness on their own, failing to engage in a close partnership with PHS officials. This, in turn, failed to provide a rich network of civic supporters that PHS officials could eventually use to increase their legitimacy and succeed in securing more congressional funding. NGO isolation from the bureaucracy essentially meant that those NGOs sharing the PHS's interests and concerns never sought to infiltrate the CDC or any other federal agency.

During this period, other civil society groups were also mobilizing. However, in contrast to the aforementioned groups, they were focused on fat acceptance and civil rights. Tired of people harassing his wife for being too overweight, in 1969 Bill Fabrey, an engineer from Queens, New York, formed the National Association to Aid Fat Americas (NAAFA). Assembled from his living room, NAAFA's primary goal was to help build self-esteem, address work-place discrimination, and increase social and government awareness. Organizing dances, speed-dating events, and focus groups, NAAFA was quickly viewed as a social refuge, a haven for people desiring to overcome depression and anxiety and to find love and friendship (Armstrong, 1981; White, 2010).

In the late-1980s, the organization's name, as well as its philosophy, changed to the National Association to Advance Fat Awareness (NAAFA). NAAFA maintained its general mission but now sought to emphasize social awareness and education (White, 2010). However, NAAFA never tried to work closely with PHS officials or even state and local health departments (White, 2010). It was not a political organization. It was isolated. It focused on its members. It focused on increasing social awareness, acceptance, and establishing a network of refuge and recreational activities (White, 2010). NAAFA's activities waned over the years, becoming essentially dormant throughout the late 1970s and into the late 1980s (Fletcher, 2009).

However, this decline in NAFA activity kindled a great deal of hostility within the organization. In 1973, the Los Angeles branch of NAAFA, well known for its radical views, such as its Fat Liberation Manifesto, demonstrations, and hostility towards government defected to form what was known as the Fat Underground (Fishman, 1998; Solovay and Rothblum, 2009). Inspired by the feminist and radical movements of the time, its leaders, Sarah Fishman and Judy Freespirit, enjoyed instigating controversy, increasing public awareness and advocating for policy change (Solovay and Rothblum, 2009). They also created an organization in New Haven, Connecticut, the New Haven Fat Liberation Front, where their activities could thrive. Fishman and Freespirit's movements were short-lived, however, failing to increase government awareness and influence policy (Fletcher, 2009).

As NAAFA gradually grew in prominence throughout the 1990s, other NGOs began to emerge. In 1997, the International Size Acceptance Association (ISAA) was formed. Led by Allen Steadham and based in Austin, Texas, with offices throughout the world, like NAAFA, ISAA's goal was to increase social awareness, combat stigma, and fight for civil rights. By the mid-to-late 1990s, NAAFA and ISAA were the two largest NGOs proactively focusing on obesity issues.

In contrast to the AIDS NGOs that emerged throughout the 1980s, obesity NGOs' interests countervailed the PHS's interests. While the PHS, as well as the aforementioned health associations, such as AHA, sought to underscore obesity's health implications while promoting individual responsibility and weight loss, NAAFA and ISAA sought to embrace obesity as a positive human trait, one worthy of respect and dignity. In fact, NAAFA was often highly critical of the CDC's efforts to underscore the negative health consequences of obesity. Furthermore, these civic organizations were small in size and were scattered throughout the nation, failing to amass a united and effective collective movement.

Initial Bureaucratic and Policy Response

An increase in attention to the obesity epidemic from civil society, the media, and the bureaucracy did not translate to an aggressive centralized bureaucratic and policy response, however. Neither the White House nor Congress was interested in creating an agency or CDC subdivision in response to obesity. Moreover, neither the White House nor Congress had an interest in increasing the CDC's budget to work on obesity programs (Jacobson, 2007; Kaplan, 2007). As mentioned earlier, Congress was at the same time riddled with special interests seeking to safeguard the corn, sugar, and fast food industry, which failed to generate incentives for augmenting the PHS's budget and/or introducing new legislation.

At the same time, no effort was made to help state and local health departments respond. During the 1990s, the amount of money allocated from Congress to the states for obesity prevention programs, especially for health education, was minimal. In 1994, for example, only $50,000 was given to the CDC to work with the states for obesity prevention (Burros, 1994). Most of the expenditures were borne by the states. Moreover, neither the White House nor Congress proposed any effort to increase the budget for health awareness and physical fitness in public schools (McCall, 1991; Jacobson, 2007).[3]

---

[3] Keep in mind that during this period, the number of children failing the President's national physical fitness examines were at an all-time high. In 1955, when the tests were first

Even the most proactive and vocal arm of the government, the PHS, was constrained in its ability to provide assistance to the states. When it came to providing financial and technical assistance, because the government did not view obesity as an important public health issue, there was no interest in helping the CDC provide grant assistance to the states. The absence of federal support during the initial years of the obesity epidemic contributed to an overall decline in nutritional educational programs and physical fitness standards in schools, in turn gradually contributing to the rise of America's obesity epidemic.

International Criticisms, Pressures, and Response

The global response to obesity first emerged in the early 1990s. Although the WHO officially recognized the health threats associated with overweight and obesity since the 1950s, because it was a problem mainly relegated to the US and the UK, the issue was not taken seriously (James, 2008). Throughout the 1970s and 1980s, the WHO nevertheless continued to monitor the health consequences of obesity, periodically sponsoring consultative panels and experts to testify on the issue (James, 2008). In part because of these efforts and the release of new data, by 1988 the WHO started to take overweight and obesity issues more seriously, though no concrete plans and efforts were being planned (James, 2008).

By 1992, however, in response to the burgeoning trend of obesity cases in the South Pacific, such as in Fuji and Samoa, a major international health conference was organized to draw awareness to the issue and to enlist the support of international organizations and governments. This occurred at the joint FAO (Food and Agriculture Organization)/WHO International Conference on Nutrition, when 159 countries recommended the development of National Plans of Action on Nutrition (NPAN) (World Health Organization, 2003a). This was soon followed up with the creation of the International

---

administered, about 55% failed; by 1991, this increased to approximately 85%; see McCall (1991) and Scarton (1993).

Obesity Task Force (IOTF) in 1995, which was created and led by a group of physicians and nutrition scientists dissatisfied with the WHO's lackluster commitment to the issue. After the IOTF organized several meetings with the WHO and FAO, the WHO eventually included the IOTF's report on the need to increase government awareness and prevention on childhood overweight and obesity issues. By 1998, the WHO executive board included the IOTF's reports as part of its Official Technical Report Series, which in turn signaled its new commitment to the issue while officially endorsing the IOTF's work, recognizing it as an influential group of international scientists (James, 2008).

By 2002, the WHO increased its efforts to work with other nations in officially recognizing and combating the obesity epidemic. That year, together with the FAO, the WHO organized a Global Forum for Food Safety Regulators. By the fall 2003, the WHO also drafted a report entitled *The 2004 Global Strategy on Diet, Physical Activity, and Health*. In it, the WHO provided a toolbox of options for nations on how to respond to obesity, which included the following: 1) an increased regulation of food advertisements, especially those aimed at children; 2) the adoption of a "snack tax" on junk food and soft drinks, as well as several other regulatory and educational programs (Buckley, 2004; Vastag, 2004; World Health Organization, 2003b). The report also suggested that there should be some financial incentives for citizens to eat more healthily and to refrain from purchasing fatty foods (Buckley, 2004).

However, the publication of this report also marked the WHO's growing frustration with the US's and other nations' lack of response to obesity. The WHO's criticisms stemmed from the report's statement that the US and other advanced industrialized nations needed to closely examine the consequences of increased sugar intake. *The 2004 Global Strategy* essentially highlighted the fact that the US and other industrialized nations had done little to regulate the fatty food industry and that it needed to increase its commitment to doing so (Norum *et al.*, 2009). While the WHO refrained from pointing fingers and blaming particular individuals within government, health agencies, and industries, it soon became clear to the US that these reports were targeted at them.

The next series of WHO criticisms did begin to blame particular individuals, however. Shortly after the release of *The 2004 Global Strategy*, Dr. Kaare Norum, a leading scientist in the WHO, criticized the Bush administration's opposition *to The 2004 Global Strategy*, which was laid out in a 30-page report from HHS Secretary Tommy Thompson to the WHO (Jacobson, 2004; Norum, 2010; Ruskin, 2004). In this report, Thompson stated that *The 2004 Global Strategy*'s accusations[4] had no merit and that its scientific evidence was inconclusive (Simon, 2004; BBC, 2004; Vastag, 2004). The HHS issued a line-by-line critique of *The 2004 Global Strategy*, which some say read as if it was drafted by the sugar industry itself (Simon, 2004). HHS, as well as the Grocery Manufacturers of America (GMA), demanded either immediate changes to *The 2004 Global Strategy* or to replace it with a message advocating for more individual responsibility and no government intervention (Doyle, 2005). Others also chastised members of the Bush administration for traveling to Geneva to meet with WHO directors with the intent of persuading them to refrain from making any further unscientifically valid claims (Center for Science in the Public Interest, 2004). This effort was perceived as just another example of how the Bush administration had reacted negatively to international criticisms and interference in US health issues. Yet, it also revealed how conservative ideology and corporate interests continued to shape the administration's international and domestic health agendas (Norum, 2010; Waxman, 2004). Of course, it did not take long for the WHO to complain and to accuse the Bush administration of siding with lobbyists from the sugar industry and other corporations (*The Guardian*, 2004; Simon, 2004).

For instance, Dr. Kaare Norum, accused the Bush administration of taking the health of millions of Americans hostage because of the

---

[4]And accuse it did. For, as Simon (2004) argues, the HHS was accused of: "(1) at least 52 times, weakening existing language, adding qualifying statements, or substituting voluntary language such as "encourage" for the stronger word "should;" (2) inserting the term "personal" or "individual" nine times (to reflect the food industry's mantra that personal responsibility is the key to solving the obesity problem, not policy regulation); and (3) striking language calling for the production and marketing of "fruit, vegetables and legumes and other health produce" (Simon, 2004: p. 406).

administration's selfish financial and political interests (Revill and Harris, 2004; Norum, 2010). Norum went on to publically state that "I think it is tragic that the US is opposing this [*The 2004 Global Strategy*] because the problem is very, very serious in the US. I think it is the multinational companies who are mainly behind this attack on the science" (Norum quoted in Boseley, 2004). Norum further argued that since 1990, several US administrations failed to take the WHO's guidelines on obesity seriously (Revill and Harris, 2004). Scientists at the IOTF supported Norum's claims (Revill and Harris, 2004).

It is important to note, however, that the WHO's criticisms did not have a serious impact on the Bush administration's policy interests. This came to light when Bush publically stated that he would never endorse the WHO's *The 2004 Global Strategy* (*Consumer Affairs*, 2006). This sent a clear message to the world, moreover, that Bush was going to tackle the obesity epidemic on his own and at his own pace (Norum, 2010). Although Bush eventually acquiesced and signed *The 2004 Global Strategy*, he did so mainly for diplomatic reasons rather than being genuinely compliant and supportive of WHO policy recommendations. In fact, Bush never adopted the WHO's recommendations, which by then included not only regulating the fast food industry but also providing assistance to states.

To make matters worse, in 2004 Bush also imposed an edict prohibiting CDC officials from accepting invitations to visit the WHO without first obtaining his expressed permission. Bush stated very clearly that CDC officials working on obesity were not allowed to freely visit the WHO, and that the oval office would have to first review who was going and what they intend to discuss (McKenna, 2004a, 2004b; Norum, 2010). This further confirmed widely held suspicions that Bush was not interested in collaborating with the WHO, neither for research nor for exploring various policy options. Incensed PHS officials called this a travesty, better yet "antithetical to the scientific process … [it] is political control in both directions … [and] it limits the WHO's opportunities to get the best people and it suppresses the domestic health agency's opportunity to provide the best people," argued Dr. Jeffrey Koplan, former CDC director and now professor at the Emory University School of Medicine (Koplan quoted in McKenna, 2004b). The White House's refusal to work closely with the WHO not only revealed the Bush administration's arrogance and political interests, but also the fact that it had no interest in increasing the government's international reputation through an aggressive domestic policy response (Norum, 2010). Instead, the White House's focus seemed to be on safeguarding the interests of the private sector, free markets, as well as consumerism.

In addition, the Bush administration's apathy towards international organizational interests in combating obesity translated to a lack of interest in providing bilateral support to combat obesity in other nations. After all, the international solution to curbing the spread of obesity, such as regulating the fast food industry, went against the Bush administration's beliefs on how to handle the issue.

Personal Interests and Commitments

While Bush may not have been interested in the global fight against obesity, domestically, he certainly displayed a personal interest and commitment to the issue. In fact, shortly after 9/11, Bush was well known for expressing his personal belief that obesity posed a serious national health threat while vehemently declaring a "war on obesity" (Kiefer, 2002; *The New York Times*, 2002; Vulliamy, 2002). As an illustration of his leadership and commitment to the issue, Bush immediately appointed a new HHS secretary, Tommy Thompson, who was just as interested and committed to responding to the epidemic because of his personal struggle to lose weight. Despite Bush's unwavering dedication to the war on terror, which understandingly usurped much of his attention (*The Washington Post*, 2002), he nevertheless remained committed to tackling obesity and pursued initiatives that reflected his personal experiences and concerns.

For example, shortly after the surgeon general's 2001 Call to Action, Bush reinvigorated the President's Council on Physical Fitness and Sports (*The Washington Post*, 2002). Created by President

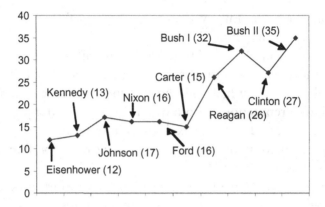

Figure 5.1 Number of presidential appointments to the president's council on physical fitness and sports (1917–present)

Source: My calculations

Dwight Eisenhower in 1956 and maintained under the Johnson and Carter administrations, the Council was essentially dormant under Clinton (*The Washington Post*, 2002). Bush strengthened the Council by appointing 20 new members while launching the HealthierUS: The President's Health and Fitness Initiative (*The Washington Post*, 2002). As Figure 5.1 illustrates, moreover, when compared to his predecessors, Bush was much more proactive in the number of members (including directors) he appointed to the Council.

Instead of focusing on sports and dieting, as prior councils did, Bush's Council was focused on encouraging Americans to become more physically active and fit. The Council emphasized activities such as daily walking while alluding to studies showing how regular exercise could help ward off obesity and other related health ailments (*The Washington Post*, 2002). Bush's Council also encouraged a gradual, small-steps plan to weight loss, which emphasized setting aside 30 and 60 minutes a day for adults and children to exercise, respectively.

Yet another initiative that Bush undertook was to sign an executive order in July 2002 requiring the directors of all health agencies to encourage physical fitness activities within their division. Specifically, the executive order required all agencies to review policies, programs, and regulations for physical activity, nutrition, and screening (*The Nation's Health*, 2002).

During this period, however, it seems that pressures from civil society were not what was motivating Bush to address the obesity issue. This mainly reflected the lack of broader concern from civil society about obesity at the time and its associated health ailments. Indeed, professors J. Eric Oliver of the University of Chicago and Taeku Lee of the University of California at Berkeley conducted a poll in the spring of 2002 and found that obesity was not a major concern for most citizens (Nagourney, 2002; Oliver, 2006a, 2006b; Oliver and Lee, 2005). Out of a random poll of 900 individuals interviewed, only one-third found obesity to be an important public health issue (Oliver and Lee, 2005).

Nor were congressional interests the key factor instigating the president's response. Evidence suggests that Congress was also apathetic about the obesity epidemic during this period, that there was no bipartisan consensus for the need to increase funding and create prevention programs (Brownlee and Wolter, 2001; Kersh and Morone, 2005; Nestle and Jacobson, 2000). Finally, the international community did not play a role in pressuring and prompting Bush to respond. As mentioned earlier, the Bush administration was not receptive to the WHO's criticisms and policy recommendations, nor was Bush concerned about increasing his international reputation through an aggressive policy response.

Bush's Personal Drive

President Bush's response to obesity mainly reflected his personal concerns and interests, which, as Figure 5.2 illustrates, motivated him to frequently talk about this issue in public. More specifically, it was his fear of gaining weight that motivated him to perceive obesity as an important issue. In addition, the fact that Bush had a prior history of staying in shape made the threat of gaining weight all the more pervasive (Kiefer, 2002). Shortly after his arrival into office, Bush recounted in an interview with *The New York Times* about telling one of his friends that he feared the possibility of gaining weight because of his busy work schedule; and that moreover, that was the main reason for why he was so committed to exercise and losing weight

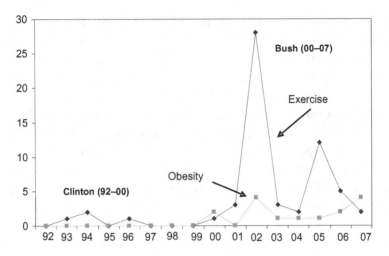

Figure 5.2   Content analysis of Clinton and Bush's public discussion of exercise and obesity

Source: Lexis Nexis; this figure measures the number of times Clinton and Bush were "quoted" in the news media as discussing their personal commitment to exercise, addressing the obesity issue and calling for a communal response to the problem. The following key words were used for this analysis: "Clinton" "Bush" and "exercise" "fitness" "obesity" "overweight" and "fat" for hundreds of newspapers and magazines throughout all regions of the US.

(Dowd, 2002). Through exercise and fitness, the president found strength and confidence: "I am convinced that running helped me quit drinking and smoking ... I quickly realized what it felt like to be healthy, and I already knew what it felt like to be unhealthy" (Bush quoted in Sweet, 2002). "He's simply a health nut! ... I've never seen anyone as committed to good exercise and health," said his good friend and HHS director, Tommy Thompson (Thompson, 2012).

In addition to Bush's personal interest, a flurry of epidemiological data also prompted his concern (*Pittsburgh Post-Gazette*, 2002). There was also a surge in media attention about the epidemic (Kersh and Morone, 2006), information that certainly contributed to Bush's interest in obesity.

Bush's personal commitment to physical fitness inspired him to ensure that others were doing the same. At his White House residence in Washington, DC, Bush expected his staff to engage in daily exercise and to watch their diet (Milbank, 2002). "It's really important for the White House team to exercise on a regular basis ... I hope you understand that's how the boss thinks," Bush once stated (Bush quoted in Jackson, 2002). Close aids claim that Bush's addiction to exercise inspired the creation of White House sports clubs, such as "Girls with Gloves" (i.e., weightlifting gloves) and the "Dixie Chicks," and daily personal exercise routines and new dietary habits. "I lost 17 pounds on the Bush plan," said Bush's deputy director for communications, James Wilkinson (Wilkinson quoted in Milbank, 2002). Other White House employees soon felt obligated to become physically fit. In a sense, Bush had created a new "culture of fitness" and nutrition within the White House. These activities, as well as his personal commitment to weight loss and fitness, won him the honor of being named the fittest president in American history (Dobin, 2003).

Nevertheless, politicians' personal interests in combating obesity did not stop at the White House. In several state governments, the fear of weight gain and its associated ailments also shaped the governors' interests in policy reform.

The initiatives pursued by former governor Michael Huckabee (Republican — Arkansas) provide a good example. Huckabee was personally affected by the consequences of excess weight. The governor finally decided to take action when on a particular evening an incident occurred which made him realize how serious and embarrassing his situation was. At the state capital meeting in Arkansas in 2003, in front of a large gathering of supporters, he broke an old wooden chair that he was sitting on. He initially shrugged it off, laughed and jokingly said: "They sure don't build them like they use to!" But later on in his book, *Quit Digging Your Grave with a Knife and Fork* (Huckabee, 2005), reflecting on the event, Huckabee stated that: "Deep down, I knew it wasn't the chair that needed rebuilding — it was me that needed a major overhaul" (Huckabee quoted in Barrett, 2005). Huckabee immediately embarked on a personal weight loss program, which he called the "12-stop" plan.[5] Within a few months, he lost 110 lbs.

---

[5] Huckabee's "12-stop" plan encourages readers to stop the following habits: 1) procrastination; 2) making excuses; 3) sitting on the couch; 4) ignoring signals from your body; 5) listening to destructive criticism; 6) expecting immediate success; 7) whining; 8) making exceptions; 9)

In addition, Huckabee was also concerned that he was going to die from a sudden heart attack. Before embarking on his successful weight loss plan, Huckabee was diagnosed with a minor — though potentially severe — heart condition. This problem, when combined with the loss of a dear overweight friend from a sudden heart attack, further magnified his concern about obesity (Barrett, 2005). Huckabee once commented: "There was [a good friend] Gov. Frank White's death from a heart attack, my own diagnosis with type 2 diabetes and a heart catheterization, which scared the daylights out of me — though [the test came out] clear, thank God. I was at my heaviest in the spring of 2003, at least 280 pounds at the time. I knew I was unhealthy and I didn't want to be this way" (Huckabee quoted in Barrett, 2005).

Governor Huckabee's worries prompted him to pursue preventative policy measures. As chairman of the National Governors Association, for example, Huckabee encouraged other governors to implement prevention programs and policies geared toward weight loss and improved health (Dewan, 2006; Tanner, 2006). He believed that the governors, mayors, and citizens needed to work together to address obesity and achieve these objectives. Through these actions, Huckabee made it clear to many that he did not want anyone going through what he experienced, and that the only way to combat the obesity epidemic was not only individualistic effort and responsibility, but also by working together as a community.

The government of Arkansas' commitment to obesity decreased substantially after Huckabee lost the governorship to Mike Bebee (Democrat — Arkansas). Federal officials became concerned with the transition because they noticed that under Huckabee, his office incessantly requested federal assistance; federal officials worried that the new Bebee administration would not seek the same level of assistance. In fact, in an interview with the director of nutrition at the USDA, Steve Carlson, he explained to me that when Huckabee was in office, he received a ton of requests for financing several of Huckabee's new

---

storing provisions for failure; 10) fueling with contaminated food; 11) allowing food to be a reward; and 12) neglecting your spiritual life.

anti-obesity initiatives (Carlson, 2007). However, as soon as Huckabee left office, the number of requests quickly declined (Carlson, 2007).

The Bureaucracy's Personal Battle

Dovetailing with the personal interests of presidents and governors were those of top-level bureaucrats. By 2002, for example, HHS Secretary Tommy Thompson's belief in the need to get serious about obesity stemmed mainly from his personal experiences of being overweight, the prospect of gaining weight and falling ill. Obesity was Thompson's "personal mission" (MSNBC, 2004). While in office, he wanted to stay in shape, live long, and prosper — a goal that he still abides by, claiming to do 50 push-ups and 100 sit-ups a day to achieve this (Browdie, 2012; Thompson, 2012). In an interview with me, Thompson commented that his father's untimely death from heart disease and smoking also motivated him to do something about obesity and its associated health ailments (Thompson, 2012). Thompson was also concerned about his close friends, many of whom were overweight, had high blood pressure, and suffered from diabetes (Thompson, 2012). But he was also startled by the number of obese individuals in the US — especially children, as well as the high level of complacency and, simply put, apathy and laziness of Americans (*The Boston Globe*, 2004).

Similar to Bush, and as Figure 5.3 illustrates, Thompson's passion and commitment to fitness and exercise prompted him to frequently talk about the issue in public. Furthermore, Thompson's personal concern with weight gain motivated him to started calling on others to take better care of themselves. He began by focusing on his own staff, encouraging them to get into better shape (Connolly, 2004; Leonard, 2004). Thompson often criticized his staff for their lack of progress in losing weight and for not taking the initiative to do so (Connolly, 2004).

Furthermore, at the HHS, he immediately ordered his staff to start taking the stairs instead of the elevator (MSNBC, 2004; Thompson, 2012), to go to the gym, and to walk during lunch (Thompson,

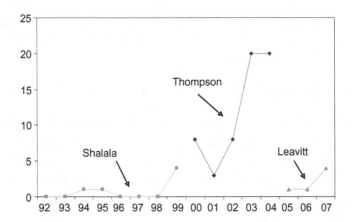

Figure 5.3 Content analysis of the number of times Shalala, Thompson, and Leavitt publicly discussed their personal commitment to exercise, fighting obesity and individual/civic responsibility (1993–2007).

Source: Lexis Nexis and Google; this figure measures the number of times all HHS secretaries since the Clinton administration were "quoted" in the media as discussing their personal commitment to "Donna Shalala" "Tommy Thompson" "Michael Leavitt" "exercise" "fitness" "obesity" "overweight" and "fat" for hundreds of newspaper and magazine articles in all regions of the US.

2012). He even went so far as to provide each of his staff with an official HHS speedometer, to be worn on the wrist, so that they could keep track of the number of calories burned every day (Thompson, 2012). In fact, Thompson was so serious about this that when visiting other countries, he provided foreign dignitaries with the official HHS speedometer (Thompson, 2012).

Thompson was so passionate about the issue that his very own staff feared him, running the other way when they saw him walking down the hallway — or even walking back into the elevator when he turned towards it (Thompson, 2012). Staff feared that Thompson would pull them aside and hound them about their progress in losing weight.

However, Thompson was not only focused on his HHS staff; he was also pointing his finger at Americans. "We're too darn fat!," he once commented (Leonard, 2004). He was focused on motivating Americans to do something about their weight, to help their kids, to change their lifestyles and to get healthy ... or else (Thompson, 2012). In short, he believed that "Americans are eating themselves to death ..." that "Americans need to understand that obesity is killing us" (Thompson quoted in CNN, 2004; Milloy, 2004a, 2004b).

Upon resigning from office in December 2004, Thompson, as well as the media (MSNBC, 2004), celebrated his achievements in having done something about obesity — in having worked with Bush to increase attention to the issue within government. He hoped that his predecessors would take the issue as seriously. Although his predecessor, Michael Leavitt, did not, Thompson was happy to see that First Lady Michelle Obama was committed to the issue. Like Thompson, Mrs. Obama took a serious, personal interest in obesity, helping further advance the government's interest in the epidemic — an issue that I will return to shortly (Thompson, 2012).

Bureaucratic Response

Aiding Secretary Thompson in his cause was the presence of bureaucratic unity and commitment to working together in response to obesity. "The USDA and the CDC are taking lead roles in the anti-obesity crusade, and many non-profit and private groups may soon join them in their battle," wrote Joyce Price of *The Washington Times* (Price, 2000; Carlson, 2007). As a matter related to the nutritional policies and guidelines that they provide, even before the surgeon general's 2001 Call to Action, the USDA had been very proactive in its response (Carlson, 2007; Price, 2000). In addition, the surgeon general's Call to Action was co-authored by CDC and NIH officials (Dietz, 2007; Carlson, 2007). While the CDC and NIH maintained their distinctive roles (the CDC providing more direct service to the states, while the NIH conducts research), since the Call to Action, CDC and NIH bureaucrats have worked together to co-sponsor several initiatives.

For example, in 2007, the CDC worked with the NIH to create a new inter-agency working group, called the IWGOOR (Internal Working Group on Obesity Research). The main reason for creating this working group was to increase research and collaboration between the agencies on obesity, and to find common ground and policy solutions that will lead to more effective policy implementation

(Carlson, 2007). The CDC and NIH have also been working on new programs to monitor and measure children's weight in schools while providing a host of educational pamphlets, guidelines, and recommendations (Dietz, 2007).

Thompson was also very much committed to working with the USDA on a host of prevention programs. Thompson worked with the USDA on joint programs aimed at working closely with the private sector, such as restaurants. In 2002, for example, Thompson and USDA Secretary Ann M. Venemamn, met with officials from the National Restaurant Association and the National Council of Chain Restaurants to initiate a dialogue about how food and beverage industries can help Americans combat obesity (US Department of Health and Human Services, 2002). Thompson once commented:

"I am calling on leaders from the food and beverage industry to aid us in our fight against obesity. Overweight and obesity are at an all-time high in America and the public health consequences are enormous. At HHS, we aim to lead by example. We must act now, and act together, in order to improve the health of our country's adults and children" (Thompson quoted in US Department of Health and Human Services, 2002).

Limited Policy Responses

For a conservative Republican administration, it is surprising to see just how responsive President Bush was to obesity. Of course, this does not mean that Bush went out of his way to help create a new federal agency and policies providing assistance to the states. Keep in mind that most of Bush's military were not obese, so there was no need to build a new agency or to even strengthen the HHS's response.

While Bush's personal interest in obesity helped to increase the government's attention to the epidemic, unfortunately this did not translate to concrete bureaucratic and policy reforms. Furthermore, Bush never pressured the House and the Senate to implement new legislation increasing the regulation of the fast food industry. These shortcomings prompted analysts to view the Bush administration as "all talk but no action." Margo Wootan, director of nutrition policy at the Center for Science in the Public Interest, commented that: "The administration gets an A-plus for talk but a D for action" (Wootan quoted in Conolly, 2003).

However, this does not mean that Bush's personal interest in obesity was insignificant. His interest was certainly better than nothing. Bush deserves credit for placing obesity on the national agenda. There is no disputing the fact that he outdid his predecessors when it came to drawing attention to obesity. Bush's personal commitment also led to a surge in political and bureaucratic attention to the issue, as well as a host of new research studies, heightened media attention, and social awareness.

Despite Bush's attention to the issue, both he and Congress did little to help HHS officials fund their obesity programs (Associated Press 2002; Tumiel, 2003). In fact, Secretary Tommy Thompson once commented: "I tell Congress to set aside dollars for prevention. They're all very encouraging, but they don't give me the dollars for it!" (*Associated Press*, 2002). And even after the surgeon general's 2001 Call to Action, the CDC managed to squeeze out of Congress a mere $100 million for obesity research and prevention activities, while the NIH received a whopping $226 million (Brownlee and Wolter, 2001). As an organization in general, and especially when compared to the NIH, the CDC's budget for obesity was extremely tight (Dietz, 2007). In fact, the CDC division in charge of obesity actually saw a *decline* in funding by 2007 (*Trust for America's Health Reports*, 2006; Dietz, 2007), while the CDC division focusing on nutrition also had a difficult time obtaining funds (Jacobson, 2004; Kersh and Morone, 2005). What's more, 2005 budget estimates suggested that the CDC would lose approximately $500 million in the next few years to work on obesity issues (Pear and Schmit, 2005; Stein, 2005). In response, CDC officials had to reshuffle funds from other departments to the department of nutrition (Herrera, 2005). The only division within the CDC that continued to receive funding during this period was bioterrorism (Dietz, 2007).

When it came to providing support to the states, the CDC once again took the lead in working closely with the governors and mayors in order to learn more about their needs. In an interview with the director for Nutritional science at the CDC, Dr. William Dietz, he stated that since 2001, the CDC has worked closely with the governors and mayors in order to learn more about obesity prevalence in their states and what the CDC can do to help (Dietz, 2007). Dietz and his staff were particularly interested in reaching out to low-income families and minorities, while providing new educational and nutritional programs in schools (Dietz, 2007). Dr. Kelly Brownell, professor of psychology at Yale University, director of the Rude Center for Food Policy and Obesity at Yale, and a long-time critic of the government's policies, supported Dietz's position (Brownell, 2007). Moreover, Brownell praised their activities and argued that of all the federal agencies under the Bush administration, the CDC was the only one doing something constructive about the problem (Brownell, 2007).

Working through the Nutrition and Physical Activity Program to Prevent Obesity and other Chronic Diseases (NPAO), which was created in 1998 and is now operating in 28 states, the CDC provided financial support for several obesity programs (Centers for Disease Control, 2007). Moreover, within three years of the surgeon general's 2001 Call to Action, the CDC implemented over 20 additional state programs, with a focus on improving nutrition and physical activity in schools (Rodgers, 2004).

And finally, in addition to providing financial and technical assistance to the states, federal health agencies can also implement policies that sustain their policy influence within a context of poorly planned decentralization processes. As we saw with Brazil's response to AIDS, these policies often entail two elements: first, the creation of federal programs providing performance-based fiscal transfers to local health agencies in need of assistance; and second, informally working with NGOs to monitor health agencies in order to increase their accountability to the center. Within a highly fragmented, decentralized context, where local health agencies are often distant from capitals, inefficient, and in need of assistance, these policies can help federal agencies to achieve their policy objectives (Rich and Gómez, 2012).

However, and similar to what we saw in Chapter 3 with the US's response to AIDS, these centralization strategies were never pursued. First, Congress has yet to authorize a federal program that provides performance-based discretionary transfers to municipal health departments working on obesity and nutrition issues. The only funding provided from Congress is for HHS agencies working on obesity prevention, which was scant under the Bush administration but nevertheless is projected to increase under President Obama's Recovery Act and the Child Nutrition Act, which was projected to increase funding for healthier school lunches by $10 billion (Fox, 2009; Woods, 2010). In the future, Congress should consider authorizing fiscal discretionary programs that can be used to reward state health agencies in compliance with the HHS and White House's Healthy America and, more recently, the First Lady's Let's Move policy guidelines. Through this process, the government can increase its influence in making sure that policies are effectively implemented and goals are met.

Second, the HHS has never tried to work closely with NGOs in order to monitor the performance of local health departments, thus holding administrators and politicians accountable for their policy actions. Nevertheless, the HHS and PHS have engaged in a series of joint partnerships with civic organizations. For instance, the HHS is working with the National Beverage Association and schools to promote better eating (HHS, 2007); partnerships with organizations committed to quality transportation — such as safer sidewalks and bike paths — and better food system deliveries to schools, as seen with the CDC's *Healthy Eating Active Living Convergence Partnership* (Bell and Dorfman, 2008); research through the CDC's National Collaboration on Childhood Obesity Research (NCCOR), created in 2008 while partnering with universities and research institutions (NCCOR, 2010); the NIH's programs to work with CBO's (community-based organizations) to promote healthy eating, such as the We Can initiative (NIH, 2003); and finally, the HHS's Take Action program, which provides seed money to CBOs to work on healthy eating and exercise (HHS, 2007).

However, the challenge is that neither the HHS nor PHS has tried to strategically use NGOs and CBOs in order to monitor and report the policy performance of local health departments. As we saw in Brazil, this kind of strategy is needed in order to increase local government accountability to the HHS and the White House's obesity initiatives.

Reforms under the Obama Administration

Though coming from different sides of the political spectrum, the Bush and Obama administrations certainly share one commonality when it comes to public health: that is, an unwavering interest in combating obesity. Nevertheless, nowhere is this more prevalent than with the First Lady, Michelle Obama. In February 2010, Mrs. Obama announced a national campaign to eradicate childhood obesity within ten years. Called the Let's Move initiative, this campaign seeks to inspire the government, families, the private sector, and local governments to work together in eradicating childhood obesity. She believes that the federal government should not be acting alone in its response to the epidemic (Obama, 2010). Instead, responding to obesity requires a shared responsibility and effort among various stakeholders, in positions that can help children lose weight and enjoy a healthier lifestyle.

The Let's Move initiative calls on federal, state, and private sector programs to achieve four key goals: 1) to help parents make healthy food choices; 2) to create healthier schools; 3) to increase physical activity; and finally 4), to increase access to healthy and affordable foods (White House, 2010a). This is the first comprehensive national campaign establishing a close partnership between the federal government, families, the private sector, and local governments.

The First Lady's motivation did not come from international or domestic pressures, but rather from the love and concern that she had for her family: specifically, the concern that she had for her daughter's health. During the unveiling of her campaign at a YMCA in the outskirts of Alexandria, Virginia, she once commented:

> We went to our pediatrician at the time ... I thought my kids were perfect — they are and always will be — but he (the doctor) warned that he was concerned that something was getting off balance ... I

didn't see the changes. And that's also part of the problem, or part of the challenge. It's often hard to see changes in your own kids when you're living with them day in and day out … But we often simply don't realize that those kids are our kids, and our kids could be in danger of becoming obese. We always think that only happens to someone else's kids — and I was in that position. (ABC, 2010a: p. 1)

In another interview, Mrs. Obama commented: "Even though I wasn't exactly sure at that time what I was supposed to do with this information about my children's BMI, I knew I had to do something … I had to lead our family to a different way…" (Associated Press, 2010: p. 1).

Mrs. Obama gradually transferred her personal concerns and experiences to the public domain. During ABC's coverage of the release of her Let's Move initiative, Mrs. Obama was quoted as saying that she had "good news to share with families … particularly with kids … that small changes can lead to big results" (ABC, 2010a). She was keen on drawing a connection between her personal family struggles and what she wanted to do for the public. Through her *Let's Move* initiative, she now had the opportunity and resources needed to do that.

President Obama supported her efforts. In May 2010, inspired by the initiative, President Obama signed an executive order creating a new Task Force on Childhood Obesity. Chaired by Dr. Melody Barnes, an attorney, prior director of domestic policy for the Obama campaign, as well as previous vice president of the Center for American Progress, the Task Force brings federal agencies, the private sector, and local governments together to achieve the following: 1) to empower parents and caregivers to have better diets; 2) to provide healthier food at schools; 3) to improve access to health and affordable foods; and 4) to increased physical activity (White House, 2010b). Similar to the Let's Move campaign, it calls on federal and state governments, as well as the private sector and families to work together in accomplishing these objectives (Black, 2010). In order to implement these initiatives, the president requested an additional $1 billion dollars from Congress. The Task Force therefore undergirds and emboldens the Let's Move initiative with clearly delegated responsibilities and more financial support.

However, the First Lady was not alone in expressing her personal interests and motivation for a response. As we saw under the George W. Bush administration, high-level bureaucrats were also personally committed to the First Lady's policies.

For example, the US surgeon general, Dr. Regina Benjamin, was committed to her policies. A well-known doctor from the rural coast of Alabama, President Obama choose Benjamin because of her extensive experience and commitment to promoting healthy living and prevention, especially among the rural poor. Despite her impressive qualifications, extensive experience, and passion for service, the media and medical professionals soon became highly critical of the fact that she was overweight. Consequently, many questioned President Obama's decision to select Benjamin, arguing that it was a bad idea to appoint someone struggling with a health issue that the government was suggesting people avoid (ABC, 2010c; Fox News, 2010). The surgeon general was supposed to be a role model — fit and strong; a bureaucratic official that people could look up to (ABC, 2010c; Fox News, 2010). Others countered by arguing that because of Benjamin's weight, she was in an even better position to address the obesity issue, as she would be personally committed to the endeavor (ABC, 2010c).

Surgeon General Benjamin was certainly committed combating the obesity epidemic. During Benjamin's first televised acceptance speech as surgeon general, she established a connection between her personal experiences and public service. In an interview with Good Morning America's Robin Roberts (ABC, 2010b), Benjamin commented that: "I'm just like 67 percent of Americans. I struggle with my weight just like they do … So I understand. And I want to have them help me, and I'll help them, and we'll work together to try to become a healthier nation." Feeling the pain of those women criticized for their weight problems, she drew a personal connection by stating: "I'm a women. Just like everyone else, I want to be attractive. You don't want to see those negative things — people calling you names. So it was very hurtful" (ABC, 2010b).

Benjamin understood the challenges that other Americans faced (Kalb, 2010). It was an empathy, a connection between the personal and the public, a connection that we first saw emerge in Chapter 2 with Roosevelt's battle with polio and his understanding and care for others because of his personal experience with this disease.

But Surgeon General Benjamin was not the only bureaucrat with a similar story. As a member of the First Lady's Let's Move campaign and the new Task Force on Childhood Obesity, Secretary of Agriculture Tom Vilsack was also motivated by his personal experiences. Similar to HHS Secretary Tommy Thompson, Vilsack is an overweight individual and cognizant of his weight, never fearing to talk about it. One could argue that in addition to his impressive qualifications and experience, President Obama's selection of Vilsack was very strategic and helpful, as Valsack's personal battle with weight gain motivated him to speak up about the issue and to take action. But rather than talk about his current health challenges, considering the First Lady's focus on childhood obesity, Vilsack has always referred to his childhood experiences. On several occasions, Vilsack established a connection between his youthful past and his current commitment to tackling childhood obesity.

Revisiting a personal experience that "haunts him to this day" (Vilsack quoted in Silicon Valley Moms Blog, 2010: p. 1), as a chubby farm boy wearing suspenders in Iowa, Vilsack remembers a time when his adopted mother plastered a cartoon picture of a rotund little boy in a beanie cap eating a cupcake on the refrigerator (Beaumont, 2010). She did this in order to remind him not to eat so much and to scare him into believing that that little cartoon boy could one day be him. It enraged him and decades later, during his time as governor of Iowa and his brief presidential campaign trail in 2008, he referred to the story, using it as one of the key reasons for why he was so committed to eradicating childhood obesity (Silicon Valley Moms Blog, 2010: p. 1). "Every time I opened the refrigerator door, I had to look at that guy," he told a crowd at the National Press Club (Vilsack quoted in Obama, 2010). As the First Lady commented in an article she wrote for *Newsweek*, it was a memory that continued to haunt Vilsack and one that to this day has motivated him to work on childhood obesity issues (Obama, 2010).

Similar to Surgeon General Benjamin, Secretary Vilsack has also realized that he shared a common struggle with the American people. On the day that the First Lady unveiled her Let's Move campaign, Vilsack was quoted as stating that: "She passionately spoke from first-hand experience as a mother of two wonderful children and the challenges that she faced as her children were growing up ... I certainly understand that passion having been one of those youngsters she talked about today who was overweight, teased at school. This is a very important initiative for us, for this country" (Vilsack quoted in Henderson, 2010).

Nevertheless, Vilsack also took his personal experiences to Congress. Motivated by his personal history and empathy for others, Mrs. Obama once commented that Vilsack is "now calling on Congress to increase meal-reimbursement rates so that schools can buy higher-priced healthier foods, including whole grains, fruits, and vegetables. He's asking for a stronger link between local farmers and cafeterias, and the authority to set standards on competitive foods" (Obama, 2010: p. 48). Vilsack is also working hard to develop partnerships with the USDA and the private sector, such as the NFL and the Dairy Council, in connection with its effort to "fuel up to Play 60" — that is, recognizing the importance of 60 minutes of active engagement by youngsters, physical activity, and getting appropriate meals (Henderson, 2010: p. 2).

Yet the First Lady's and these bureaucrats' personal experiences, fears and interests have not led to concrete policy reforms. As mentioned earlier, Obama has sought to expand the NIH and CDC's work on childhood and adult obesity, providing more funding and expanding its employment force. At the same time, new federal programs have provided funding to the states. But key elements of an effective centralized response, such as either the creation of a new federal agency or a subdivision within the PHS focused exclusively on obesity, the strategic usage of close partnerships with NGOs to monitor local governments and hold them accountable, as well as the creation of discretionary, performance-based grants to the states, are still absent. In short, there are no new bureaucratic and policy initiatives that embolden and sustain the White House, Congress, and the PHS's policy influence within a context of healthcare decentralization.

Nevertheless it seems that this type of centralized response is needed in order to ensure that the goals outlined in the Let's Move and the presidential Task Force are achieved. Ensuring that the states and even the private sector meet their half of the bargain will require innovative policy initiatives that ensure that all the stakeholders involved are complying with the First Lady's policy recommendations.

International Cooperation and Obesity's National Security Threat

Under President Obama, however, two issues have emerged that may lead to a shift in US international cooperation and a more aggressive, centralized bureaucratic and policy response to obesity. First, Obama is striving to transform the government's relationship with the international community. According to Dr. Kaare Norum, in contrast to the previous presidential (George W. Bush) administration, Obama is fully committed to working with the WHO to address childhood nutrition and obesity issues (Norum, 2010). Moreover, Obama has encouraged CDC and NIH officials to visit and work with the WHO (Norum, 2010), an endeavor that was never allowed under the Bush administration. In the future, the CDC's ability to work closely with the WHO and other international health agencies may lead to the creation of a new partnership that further increases its credibility and influence, thus potentially enhancing the CDC's ability to obtain more funding from Congress.

Second, the perception of obesity posing a new national security threat may incentivize efforts to heighten the government's response. Similar to what we saw in Chapter 2 with malnutrition's negative effect on the military's ability to recruit soldiers for the two world wars, a similar problem is occurring with obesity today. In 2010, First Lady Obama started to refer to the obesity epidemic as a national security threat (Huffman, 2010; Starr, 2010). Furthermore, in April 2010, Secretary Valsack met with retired military officials at a Capitol Hill news conference to discuss how childhood obesity is posing a serious threat to military recruitment (Park, 2010). In particular,

Vilsack stated: "the reality that so many youngsters are not fit for military service is a wake-up call for this country" (Park, 2010: p. 1).

By 2010, in an op-ed written for *The Washington Post*, military officials claimed that as of 2005, "at least 9 million young adults — 27 percent of all Americans ages 17 to 24 — were too overweight to serve in the military ... and since then, these numbers have remained largely unchanged" (Shalikashvili and Shelton, 2010: p. 1). This same article claimed that being overweight or obese have become the "leading medical reason recruits are rejected from military service" ... and that "since 1995, the proportion of potential recruits who failed their physical exams because of weight issues has increased nearly 70 percent, according to data reported by the Division of Preventative Medicine at the Walter Reed Army Institute of Research" (Shalikashvili and Shelton, 2010: p. 1). When commenting on why American's youth were failing to qualify for military service, retired US Air Force Lt. General Norman Seip stated: "it's not drug abuse, it's not asthma, it's not flat feet — by far the leading medical reason is being overweight or obese" (Seip quoted in Park, 2010: p. 1).

In addition, weight and obesity issues are leading to a gradual decline in soldier retention and completion of service. According to General Seip: "We lose upwards to 12,000 young men and women per year before they even finish up the first term of enlistment" ... "That's another person, who has been recruited, trained and left because they're not able to maintain standards and can't pass the physical fitness test" (Seip quoted in Park, 2010: p. 1). More than ever, it is gradually becoming clear that obesity is perceived as a serious threat to a core aspect of US national security, that is, military readiness.

Former retired military officials have also come out of retirement to try and help the government respond to this situation. In May 2010, for example, two retired generals, John Shaklikashvili and Hugh Shelton, both former chairmen of the US Joint Chiefs of Staff, claimed that obesity threatens America's overall health as well as the future strength of the military (Park, 2010). Seeing the need to mobilize in response, Generals Shaklikashvili and Shelton went on to claim that: "We consider this problem so serious from a national security perspective that we have joined more than 130 retired generals, admirals and senior military leaders in calling on Congress to pass new child nutrition legislation" (Shaklikashvili and Shelton quoted in Park, 2010: p. 1). These retired generals have joined other veterans and current senior military leaders in creating a non-profit organization called Mission: Readiness (Park, 2010, p. 1). This NGO is urging Congress to pass new legislation that ensures better nutrition in schools (Park, 2010).

Mission: Readiness' cause gradually spread throughout the nation, inspiring military leaders to work with state representatives to improve children's nutrition and health. On June 2, 2010, for example, several of Mission: Readiness' members held a news conference in the state of Maine to discuss DOD (Department of Defense) statistics, showing that 75% of American young adults aged 17–24 are unable to enlist in the military because they either failed to graduate high school, have a criminal record, or are physically unfit, while urging Maine lawmakers to provide pre-kindergarten and early care services to help ensure that children are fit for future military service (Mission: Readiness, 2010b). Furthermore, on June 14, 2010, in Philadelphia, three of Mission: Readiness' retired generals, joined by District Attorney R. Seth Williams and Dr. Eugene J. Richardson, an original Tuskegee airman, came together to urge lawmakers to create high-quality early education programs to help students stay in school, avoid crime, and have access to better nutrition (Mission: Readiness, 2010c). Mission: Readiness' efforts are therefore gradually radiating throughout the states, leading to a coalition of military leaders and public officials committed to reducing childhood obesity and preparing children for future military service.

At the national level, Mission: Readiness also fully endorsed President Obama's Task Force on Childhood Obesity. Mission: Readiness urged Congress to follow up with the following tasks:

1) To get junk food out of schools by adopting new standards for food and drinks sold, which are currently 15 years old and need to be updated;
2) To support the Obama administration's proposal for an increase in $1 billion dollars per year for ten years for child nutrition programs

improving nutrition standards, enhancing the quality of meals served in
schools and increasing access to them;

3) And finally, to develop research-based strategies, implemented
throughout our schools, that help parents and children develop
better eating habits (*Mission: Readiness*, 2010a).

In addition, one of Mission: Readiness' members, retired US Army
general called Paul Monroe, met with and urged Congress to implement these goals. Testifying before the House Education & Labor
Committee, Monroe stated the following: "Make no mistake. Child
obesity threatens our nation's security ... when 1 out of 4 adults is too
overweight to defend our country, then something is seriously
wrong" (Mission: Readiness, 2010a). Monroe closed by noting that
Congress needs to respond like they did in the past, arguing that "In
1946, Congress passed the National School Lunch Act as a matter of
national security ... In the past retired admirals and generals have
stood up to make it clear that America is only as healthy as our
nation's children. Childhood obesity is now undermining our national
security, and we need to start turning it around today" (Mission
Readiness, 2010a: p. 1).

Therefore, as we saw in Chapter 2 with the response to malnutrition and its ramifications for military recruitment, the military is once
again rising to the occasion by gradually seeking the creation of a new
reform coalition between military officials, the federal government,
and local government officials in order to implement policies aimed
at combating childhood obesity. While no new federal agencies have
been proposed, this is not an unrealistic possibility. As obesity
becomes even more prevalent in high schools, and as the military sees
a consistent drop in enlistees, we may see new calls for a centralized
agency focused exclusively on obesity.

Conclusion

As we saw in the past, it is interesting to note that once again, the US
government did not immediately respond to the emergence of a new
public health epidemic. Despite the HHS's and PHS's warnings and

declarations that obesity reached epidemic proportions, neither the presidents nor Congress took their declarations seriously. During the first few years of the epidemic, the absence of obesity's threat to US national security and a Congress heavily influenced by private sector interests, all coupled with President Clinton's lack of interest, failed to provide any effort in creating a national strategy and, needless to say, a centralized response. As we saw with the government's response to AIDS, though adamant in their insistence that something be done, PHS officials once again worked alone, always struggling to obtain more funding and political support. To make matters worse, they had no access to civic supporters. The few NGOs that existed were divided in their purpose and mission, failing to advocate policy ideas and beliefs in a centralized response to epidemics, while deciding not to work closely with PHS officials. Without civic supporters, PHS officials would not have the legitimacy and influence needed to pursue their policy interests.

With the emergence of international criticisms and pressures, there seemed to be some hope that the government would strengthen its policy response. However, this never occurred. As we saw with AIDS, President Bush was not only apathetic towards international criticisms and pressures, but he also criticized the WHO's critique of the government's lackluster response. The HHS was ordered to clandestinely convince the WHO to revise its 2004 Global Strategy, while CDC officials were literally forbidden to work with WHO officials.

The government's interest in obesity ultimately depended on the interests of the president and senior HHS officials; despite failing to provide support for HHS and CDC expansion, their personal experiences and fears helped to put obesity onto the national agenda. Yet, despite their interests, there were no concrete efforts to introduce legislation. Furthermore, despite starting to work closely with the states, the HHS and CDC still did not receive adequate support from the presidents and Congress to engage in a policy response.

While international criticisms of the US's response to obesity remain, the Obama administration is nevertheless committed to working closely with the WHO to address obesity. In addition, the military is now proactively involved. If we have learned anything from history, we know that the military in the US can have a major impact on building new institutions and programs in response to health epidemics. A military-based civic organization, Military: Readiness, has emerged to create a new government coalition aimed at reducing childhood obesity. As we saw in Chapter 2, given the rich history of military movements, ideas, and beliefs immediately working with the government to engage in a centralized response whenever epidemics threaten military recruitment, perhaps Military: Readiness will provide the civic supporters that the CDC needs to muster the legitimacy and influence needed to expand its initiatives on obesity.

Until this occurs, however, the US government must rely on a particular causal force that continues to reemerge and shape how it responds to contested epidemics: that is, personal experiences and fears in the highest echelons of government. Once again, as we saw with Roosevelt in Chapter 2, and as we saw with President George W. Bush, HHS officials and state governors, the personal fear and commitment of First Lady Michelle Obama and her HHS officials has placed obesity even further onto the national agenda. Similar to President Bush and the First Lady, the bureaucrats, namely Surgeon General Regina Benjamin and Secretary of Agriculture Tom Vilsack have been openly candid about their personal experiences and fears, while using this to establish a bridge between their experiences and the needs of civil society. Their personal experiences with obesity have generated a great deal of empathy and awareness that all citizens, including the most prestigious politicians and bureaucrats, can suffer from the same types of health ailments.

In the future, we can only hope that the personal experiences and fears of government leaders are combined with serious commitments to institutional and policy reform. More than ever, the US government needs to unify personal fears and empathy with a stern political and policy commitment to tackling obesity. Until then, while the government and civil society may continue to talk about the problem, write articles, and broadcast interesting TV shows, local governments, schools, families, and children will continue to suffer from the ongoing and highly contested obesity epidemic.

References

ABC (2010a). First Lady Gets Personal on Obesity Issue. Available on-line: http://abcnews.go.com/video/playerIndex?id=9690831. Accessed March 22, 2014.

ABC (2010b). Surgeon General Exclusive: 'I Struggle with my Weight' Like Most Americans. Available on-line: http://abcnews.go.com/GMA/OnCall/surgeon-general-exclusive-struggle-weight/story?id=9526674. Accessed March 22, 2014.

ABC (2010c). Critics Slam Overweight Surgeon General Pick, Regina Benjamin. Available on-line: http://abcnews.go.com/Health/story?id=8129947&page=1. Accessed March 22, 2014.

Aggleton, P. (2001). HIV/AIDS in Europe: The Challenge for Health Promotion Research, *Health Education Research*, 16, 403–409.

Ahmad, S. (1997). How to Slim Down the World's Fattest Society, *US News & World Report*, December 29, p. 62.

Altman, D. (1986). *AIDS in the Mind of America*, Doubleday Press, New York.

Armstrong, K. (1981). Fat Americans Form National Association, *Lawrence Journal-World News*, November 13, p. 6.

Associated Press (1998). Satcher Discusses the Childhood Obesity Epidemic, November 17.

Associated Press (2002). An Ounce of Prevention with a Pound of Cure, March 2.

Associated Press (2010). Michelle Obama Worried about Daughter's BMI, January 29, p. 1.

Baldwin, P. (2007). *Disease and Democracy: The Industrialized World Faces AIDS*, University of California Press, Berkeley.

Barrett, J. (2005). Campaigning for a Healthier America, *Newsweek*, May 5, p. 1.

BBC (2004). US Forces Changes to Obesity Plan, January 20. Available onlin: http://news.bbc.co.uk/1/hi/world/americas/3414741.stm. Accessed March 22, 2014.

Beaumont, T. (2010). On Fight with Child Obesity, Vilsack has Personal Story, *Iowa Politics Insider*, February 9.

Bell, J. and Dorfman, L. (2008). *Introducing the Health Eating Active Living Convergence Partnership*, PolicyLink Press, Oakland.

Black, J. (2010). Michelle Obama on Obesity: Time for a Wake up Call, *The Washington Post*, February 9, p. 1.

Booth, W. (1991). Americans Fail to See the 'Lite', *The Washington Post*, July 13, p. Al.

Browdie, B. (2012). 70-year-old Tommy Thompson does 50 Push-ups in One Minute to Prove his Fitness for the Senate, *New York Daily News*, August 9, p. 1.

Brownlee, S. and Wolter, P. (2001). Supersize Country, *The Washington Post*, December 15, p. A29.

Boseley, S. (2004). US Accused of Sabotaging Obesity, *The Guardian*, Friday 16, p. 1.

Brownell, K. (2007). Personal interview. February 19.

Buckley, N. (2004). WHO Advocates Taxes to Combat Obesity, *The Financial Times*, April 20, p. 8.

Burros, M. (1994). Despite Awareness of Risks, More in US are Getting Fat, *The New York Times*, July 17, p. 1.

Capital Times (1994). 3rd of Americans are Fat, Study Confirms, Nation/World, July 19, p. 1D.

Carlson, S. (2007). Personal interview. February 22.

Centers for Disease Control (2007). *Overweight and Obesity: State-Based Programs*, Centers for Disease Control, Atlanta.

Center for Science in the Public Interest (2004). *Bush Administration Trying to Bury WHO Report: Behind the Scenes Lobbying at Odds with Anti-Obesity Rhetoric*, January 16. Available on-line: http://cspinet.org/new/200401161.html. Accessed March 22, 2014.

CNN (2004). White House takes aim at Obesity, November 19. Available on-line: http://edition.cnn.com/2004/HEALTH/diet.fitness/03/12/obesity.campaign/. Accessed March 22, 2014.

Connolly, C. (2004). Obesity Fight Now Personal for HHS Chief; Thompson Puts Himself, Department on Diet, *The Washington Post*, March 12, p. A21.

Consumer Affairs (2006). HHS Gives Short Shrift to Obesity, CSPI Charges, April 28. Available on-line: http://www.obesitydiscussion.com/forums/f10/hhs-gives-short-shrift-obesity-1050.html. Accessed March 22, 2014.

Dewan, S. (2006). 100 pounds Lighter, with Advice to Share, *The New York Times*, September 10, p. 22.

Dietz, W. (2007). Personal interview. January 25.

Dobin, M. (2003). Fit to be President: Many of our Nation's Leaders have made Exercise a Priority, but George W. Bush Outruns them All, *McClatchy Newspapers Inc.*, January 8.

Dowd, M. (2002). Hans, Franz, and W, *The New York Times*, June 23, p. 13.

Doyle, S. (2005). Great Communicating: Learning from Ronald Reagan's Public Appeals to Address the Obesity Epidemic in America, *John F. Kennedy School of Government*, Working Paper, May 4.

Elder, L. (1999). A Fat Tax in our Future? *The Washington Times*, November 6, p. 10.

Finkelstein, E., Ruhm, C., and Kosa, K. (2005). Economic Causes and Consequences of Obesity, *Annual Review of Public Health, 26*, 239–57.

Fishman, S. (1998). Life in the Fat Underground, *Radiance: The Magazine for Large Women*. Available on-line: http://www.radiancemagazine.com/issues/1998/winter_98/fat_underground.html. Accessed March 23, 2014.

Fleck, F. (2004). Rich and Poor to Clash over Sugar in WHO's Health Diet Plan, *British Medical Journal, 328*, 730.

Flegal, K., Carroll, M., Ogden, C., and Johnson, C. (2002). Prevalence and Trends in Obesity Among US Adults, 1999–2000, *Journal of the American Medical Association, 2888*, 1723–1727.

Fletcher, D. (2009). The Fact-Acceptance Movement, *Time Magazine*. Available on-line: http://news.google.com/newspapers?id=BaUyAAAAIBAJ&sjid=c-cFAAAAIBAJ&pg=4304,2326994&hl=en. Accessed March 23, 2014.

Fox, M. (2009). US States to Get 'Significant' Obesity Money, *Reuters*, July 28, p. 1.

Fox News (2010). Is Obama's Pick for Surgeon General Too Fat? *The O'Reilly Factor*, July 24, p. 1.

Gustaitis, J. (2005). Special Feature: Obesity — A Killer at Large, *The World Almanac E-Newsletter, 5*, 1.

Henderson, O. (2010). Vilsack Part of Childhood Obesity Initiative, *Radioiowa.com*. Available on-line: http://www.radioiowa.com/2010/02/09/vilsack-part-of-childhood-obesity-initiative/. Accessed March 23, 2014.

Herrera, C. (2005). Some Fat Lies, *The Washington Times*, July 5, p. A16.

HHS (2007). *Department of Health and Human Services (HHS) Community-Based Organizations*, Prevention Report, **21**, HHS Press, Washington, DC, pp. 1–4.

Huckabee, M. (2005). *Quit Digging Your Grave with a Knife and Fork*, Center Street Publications, Lebanon.

Huffman, K. (2010). Michelle Obama's Anti-obesity Initiative Generates a Childish Backlash, *The Washington Post*, February 20.

Jackson, D. (2002). Dash for Fitness: Bush Takes on Staff to Promote Exercise, *The Seattle Times*, June 23, p. A6.

Jacobson, M. (2004). Obesity: We've Got to Do a Lot More! Executive Director, Center for Science in the Public Interest.

Jacobson, M. (2007). Personal interview. February 16.

James, W. (2008). WHO Recognition of the Global Obesity Epidemic, *International Journal of Obesity*, **32**, 120–126.

Kaplan, J. (2007). Personal interview. July 6.

Kersh, R. and Morone, J. (2002). The Politics of Obesity: Seven Steps to Government Action, *Health Affairs*, **21**, 142–53.

Kersh, R. and Morone, J. (2005). Obesity, Courts, and the New Politics of Public Health, *Journal of Health Politics, Policy and Law*, **30**, 839–868.

Kiefer, F. (2002). Bush Joins New War: Battle of the Bulge, *Christian Science Monitor*, June 20, p.01.

Krucoff, C. (1997). In the Battle of the Bulge, Better Diet and More Exercise Remain Safe Alternatives, *The Washington Post*, September 16, p. Z14.

Kuczmarksi, R., Flegal, K., Campbell, S., and Johnson, C. (1994). Increasing Prevalence of Overweight among US Adults. The National Health and Nutrition Examination Surveys, 1960 to 1991, *JAMA*, **272**, 205.

Lasalandra, M. (1999). Land of the Fat and Lazy: Surgeon General's Report has Good News, Bad News about America's Health, *The Boston Herald*, June 11, p. 03.

Lee, P. (2007). Personal interview. July 3.

Leonard, M. (2004). US Launches a Fight Against Obesity, *The Boston Globe*, March 10, p. A1.

McCall, C. (1991). Yuck!; School Lunches, *The Washington Times*, September 15, p. E1.

McFeatters, D. (1999). Tubbier with Tellies in Interactive Age, *The Washington Times*, October 31, p. B4.

McGinnis, M. (2007). Personal interview. July 12.

McKenna, M. (2004a). Feds Curb Access to CDC Experts, *Cox News Service*, June 30.

McKenna, M. (2004b). Government to limit access to CDC experts, *Ventura County Star*, July 1, p. 14.

McMurtrie, B. (1994). *Salt Lake Tribune*, Nation-World Section, July 21, p. A15.

Milbank, D. (2002). Fit to Govern, and Then Some, *The Washington Post*, June 17, p. C03.

Milloy, S. (2004a). Obesity Obsession, *The Washington Times*, May 10, p. A16.

Milloy, S. (2004b). Overblown Obesity Scare, *The Washington Times*, September 10, p. A16.

Mission: Readiness (2010a). Retired Admirals and Generals Urge Congress To Get Junk Food Out of Schools: Former Head of California Army National Guard Tells House Panel Child Obesity Poses a Threat to National Security, July 1. Available on-line: http://www.missionreadiness.org/wp-content/uploads/HearingPR.pdf. Accessed March 23, 2014.

Mission: Readiness (2010b). Main's Young Adults: Reading, Willing, and Unable to Serve: 75 percent of Young Adults cannot join the Military; Early Education across Main is needed to Ensure National Security. Available on-line: http://www.missionreadiness.org/wp-content/uploads/ME_Early_Ed_Report.pdf. Accessed March 23, 2014.

Mission: Readiness (2010c). Unable to Serve: Why Military Service is out of Reach for Most Young Philadelphians. Available on-line: http://www.missionreadiness.org/wp-content/uploads/Philadelphia_Early_Ed_Report.pdf. Accessed March 23, 2014.

MSNBC (2004). Thompson Resigns with Grim Warning, December 3, page 1.

Nagourney, E. (2002). Vital Signs: Perception; Excess Fat? Ho-Hum, Many Say, *The New York Times*, June 4, p. 8.

Nathanson, C. (1996). Disease Prevention as Social Change: Towards a Theory of Public Health, *Population and Development Review*, **22**, 609–637.

NCCOR (2010). Official website. Available on-line: http://www.nccor. org/. Accessed March 23, 2014.

Nestle, M. and Jacobson, M. (2000). Halting the Obesity Epidemic: A Public Health Policy Approach, *Public Health Reports*, **115**, 12–24.

NIH (2003). *Community-Based Organizations.* Available on-line: http:// www.nhlbi.nih.gov/health/public/heart/obesity/wecan/partner-with-us/cbo.htm. Accessed March 23, 2014.

Norum, K., Waxman, A., Selikowitz, H., Bauman, A., Puska, P., Rigby, N., James, P., and Yach, D. (2009). 'The WHO Global Strategy on Diet, Physical Activity and Health', in Tellnes, G. (ed.), *Urbanisation and Health: New Challenges in Health Promotion and Prevention*, Oslo Academic Press, Olso.

Norum, K. (2010). Personal interview. June 16.

Obama, M. (2010). Michelle on a Mission: How we can Empower Parents, Schools, and the Community to Battle Childhood Obesity, *Newsweek*, March 22, pp. 40–48.

Obesity, Fitness & Wellness Week (2002). Fitness: HHS Encourages Kids to Exercise, August 24, p. 11.

Obesity, Fitness & Wellness Week (2002). Overweight and Obesity Threaten US Health Gains, p. 1, January 12.

Oliver, E. (2006a). *Fat Politics: The Real Story Behind America's Obesity Epidemic*, Oxford University Press, New York.

Oliver, E. (2006b). The Politics of Pathology: How Obesity became an Epidemic Disease, *Perspectives in Biology and Medicine*, **49**, 611–627.

Oliver, E. and Lee, T. (2005). Public Opinion and the Politics of Obesity in America, *Journal of Health Politics, Policy & Law*, **30**, 923–54.

Park, M. (2010). Ex-military Leaders: Young Adults 'Too Fat to Fight,' CNN, April 20. Available on-line: http://www.cnn.com/2010/HEALTH/04/20/military.fat.fight/index.html. Accessed March 23, 2014.

Pear, R. and Schmit, E. (2005). Bush Budget Calls for Cuts in Health Services, *The New York Times*, February 5, p. 10.

Piani, A., and Schoenborn, C. (1990). Health Promotion and Disease Prevention: United States, 1990, *Vital Health Stat*, **10**, 1–90.

Pittsburgh Post-Gazette (2002). Making Americans Shape Up: Bush Wants a New Surgeon General to Deal with the Fat of the Land, March 31, p. C-3.

Price, J. (1994). Fat People to Protest for Say in Health Plan, *The Washington Times*, August 25, p. A6.

Price, J. (2000). War on Widening Waistlines; Government hopes to Spur Leaner Diets, More Exercise, *The Washington Times*, January 30, p. C-1.

Price-Smith, A. (2002). *The Health of Nations: Infectious Disease, Environmental Change, and their Effects on National Security and Development*, MIT Press, Cambridge.

Price-Smith, A., Tauber, S., and Bhat, A. (2004). State Capacity and HIV Incidence Reduction in the Developing World: Preliminary Empirical Evidence, *Seton Hall Journal of Diplomacy*, Summer/Fall, 149–160.

Revill, J. and Harris, P. (2004). US Sugar Barons 'Block Global War on Obesity, *The Observer*, January 18. Available on-line: http://www.guardian.co.uk/world/2004/jan/18/health.usa. Accessed March 23, 2014.

Rodgers, B. (2004). A Marathon Effort to Slim Down America, *The Boston Globe*, April 19, p. A13.

Rosenbrock, R. and Wright, M. (eds) (2000). *Partnership and Pragmatism: Germany's Response to AIDS Prevention and Care*, Routledge Press, London.

Rosin, H. (1994). Solid Citizens on the March, *Pittsburgh-Post Gazette*, September 11, p. D1.

Rovner, S. (1985). Obesity is a 'Killer Disease' Affecting 34 Million Americans, *The Washington Post*, February 14.

Rubinowitz, S. (1999). Chub club expanding; obesity in the U.S. is on the rise, *New York Post*, October 27, Page 9.

Ruger, J. (2005). Democracy and Health. *Quarterly Journal of Medicine*, **98**, 229–304.

Runge, C. (2007). Economic Consequences of the Obese, *Diabetes*, **56**, 2668–72.

Ruskin, G. (2004). Secret Document Shows Bush Administration Effort to Stop Global Anti-Obesity Initiative, *Commercial Alert*, January 15, p. 1.

Russell, C. (1994). The Young and the Rested: CDC Study Shows Teens Get Little Exercise, *The Washington Post*, November 8, p. A1.

Scarton, D. (1993). Kids' Health Going Down the Tube, *Pittsburgh Post-Gazette*, March 31, p. C5.

Schnurr, C. (1992). Officials: Even a little exercise will help a lot of sedentary lifestyles lead to many health problems, experts warn, *The Atlanta Journal-Constitution*, July 16.

Sen, A. (1999). *Development as Freedom*, Knopf Press, New York.

Shalikashvili, J. and Shelton, H. (2010). The Latest National Security Threat: Obesity, *The Washington Post*, April 30. Available on-line: http://www.washingtonpost.com/wp-dyn/content/article/2010/04/29/AR2010042903669.html. Accessed March 23, 2014.

Shut, N. (2011). Bill Clinton's Life as a Vegan, *NPR News*, August 20. Available on-line: http://www.npr.org/blogs/health/2011/08/20/139782972/bill-clintons-life-as-a-vegan. Accessed March 23, 2014.

Silicon Valley Moms Blog (2010). Secretary of Agriculture Vilsack Speaks with Mom Bloggers, February 22. Available on-line: http://technorati.com/women/article/svmoms-2010-02-secretary-of-agriculture-tom-vilsack-speaks-with-mom-bloggers/. Accessed March 23, 2014.

Simon, M. (2004). Bush Supersizes Effort to Weaken the World Health Organization, *International Journal of Health Services*, 35, 405–407.

Solovay, S. and Rothblum, E. (2009). No Fear of Fat, *The Chronicle of Higher Education*, November 8. Available on-line: http://chronicle.com/article/No-Fear-of-Fat/49041/. Accessed March 23, 2014.

Somerson, M. (1995). Obesity in Children, Teens Doubles; Weight Gains Since '85 Raise Heat Disease Risk, *Columbus Dispatch*, October 3, p. 1B.

Squires, S. (1998). Obesity-Linked Diabetes Rising in Children; Experts Attending Agriculture Department Forum Call for New Strategies to Reverse Trend, *The Washington Post*, November 3, p. Z07.

Starr, P. (2010). First Lady Links Childhood Obesity to National Security in Launch of 'Let's Move' Campaign, *CNSNEWS*, February 9. Available on-line: http://www.cnsnews.com/news/article/first-lady-links-childhood-obesity-national-security-launch-let-s-move-campaign. Accessed March 23, 2014.

Stein, R. (2004). U.S. Says it Will Contest WHO Plan to Fight Obesity; But Claim of Faulty Science is Rejected by Nutritionists, *The Washington Post*, January 16, p. 1.

Stein, R. (2005). Internal Dissention Grows as CDC Faces Big Threats to Public Health, *The Washington Post*, March 6, p. A09.

Strumpf, E. (2004). The Obesity Epidemic in the United States: Causes and Extent, Risks and Solutions, *The Commonwealth Fund/John F. Kennedy School of Government*, Issue Brief, November 2004.

Sujo, A. (2005). Fed Diet Advice 'Fit' to be Tried; Eat your way to a Healthy, Long Life, *The New York Post*, January 15, p. 20.

Suplee, C. (1997). American Adults, Children Significantly Fatter since 1980, *Washington Post*, March 7, p. A16.

Sweet, L. (2002). Bush hits Hard on Fitness, *Chicago Sun Times*, August 28, p. 33.

Tanner, R. (2006). Governors say Follow their Lead get Healthy, Cut Health Care Costs, *The Associated Press*, February 25.

The Boston Globe (2004). Mixed Messages on Obesity, March 15, p. A14.

The Guardian (2004). US Accused of Sabotaging Obesity Strategy, *Buzzle. com*, January 15. Available on-line: http://www.theguardian.com/society/2004/jan/16/usnews.food. Accessed March 23, 2014.

The Hill (1999). Surgeon General David Satcher; much has been done to improve health quality, but there's still much to do, October 6, p. 19.

The Nation's Health (2002). White House takes on U.S. obesity epidemic: Initiative unveiled, American Public Health Association, pp. 1 and 32.

The New York Times (2002). A Better War to Fight, October 3, p. 26.

The San Francisco Chronicle (2004). Overstating the obesity epidemic, November 29.

The Washington Post (1995). Ten Health Resolutions: New Year's Advice from Secretary Shalala, January 3, p. 27.

The Washington Post (2002). The President's Council on Fitness: Once More, with Vigor, p. F03.

Thompson, G. (1998). With Obesity in Children Rising, More Get Adult Type of Diabetes, *The New York Times*, December 14, p. 1.

Thompson, T. (2012). Personal interview. December 21.

Tillotson, J. (2004). America's Obesity: Conflicting Public Policies, Industrial Economic Development, and Unintended Human Consequences, *Annual Review of Nutrition*, **24**, 617–643.

Trust for America's Health Reports (2006). TFAH Response to President's FY07. Budget. Available on-line: http://healthyamericans.org/reports/budget06/. Accessed March 23, 2014.

Tumiel, C. (2003). Speakers endorse preventive health; economic link cited at forum in state capital, *San Antonio Express-News*, January 24, p. 3B.

US Department of Health and Human Services (2002). *HHS, USDA Take Next Steps in Obesity Fight, Secretaries Thompson and Venemamn Meet with Leaders from Food Industry,* News Release, October 15. Available on-line: http://archive.hhs.gov/news/press/2002pres/20021015c.html. Accessed March 23, 2014.

US Department of Health and Human Services (2008). Childhood Overweight and Obesity and Underage Drinking: Common Interests, Common Challenges, Presidential lecture given by RADM Steen K. Galson, Acting Surgeon General, Stony Brook, NY, May 1. Available on-line: http://www.surgeongeneral.gov/news/speeches/sp20080501a. html. Accessed March 23, 2014.

Vallgarda, S. (2007). Problematizations and Path Dependency: HIV/AIDS Policies in Denmark and Sweden, *Medical History*, **51**, 99–112.

Vastag, B. (2004). Obesity is Now on Everyone's Plate, *The Journal of the American Medical Association*, **291**, 1186–1188.

Vulliamy, E. (2002). Bush Declares War on Fat America, *The Observer*, June 23, page 1.

Waxman, H. (2004). Politics of International Health in the Bush Administration, *Development*, **47**, 24–28.

White, F. (2010). Personal interview. June 25.

White House (2010a). *Let's Move: America's Move to Raise a Healthier Generation of Kids*. Available on-line: http://www.letsmove.gov/. Accessed March 23, 2014.

White House (2010b). *White House Task Force on Childhood Obesity*. Available on-line: http://www.whitehouse.gov/the-press-office/child-hood-obesity-task-force-unveils-action-plan-solving-problem-childhood-obesity-. Accessed March 23, 2014.

Woods, T. (2010). Let's Move; Michelle Obama on a Mission to Help Childhood Obesity, *EmaxHealth*. Available on-line: http://www.emax-health.com/1357/109/36038/lets-move-michelle-obama-mission-help-childhood-obesity.html. Accessed March 23, 2014.

World Health Organization (2003a). FAO/SPC/WHO Pacific Island Food Safety and Quality Consultation, Regional Office for the Western Pacific, Manila, Philippines.

World Health Organization (2003b). *Global Strategy on Dietary, Physical Activity, and Health*, World Health Organization, Geneva.

Chapter 6

Contesting Tuberculosis in Brazil

As a byproduct of the rise of the HIV virus, heightened economic growth, urbanization, and poverty, by the early 1980s tuberculosis (TB) reemerged as a health epidemic in Brazil. Considering political scientists' depictions of Brazil as having very little experience with democratic institutions, electoral accountability, the incorporation of the interests of civil society, policy recommendations into national healthcare committees, and minimal per capita healthcare spending and infrastructure, one would expect Brazil not to have successfully responded to TB (Lieberman, 2009; Patterson, 2005; Parker, 2003). Likewise, the presence of these favorable conditions in the US and other advanced industrialized nations should, at least in theory, lead to a more aggressive centralized bureaucratic and policy response to similarly contested epidemics (Aggleton, 2001; Altman, 1986; Baldwin, 2007; Nathanson, 1996; Price-Smith, 2002; Price-Smith *et al.*, 2004; Rosenbrock and Wright, 2000; Ruger, 2005; Sen, 1999; Vallgarda, 2007); however, as we saw with the US's lackluster responses to AIDS and obesity, this never occurred. In further contrast to what these scholars would expect, Brazil's response to TB was quite aggressive, leading, as this chapter explains, to a centralized — albeit delayed — bureaucratic and policy response, although at a level that was not as innovative as we saw with the government's response to AIDS.

Similarly to what we saw with AIDS in Chapter 4, Brazil's government was initially delayed in its response to TB. This mainly had to do with the fact that TB was initially perceived as an old disease, successfully contained through aggressive public health programs under the Getúlio Vargas administration (1930–1945). At the same time, and similarly to what we saw during the early 20th century in Brazil, the presence of multiple diseases and health system challenges convinced policymakers that the government did not need to treat TB any differently. Moreover, this occurred despite TB officials' insistence in immediately responding to TB by strengthening the National TB Program (NTBP) within the Ministry of Health (MOH), increasing its financial resources and technical staff, while providing assistance to the states. Instead, in 1990 the president and senior MOH bureaucrats decided to *decrease* the NTBP's size and responsibilities by decentralizing all TB administrative and policy responsibilities. Moreover, this occurred even when TB cases and deaths were at an all-time high, triggered by escalating HIV/AIDS cases (through co-infection), and when local health departments were bereft of adequate funding, and administrative and technical experience in implementing TB programs.

Similar to what we saw with AIDS, however, the government eventually became committed to strengthening the NTBP and, in fact, recentralizing its policy responsibilities. However, rebuilding the NTBP was not the product of vehement civic protests and non-governmental organization (NGO) pressures. Instead, this process was triggered by the emergence of international criticisms, pressures, and the president's interests in increasing Brazil's international reputation as a nation capable of eradicating disease.

Indeed, by 1994, in response to heightened international criticisms and pressures, the government created the National Emergency Plan for TB, followed by the NTBP's resurrection through a recentralization of funding and policy responsibilities in 1998. While the NTBP began to engage in several bureaucratic and policy initiatives, such as expanding its staff and programs with the states, the NTBP was soon perceived as poorly organized and ineffective in achieving its objectives. By the mid-2000s, the NTBP had failed to provide adequate and consistent technical support to the states, such as following up treatment with meetings and providing an adequate supply of TB drugs. Meanwhile, the social health movements emerging in response to TB, namely the Fórum Estadual das ONGs na Luta contra a Tuberculose no Rio de Janeiro (State Forum of NGOs fighting against

Tuberculosis) and the Rede para o Controle Social da TB no Estado de São Paulo (Tuberculosis Social Control Network of São Paulo), were too small and lacked adequate funding to effectively collectivize and pressure the government for policy reform.

In contrast to what we saw with the government's response to AIDS in Chapter 4, all of these problems seemed to be attributed to the absence of civic supporters and, consequently, national TB bureaucrats' inability to strategically use them in order to increase bureaucratic legitimacy and influence when seeking ongoing support for policy reform. This chapter therefore illustrates that while presidential sensitivity to international criticisms and reputation building can be an important catalyst for a centralized bureaucratic and policy response, in the absence of civic supporters, national public health programs will not be able to deepen their centralized influence within a context of poorly planned decentralization processes.

The First Few Years of the TB Epidemic

TB did not reemerge in Brazil as suddenly and as mysteriously as the AIDS virus, and it did not trigger immediate fear and uncertainty. The gradual spread of TB throughout the 1970s and 1980s was attributed mainly to urbanization, free market reforms, economic crisis, and unemployment (Adeodato, 1991; Barrozo, 1993; *Jornal do Brasil*, 1993; Marques, 1992). The inefficiencies of decentralization stemming from the military government's decentralized SUS (Sistema Unico de Sáude) program and its repeated inability to adequately monitor and respond to TB also contributed to the latter's spread (Adeodato, 1991, *Jornal do Brasil*; Santos Filho, 2006a).

Others nevertheless attributed TB's resurgence to AIDS (*Jornal do Brasil*, 1989; *Folha de São Paulo*, 1991). Because individual immune systems are weakened by the HIV virus, TB quickly spread among HIV positive individuals. This was most commonly seen within highly congested urban centers, such as in Rio and São Paulo.

In the city of Rio, for example, the number of TB cases essentially ran parallel to the surge in AIDS cases throughout the 1980s and 1990s (Gómez, 2013). This was mainly attributed to the difficulty of diagnosing AIDS patients with TB. The coughing, vomiting of blood, and rapid weight loss commonly seen with TB patients is not present with those individuals simultaneously infected with HIV and TB (Santos Filho, 2006b; Delcalmo, 2006). As a result, those that were TB–HIV positive often did not realize that they had TB and therefore did not seek immediate medical attention.

Similar to AIDS, during this period there was also a relatively high level of social stigma towards those with TB. As in the past, it was a disease that is mainly seen among the poor. In Brazil, having TB also reveals one's low income and low social status, which in Brazil often conjures up issues of racism and discrimination (Gómez, 2013). As Gómez (2013) has written, while AIDS attacked the gays, TB attacked the poor *and* the gays, due to the spread of HIV. However, one key difference between the two epidemics was that AIDS dovetailed with the preexisting movement for gay and human rights throughout the redemocratization period. Further, AIDS garnered a lot of media attention because of its prevalence among influential white elites (Parker, 2003). In contrast, few civil society elites were TB positive during this period, while those that were TB positive could not benefit from preexisting pro-TB/HIV or pro-poor social movements pressuring the government for a policy response.

Prior to the reemergence of TB in the 1980s, neither the president nor Congress was convinced that TB posed a serious national health threat. As in the past, the government's focus was instead on taking care of what it perceived to be more imminent health threats, such as samparo, dengue, and malaria. The president and the MOH believed that there were too many health problems in Brazil and that TB did not warrant special attention. This view became clearer when in 1985, Brazil's President, José Sarney, publicly announced that TB was no longer a health problem, that there was nothing to worry about, and that there were other, more pressing health matters that the government needed to tend to (Fihlo, 2006).

Several conditions contributed to these government perceptions. The first was the well-known history of successfully controlling TB under prior military regimes. During the redemocratization period (1980–1985), government officials recalled the Getúlio Vargas administration's success at eradicating TB. As we saw in Chapter 2, beginning with the Ministerio de Educação e Saúde Publico in 1931 and the creation of the NTBP under Vargas in 1941, the government was fully committed to financing and expanding the NTBP in order to eradicate the epidemic. International philanthropic organizations, such as The Rockefeller Foundation, also contributed to these efforts. This centralized response, when combined with the introduction of medical treatments such as Streptomycin in 1944, Para-aminosalicylic, and Isoniazid in 1952, as well as the resulting decline in prevalence of and death rates attributed to TB helped to form the general perception within government that TB was under control and that it would never reemerge (Fihlo, 2006).

Because the government felt confident that TB was now under control, it did not feel the need to sustain a centralized bureaucratic and policy response. Consequently, the MOH decided to decentralize the management and implementation of TB policy to the municipalities. As was the case with AIDS, by the early 1980s pressures from below, mainly from the governors and mayors, for greater control over health policy and management were too overwhelming to ignore (Gómez, 2013). In 1990, the president and Congress decided to devolve all aspects of TB management, policy, and treatment to the municipalities. The only responsibilities retained at the federal level was the creation of technocratic norms for TB treatment from the MOH and the financing of medications provided through the national TB reference centers, which are located in cities throughout Brazil.

Health policy devolution nevertheless equated to a weakening of the NTBP. While decentralization could have easily been perceived as a more efficient institutional response (mainly through increased local accountability), the problem was that decentralization was poorly planned and implemented; that is, it occurred at a very fast pace, without the government ensuring that municipal heath agencies were adequately prepared to manage and implement policy (Franco, 1991; Gómez, 2008).

What this suggested is that the government was apathetic about making sure that municipal health agencies had the administrative and technical capacity needed to implement policy. Most municipal health departments were simply unprepared, administratively, medically, and financially, to render treatment services, such as DOTS (directly observed treatment, short course) (Franco, 1991; Ruffino-Netto and Figuerido de Souza, 2001). As a result, the quality of TB policy suffered (Antunes and Waldman, 1999; *O Globo*, 1998). This was in large part a direct consequence of the fast-paced timing of decentralization and the state governments' reluctance to work with municipal health agencies (Gómez, 2008).

During this period, problems within the MOH further delayed the government's response. Similar to what we saw with the first few years of the AIDS epidemic, MOH bureaucrats were initially divided over whether or not a new TB epidemic had emerged. Health Minister Carlos Santa'Anna and his bureaucratic officials did not believe that TB had resurfaced as an epidemic (Serra, 2000), thus siding with the president's views that TB did not pose a serious national health threat. This contrasted with the views of TB officials in the MOH. Moreover, prior to 1990 TB officials were entirely opposed to the idea of dismantling the NTBP through decentralization. Instead, they preferred that it remain centralized and strengthened (Delcalmo, 2006).

The Absence of Civic Mobilization

An additional factor facilitating the decentralization process was the absence of a proactive social health movement and NGOs pressuring the national government for a response. However, because there never existed a well-organized civic movement for TB during the 1980s and 1990s (Basilia, 2006a; Gómez, 2013; Raimundo do Nascimento, 2005; Santos Filho and Gomes, 2007), this kind of response never emerged for TB.

But why did this occur? When it came to TB, the civil society elites needed to construct effective social health movements and NGOs were missing. At first these elites viewed TB's resurgence as lingering remnants of an old disease, a problem that had already been controlled through aggressive federal programs and medical treatment (Basilia, 2006b). This perception mirrored the president's initial views. TB was also perceived by civil society elites as something that only the poor received. As a result, the medical profession did not perceive TB as an urgent national health threat (Basilia, 2006b).

Another issue that precluded the rise of a new social movement and NGOs was the fact that TB simply did not have the same "sex appeal" that AIDS did. This perception had several consequences. First, when confronted with the choice to either work on TB or AIDS, few medical scientists had incentives to work on TB. Most of the medical talent and interest was going to AIDS, which was a new, mysterious, unexplored virus that could help make one's career over night. TB, in contrast, was an old virus. It had no such appeal. A cure had already been found. As a result, working on TB offered no career benefits (Basilia, 2006b). Moreover, by the time TB reemerged, chronic, non-communicable diseases, such as cancer, diabetes and heart disease, as well as biomedical research, took most of the laboratories' attention. Because of this the medical and academic community was not very well equipped, nor did they have the experience needed, to establish a strong connection with civil society (Basilia, 2006b).

Initial Centralized Bureaucratic and Policy Outcomes

The government's lack of interest in responding to TB had serious ramifications. While TB officials consistently appealed to Presidents Sarney, Collor, and Franco for additional funding and technical support, they never responded (Gómez, 2013). As mentioned earlier, the government did not perceive TB to be an urgent public health issue. Consequently, a centralized response to TB never emerged.

It is important to keep in mind, however, that while the decentralization of TB administration and policy did not occur until 1990, the government's commitment to a decentralized approach to healthcare gradually increased throughout the early-to-mid 1980s, precisely when the AIDS epidemic emerged (Gómez, 2013). Because of this, the president and Congress did not take the NTBP's requests for additional funding very seriously. All of the funding was going to the states, mainly through SUDS (Sistema Unificado e Descentralizado de Saúde) and later the SUS health decentralization program of 1988 (Gómez, 2013). This made it clear to many that the NTBP was losing the interest and support of the executive branch. Without this support, the NTBP could not expand. In addition, because the momentum in favor of decentralization was so overwhelming, and because the NTBP's influence within government waned, there were few incentives for the MOH to provide financial and technical assistance to the states (Gómez, 2013; Santos Filho, 2006b).

International Criticisms, Pressures, and the Incentives for Reform

By the late 1980s, the international community was becoming increasingly attentive and responsive to the resurgence of TB in Brazil and other nations (*Jornal do Commercio*, 1998). The situation could no longer be ignored. And it was becoming increasingly apparent to the international community that TB's resurgence was highly correlated with the HIV virus (*Jornal do Brasil*, 1995; Neto and Pasternak, 1995; *O Fluminense/RJ*, 1997; Tarantino, 1994).

By 1993, the HIV/AIDS–TB co-infection problem prompted the World Health Organization (WHO) to officially declare TB a new pandemic threat (*Revista Global Cienca*, 1993; *Tribuna da Impresna*, 1998). By 1996, the Global Stop TB Partnership was formed, further increasing international attention and commitment to addressing the issue. The Brazilian government and the media noticed these activities (Freitas, 2000; Gómez, 2013).

Shortly after the WHO's declaration in 1993, international organizations began to critique country responses to TB. However, it is important to keep in mind that even before the WHO declaration, the World Bank was already criticizing Brazil for its biased attention to AIDS at the expense of overlooking TB (*Jornal do Brasil*, 1994; Santos Filho, 2006a; Wodtke, 1989;). For example, at the 10th annual International AIDS Conference held in Japan in 1994, the WHO pointed out that government officials in Brazil and other nations were not recognizing the HIV–TB co-infection problem and that it would kill an estimated 3.5 million people by the year 2000 (*Jornal do Brasil*, 1994; *Gazeta Mercantil*, 1994b; *O Globo*, 1994). In 1998, the WHO followed up these statements with yet another critique of Brazil's lackluster policy response to TB (*O Globo*, 1998; *Tribuna de Impresa*, 1998). Academics from the US and abroad began meeting with Brazilian health officials to discuss why the government was not responding (Biancarelli, *Folha de São Paulo*, 1996). Some MOH officials were becoming increasingly concerned with the NTBP's inability to adequately monitor the spread of TB and respond (*Jornal do Commercio*, 1994).

These criticisms had a profound impact on the government's perceptions and response. Striving to increase the government's international reputation as a nation capable of controlling the spread of TB, President Luis Ignacio "Lula" da Silva and senior MOH officials publically declared TB to be a national crisis in 1994 (Gómez 2007, 2013; Rich and Gómez, 2012). For the first time since the Getúlio Vargas administration, the government officially recognized TB as a national health threat (Gómez, 2007, 2013; Santos Filho, 2006a). MOH officials finally admitted that they had overlooked the TB situation and that they needed to respond (Santos Filho, 2006a; Serra, 2000).

In an effort to further increase the government's international reputation, the government engaged in several activities. For instance, the MOH began hosting several international conferences on TB (Barreira, 2009). And in March 2009, the Brazilian national Stop TB Partnership, co-founded with the MOH and organized by the Lula administration, hosted the International TB Partners Forum in Rio (Stop TB Partnership, 2009). Because the purpose of the Forum is to bring together partners in the fight against TB, which includes health officials, civic organizations, and the private sector, with the goal of sharing success stories, learning from and inspiring one another (Stop TB Partnership, 2009), TB officials were able to reveal their success and policy commitments to the international community. Moreover, in recent years the NTBP has organized several conferences and meetings with officials from the WHO and the Global Fund to Fight AIDS, Tuberculosis and Malaria (henceforth the Global Fund), as well as academics, to discuss the NTBP's policies and to learn new ways for improving the program's policies (Barreira, 2009).

Centralized Bureaucratic and Policy Outcomes

In a move that essentially commemorated the national government's initial response to TB, in 1994 the MOH created the Emergency Plan for TB Control (Junqueira, 1998; Santos Filho, 2006a). The Plan included a monetary transfer of approximately R$100 (Brazilian reais) for each individual case of TB to municipal health agencies (Ruffino-Netto and Figuerido de Souza, 2001). Any additional allocation of money would be based on agreements between the municipalities and the National Foundation of Health, which was part of the MOH. In addition, government scientists, mainly in the federal Instituto Oswaldo Cruz (a branch of the MOH focused on public health research) started to conduct studies on the HIV–TB co-infection problem (*Gazeta Mercantil*, 1994b; *Jornal do Brasil*, 1994).

In a further effort to strengthen the government's centralized response, in 1998 the National Council of Health decided to reestablish the national TB program (NTBP) (Cioccari, 1999). MOH officials — and even the director of the national AIDS program at the time, Pedro Chequer — realized that because the states were having a difficult time financing and implementing TB policy throughout the 1990s, that these policy responsibilities needed to be re-centralized; this, in turn, was perceived as marking the government's renewed commitment to eradicating TB (Leali, 1999; Serra, 2000).

The NTBP's goal was to detect, by 2001, 92% of all cases and to cure at least 85% of them (Leali, 1999). In addition to decreasing TB incidence through DOTS to 50% by 2007 and mortality rates by two-thirds, the NTBP was given the responsibility "for establishing official standards for TB control, procuring and providing drugs, developing laboratory and treatment guidelines, coordinating the surveillance system, furnishing technical support to the states and municipalities, and providing inter-sectoral coordination. It [was also] keen on trying to insure inter-sectoral harmony between the federal, state, and municipal level for TB while advocating increased community participation in policy-making" (Ruffino-Netto and Giguerido de Souza, 2001).

Further initiatives were taken by the Lula administration. In 2003, the government mobilized a congressional and MOH coalition intensifying the government's commitment to TB. The goal was to reach and maintain a detection rate above 70%, to cure at least 85% of all new cases, continue to implement DOTS treatment, and to maintain a decentralized form of healthcare treatment. By 2004, the administration appeared to have met its goals: detections rates were above 70%, cure rates above 73%, and 30 new public health professionals were hired and approximately 9,000 new ones in the process of being trained (Basília and Santos, 2005).

To further its commitment, in November 2004 the Lula administration created the national Stop TB Partnership. Comprised of MOH officials, the business sector, and NGOs, this initiative mimicked the Global Stop TB Partnership, which, as mentioned earlier, was created in 1996. So far the national government version has been very successful at marketing TB as a new public health threat. One of the ways it has done this is by enlisting the support of famous television and movie stars. In fact, at a national TB awareness day in Brasília that year, a famous movie star was named the national "TB Ambassador" (Basília and Santos, 2005). Moreover, this dovetailed with President Lula's commitment to his ongoing war against poverty, ushering in a host of new family-based programs for the poor. These types of initiatives are vital for increasing TB awareness and drawing more attention to the epidemic.

Despite these initiatives, several problems began to emerge. The first had to do with the timing of the government's response, while the second had to do with its quality. When it came to the timing of reform, it became increasingly apparent that the government's response was too late. The NTBP should have been resurrected as soon as TB resurfaced. As noted earlier, during the 1980s the media and several government officials were cognizant of the fact that TB had resurfaced because of HIV and increased urbanization rates (*Folhã do São Paulo*, 1991; *Jornal do Brasil*, 1989; *O Globo*, 1991; Safatle, *Gazeta Mercantil*, 1994a). Nevertheless, and as we saw with the government's response to AIDS, it was not until international criticisms and pressures emerged and the WHO's declaration in 1993 that the national government began to respond.

But the government also began to be criticized for its half-hearted attempt at resurrecting and strengthening the NTBP. By the year 2000, officials from the WHO and the Pan American Health Organization (PAHO) declared that the NTBP was poorly organized and ineffective in meeting its policy objectives (Ruffino-Netto and Giguerido de Souza, 2001). The program was also critiqued for not having a long-term strategy, possessing few technical and financial resources and for its lack of commitment to working with the states (Ruffino-Netto and Giguerido de Souza, 2001).

But the important question to ask is the following: if the government was so interested in once again increasing its international reputation, then why did these lackluster policy initiatives take place? Why was the NTBP incapable of expanding and engaging in concrete initiatives in order to help the states combat TB?

As I explain in more detail shortly, it seems that the answer can be found in the NTBP's lack of access to well-organized social health movements and NGOs — in other words, civic supporters. For, as mentioned earlier, and in sharp contrast to what we saw with AIDS, by the 1990s, even after international criticisms, reputation-building interests, and the president's new commitment to reforms had emerged, not one single social health movement or NGO emerged to work with TB officials in order to increase awareness, combat stigma, seek drugs and medical treatment, and ensure that policies were effectively implemented at the local level (Gómez, 2013; Santos Filho, 2006a).

In this context, national TB officials were in desperate need of funding and support. But where could they turn to for help? As we saw with the national AIDS program during the early 1990s, NTBP turned to the international donor community for assistance.

The Global Fund to Fight AIDS, Tuberculosis and Malaria

In 2001, a potential source of international funding for TB emerged with the creation of the Global Fund. Based in Geneva, Switzerland, the Global Fund was formed as an international consortium of nations donating money to fund prevention and treatment policies for these three diseases. In contrast to the World Bank, the Global Fund provides grants, not loans, yet in exchange for assistance demands that funding applicants include the participation of civil society in the grant application, polic-making, and implementation process. This is done through the creation of country coordinating mechanisms (CCMs), a required formal meeting where civil society actors, government officials, and the private sector convene to create a grant proposal and propose policy initiatives.

Seeking support for their initiatives, in 2003 the NTBP approached the Global Fund for help. In 2005, TB officials, through the CCM, submitted an application. Although the CCM's application was not approved the first time around, due to the fact that the Global Fund was not convinced that the interests of civil society were adequately represented on the CCM (Fihlo, 2006; Winters, 2009), the NTBP reapplied in 2006 and was approved for a grant of $23,021,005. Titled Strengthening of the TB-DOTS Strategy in 10 Metropolitan Areas and in the City of Manaus in Brazil, the grant's overall objective has been to expand DOTS coverage, increase social mobilization (thus working closely with NGOs), information and awareness, reduce stigma, and to establish joint programs with the HIV/AIDS program (The Global Fund to Fight AIDS, Tuberculosis and Malaria, 2005). The Global Fund gave the full amount requested by Brazil (Global Fund to Fight AIDS, Tuberculosis and Malaria, 2005).

However, the MOH, which was responsible for distributing the money to the principle recipients (PRs) of the grants, namely the Foundation for Scientific and Technological Development in Health (Fundação para o Desenvolvimento Científico e Technológico em Saúde — FIOTEC) and the Ataulpho de Paiva Foundation (Fundação Ataulpho de Paiva — FAP), did not receive all of the grant money at once. The grant money was divided into five phases, with the first and second phases providing for the first two years. The remaining three phases were contingent on how well the government and its PRs used the money. Every year after the second phase, a private auditing firm, contracted by the Global Fund, conducts an evaluation and reports back to the Global Fund in Geneva. This is done in order to ensure a high degree of accountability and that the money is used effectively. By 2010, the PRs had received a total of $15,194,557 and were scheduled to receive the remaining portions.

Once again, however, and similar to what we saw with the World Bank's impact on AIDS in Brazil, the availability of international funding helped to develop a stronger civil society response to TB (Gómez and Atun, 2012). While the Global Fund did not instigate a civil society response, it did help to strengthen it (Gómez and Atun, 2012).

The Emergence of a Civic Response

Indeed, prior to the Global Fund's arrival, the first attempt to organize a civil society response to TB emerged in 2003, in the city of Rio de Janeiro. Called the Fórum Estadual das ONGs na Luta contra a Tuberculose no Rio de Janeiro (Forum of State NGOs against Tuberculosis in Rio de Janeiro), the Forum was dedicated to increasing awareness of the TB situation, promoting access to information, while defending the human rights of the TB afflicted (Basilia, 2006a). A similar forum was organized in the city of São Paulo two years later, which was called the Rede para o Controle Social da TB no Estado de São Paulo (Tuberculosis Social Control Network of São Paulo).

In Rio, NGOs focusing on nutrition and wellbeing and human rights, academic researchers, health professionals, TB activists, and victims came together to create these forums. Moreover, activists from well-known AIDS NGOs, such as PellaVida and ABIA, as well as a host of other smaller AIDS and health NGOs joined in to provide advice and support (Santos Filho and Gomes, 2007).

Ever since its inception in 2003, Rio's Forum has been committed to working with the NTBP to obtain more technical and financial support, both for the distribution of treatment and prevention policy. In addition, the Forum has worked diligently to convince the NTBP that providing medications and services for TB patients is a fundamental aspect of their human rights. Forum leaders have made frequent reference to the 1988 constitution, which is grounded in these very principles (Basilia, 2006b).

In São Paulo's Forum, a host of community-based NGOs focusing on nutrition and human rights, TB victims, activists, and researchers have been proactively involved. In addition, pastors from large evangelical churches and the Catholic Church have contributed to the Forum's growth and influence (Basilia, 2006b).

In addition to working closely with the government, the forums in Rio and São Paulo have effectively used the media to increase awareness about the TB situation (Santos Filho and Gomes, 2007). The forums have done so by broadcasting their message over the internet (mainly through email messages), the media, organizing workshops and conferences, and even providing information at train and bus stations (Santos Filho and Gomes, 2007). The Rio and São Paulo Forums have also worked with the Global Fund to publish its information on YouTube, an open-source website where commercials and movies can be displayed.[1] The forums have also sponsored conferences with the municipal and state health secretariats, such as the Encontro Comunitário das ONGs na Luta contra a Tuberculose no Estado do Rio de Janeiro (the National Meeting of NGOs Fighting Against Tuberculosis in the State of Rio de Janeiro), which has met five times since 2003, while collaborating with the NTBP through the national Stop TB Partnership, formed in 2004, and which hosts yearly conferences in Brazil. Because of these activities, the forums have helped increase awareness about TB in the press and have motivated the government and community-based organizations to talk more about the issue (Santos Filho and Gomes, 2007).

The Global Fund's emergence and the prospects of obtaining funding helped to strengthen civic mobilization and support for the forums (Werlang, 2011). Because the forums were aware of the Global Fund's mandate of incorporating civil society into the grant application process, additional NGOs and civic organizations started to join the Rio and São Paulo Forums in order to work with the

---

[1] For a listing of all the movies that the Rio and São Paulo Forums have published on YouTube, both independently and in conjunction with the Global Fund, please visit the following youtube.com website: http://www.youtube.com/results?search_query=Global+Fund+Brazil+TB&search_type=&aq=f.

Global Fund and propose new policy initiatives (Barreira, 2011; Gerhardt, 2006; Gómez and Atun, 2012; Sanchez, 2011; Kritski, 2006). In need of funding due to a decline in the need to mobilize for AIDS prevention and treatment services, given that the national AIDS program had met most of the AIDS NGOs' needs by the late 1990s (Massé, 2009; Rich, 2009), a spate of AIDS NGOs also joined the forums. Since their formation, the forums have burgeoned in size, spanning across Rio, São Paulo, and other cities (Basilia, 2009; Gómez and Atun, 2012; Santos Fihlo, 2006).

However, it is important to emphasize that the Global Fund's mandate that applicants create CCMs also generates incentives for civil society to mobilize (Barreira, 2011; Gómez and Atun, 2012; Sanchez, 2011; Werlang, 2011). Moreover, this has occurred precisely because CCMs guarantee civic representation within the NTBP. Furthermore, the Global Fund requires that the NTBP work closely with civil society, state, and municipal health agencies in order to ensure that the grant money is being used effectively (Barreira, 2009; Barreira, 2011; Delcalmo, 2006; Gómez and Atun, 2012; Gerhardt, 2006; Sanchez, 2011; Werlang, 2011). Prior to the Global Fund's emergence, civil society's representation in the NTBP was non-existent.

With additional resources from the Global Fund and the rise of a social movement through the forums, the NTBP once again tried to expand and provide additional assistance to the states. In addition, scholars note that by the mid-2000s, TB officials were frankly embarrassed with their lackluster response to TB and were eager to start anew and to engage in effective centralized bureaucratic and policy reforms (Gómez, 2013; Santos Filho, 2006a).

One of the first initiatives that the NTBP pursued was targeted at strengthening its relationship with the national AIDS program and thus, in turn, increasing inter-agency collaboration in order to acquire additional funding and technical assistance. In 2005, the NTBP created a special division, the Coordenador Adjunto, Programa Nacional de Controle de Tuberculose (Adjunct Coordinator of the NTBP), to solidify its partnership with the AIDS program (Maherdai, 2006; Santos Fihlo, 2006). Since then, relationships between AIDS and TB officials have strengthened, facilitating their work on a variety of conferences, prevention and treatment programs for HIV–TB co-infection. Facilitating this process is the fact that the current NTBP director, Dr. Draurio Barreira, worked for several years in the national AIDS program (Barreira, 2009). Barreira's extensive networks, experience, and commitment to working with the national AIDS program have strengthened the programs' partnership.

In 2004, the NTBP also decided to scale up its assistance to the municipalities. First, it announced that it would hold regional meetings, twice a year, with all municipal health secretariats. To formally consolidate this process, that year the government created the Stop TB Partnership (which is, as mentioned earlier, the domestic equivalent of the Global Stop TB Partnership). In addition to incorporating the views of civil society, through the Stop TB Partnership the government sought to engage in a persistent dialogue with the mayors while providing more technical and administrative assistance. For those municipalities with the highest infection rates, such as Rio and São Paulo, these regional meetings were very important for obtaining information about what health agencies needed to do to better serve the sick (Galesi, 2006).

There were other benefits to holding these meetings. First, meeting with the mayors continued to reinforce the need for more effective DOTS training and implementation. Through these meetings, bureaucrats and doctors working in the NTBP meet with local TB managers to ensure that they are adhering to the DOTS regimen (Santo Fihlo, 2006). These meetings also provide the technical assistance needed to help TB mangers (especially in the more rural, hard-to-reach areas, such as the Amazon) learn and understand how DOTS treatment works and the various strategies they can take to ensure that patients are adhering to their drug regimen.

In 2004, the NTBP also implemented a host of new guidelines for the states on how to administer DOTS treatment, the type of treatment given, and what municipal health secretariats need to do in order to ensure that the poor have access to medicine. The program also established new goals, such as promising to assist 315 municipalities with

80% of the TB problem by 2007, diagnosing 70% of all pulmonary TB infections with bacillary TB diagnostic tests (sputum tests), while continuing to maintain TB treatment and cure rates above 80%.

Since 2004, the government also promised to finance the distribution of all TB medicine free of charge. In a context where many state and municipal departments are often lacking adequate funding, this support is vital for ensuring that TB policies are properly managed and implemented. The MOH currently finances the manufacturing and distribution of all TB drugs, including drugs for MDR-TB, and works through the Centro de Referencia Profesor Helio Fraga (the Brazil National TB Reference Center, henceforth CRPHF), which is located in Rio, to provide these drugs. Neither the states nor municipalities are allowed to purchase and provide these drugs on their own. The only time they are allowed to do this is when infection rates are spiraling out of control and when the TB program cannot distribute the medications on time. Furthermore, the program makes sure that all drugs are provided through public municipal hospitals falling under SUS guidelines. Everyone, rich or poor, has to go to the same local SUS hospital to receive their medications. There are no exceptions. This not only reflects a strong central government presence, but it also establishes a sense of equality and fairness in drug distribution (Dalcalmo, 2006).

In addition to distributing drugs, the NTBP also provides money for training programs, information, and the procurement of equipment. This assistance has been critical for the larger cities with hundreds of poor neighborhoods. In São Paulo, for example, which next to Rio has the highest incidence of TB cases, municipal officials believe that this federal assistance was vital for helping them respond to TB, especially among the HIV–TB co-infected (Galesi, 2006).

The provision of a Global Fund grant has further increased the NTBP's efforts to work with municipalities (Barreira, 2009, 2011; Gómez and Atun, 2012; Projecto Fundo Global Tuberculose, 2009; Sanchez, 2009; Sanchez, 2011; Werlang, 2011). This is mainly because the Global Fund stipulates that as a condition for ongoing grant assistance, the NTBP needs to work closely with municipal health agencies, NGOs, and philanthropic organizations (Barreira, 2009; Barreira,

2011; Gómez and Atun, 2012; Projecto Fundo Global Tuberculose, 2009; Sanchez, 2009; Sanchez, 2011; Werlang, 2011). As a result, more meetings between the NTBP and municipal health agencies, NGOs, and philanthropic organizations have been scheduled for the duration of the grant, which is five years (Barreira, 2009; Barreira, 2011; Gómez and Atun, 2012; Projecto Fundo Global Tuberculose, 2009; Sanchez, 2009; Sanchez, 2011; Werlang, 2011). Since the NTBP is periodically reviewed by private auditing firms assigned by and working through the CCM, the TB program will have more incentives to continually work with the co-recipients of the grant.

Initially, some municipal TB officials acknowledged an increase in the NTBP's commitment to meeting with them. In Rio, for instance, the Global Fund motivated the NTBP to listen more to the needs of previously stigmatized and ignored TB victims (Durovni, 2006; Gómez and Atun, 2012). The director of Rio's municipal health program on TB, AIDS, and leprosy, Dr. Bettina Durovni, stated in an interview with me that the Global Fund allowed her to better communicate with the NTBP (Durovni, 2006). She claims that the Global Fund also sought her advice on policy issues and that they were committed to working with her for more financial assistance, training, and programs (Durovni, 2006). Other health officials confirmed this trend, noting that the Global Fund grant helped to increase direct lines of communication and assistance between the NTBP and various other states and municipalities (Delcalmo, 2006; Gerhardt, 2006).

Despite these new initiatives, further investigation reveals that the NTBP is still not fully committed to following through its policy commitments and that it needs to improve in the following areas: (1) regularly meeting with state and especially municipal health officials; (2) ensuring that municipal health agencies have adequate financial resources for technical training, staff build up, and general administrative capacity; and (3) the development and distribution of free drugs.

When it comes to regularly meeting with local health officials, pundits of the government as well as government officials themselves noticed that the NTBP did not remain committed to meeting with municipal health secretariats in a consistent manner. Dr. Vera Gelasi, the director of the São Paulo TB program, stated in an interview with me that the regional meetings held in 2004, which were originally held twice a year with state and municipal health secretariats, were not done in a consistent manner (Gelasi, 2006). A follow-up interview with Gelasi confirmed this ongoing problem (Galesi, 2009). Furthermore, Gelasi notes that NTBP assistance is sporadic and unpredictable (Galesi, 2009). So what is the problem?

"It's politics," Gelasi commented to me (Galesi, 2009). She claims that the NTBP only met with her when the agency director and President Lula felt that TB was an important political issue. If Lula felt on any given day that for some reason the TB issue was suddenly important, then the NTBP met with her and continued to schedule meetings; otherwise, for reasons that she could not disclose, it does not. Thus it seems that the NTBP's response had nothing to do with political party allegiance and electoral competition — consider that both the governor and mayor of Rio hailed from the same governing party as Lula. Rather, these meetings were influenced by the president and the NTBP's interests and perception of what was going on, which was fickle and inconsistent.

Activists also noticed a lack of NTBP commitment to meeting regularly with the forums. Carlos Basilia, director of Rio's TB Forum and the national Stop TB Partnership, stated in an interview with me that the NTBP did not try to engage in a consistent dialogue with the forums in Rio and São Paulo (Basilia, 2006b). A subsequent follow-up interview with Basilia in 2009 confirmed that this was still a problem (Basilia, 2009). Furthermore, he also believed that the NTBP was often apathetic to learning more about what the Rio and São Paulo Forums needed and had to say. This made it difficult for the Forum to know when and how they could meet with NTBP officials (Basilia, 2006b, 2009).

When it came to providing financial and technical assistance to the municipalities, some were also of the opinion that the NTBP was not fully committed. Some municipal health officials that I interviewed stated that they were still in need of financial assistance. For example, São Paulo's director of the municipal TB program, Dr. Vera Galesi, claimed that despite all the promises the NTBP made, she still did not receive enough funding to support DOTS treatment (Galesi, 2006). A follow-up interview with Galesi in 2009 confirmed this ongoing problem (Galesi, 2009). Galesi also claimed that the state health secretariat was not providing financial support. Consequently, she had to find alternative means of funding, such as working with the donor community, e.g., the USAID (US Agency for International Development) and PAHO, for smaller projects in remote municipalities where access to medicine and successful DOTS treatment is difficult to achieve (Galesi, 2006).

The same situation occurred in Rio. There, the director of the TB program, Bettina Durovni, also complained that the NTBP was inconsistent in its provision of financial assistance. Some years it was great, some other years it was not, she claimed (Durovni, 2006). Durovni further argued that it all had to do with politics: when the TB epidemic was perceived as important and when there was sufficient international and domestic pressures, she received financial support; but, in the absence of these conditions, she did not (Durovni, 2006).

Furthermore, despite all the effort to provide TB medication free of charge, ironically it was the most troubled cities where TB incidence rates were the highest that still did not receive sufficient medication for DOTS treatment. Again, in Rio, Durovni claimed that the NTBP had not provided sufficient medicine and that the state government was behind in manufacturing and distributing certain types of medications (Durovni, 2006). Because of this, Durovni was forced to obtain medication from other countries, going as far as Bolivia to obtain assistance. As noted earlier, the law permits municipal health departments to purchase foreign medication when TB case rates are increasing at an alarming speed.

An important question to ask, however, is why Durovni had to do this, especially when medications for AIDS treatment have always been produced on time and distributed in an equitable and effective manner? However, perhaps an even better question to ask is why the city with the highest TB prevalence and growth rate had this difficulty in the first place? This seems to suggest that while the government had created a generous program for access to TB medication, it still was not fully committed to ensuring that the most afflicted areas had the medicine that they needed.

Finally, in addition to these sporadic meetings, financing, and, in some instances, lack of medication, even after 18 years of administrative decentralization (which began in 1988), most municipalities still lacked the human resources needed to implement successful TB programs. While the NTBP provided money for personnel training, it was sporadic and insufficient, leaving many municipal hospitals understaffed and poorly paid (Barreira, 2011; Gómez, 2013; Kritski, 2006; Santos Fihlo, 2006). Salaries for TB healthcare workers were low. In Rio, for example, Santos Fihlo (2006) notes that a TB healthcare worker only receives R$1,200 a month (approximately $580), a pay rate which is also common in other states. Low pay provides few incentives to remain in the healthcare industry. In the future, the NTBP will need to focus on increasing the salaries of municipal healthcare workers in order to retain staff and motivate them to work harder.

Some analysts are optimistic that the Global Fund grant will help ameliorate these issues (Gómez and Atun, 2012). However, this raises an important question: why has the NTBP waited on external funding to accomplish these tasks? What was it waiting for? Moreover, if international criticisms and reputation building was important, why did the NTBP not respond as effectively then?

While the argument could certainly be made that it was a lack of sufficient financial resources and that the NTBP had to wait for additional external support, and while this may have certainly helped to explain the delay in the financing and production of medication, it still cannot explain why the NTBP neglected to meet with municipal health officials in a consistent manner; furthermore, it still cannot explain why the NTBP was not fully committed to working closely with civil society, especially when compared to the national AIDS program's ongoing partnership with AIDS NGOs.

Some serious consequences have emerged because of the NTBP's lackluster response. The first has to do with donor support. While Brazil was eventually able to obtain a general grant from the Global Fund in 2005, it was denied round nine funding in December 2009.

Yet again, the NTBP failed to demonstrate a strong commitment to working with civil society. The CCM application barely had enough representatives from the TB forums on it (Basilia, 2009). Additionally, the MOH was not careful about which civic organizations to place on the CCM. Members of several AIDS NGOs working with the TB Forums were included in the CCM and grant proposal. While they worked closely with the TB community, this gave the impression that the MOH was trying to get money for AIDS and not TB. This provided further evidence that the MOH and NTBP was not fully committed to working closely with civil society.

Furthermore, pundits note that Minister of Health José Tamporão, did not do a good job of putting together a strong CCM proposal, lacking in quality indicators and policy objectives (Basilia, 2009; Formenti, 2009). This suggested a lack of commitment on the part of the health minister to ensure that Global Fund support continued. On the other hand, others claim that Brazil's emerging financial prowess, as evident through its recent payoff of debts owed to the World Bank and IMF (International Monetary Fund), as well as its recent contributions to these institutions and even to the Global Fund — for AIDS — puts Brazil in a unique category. As an emerging middle-income nation, it seems that the Global Fund board believed that Brazil had enough money to finance its response to TB and that it no longer needed the Global Fund's support (Faraone, 2010).

And finally, in spite of the Cardoso and Lula administrations' proclaimed commitment to combating TB, reinforced and inspired by their international reputation-building interests, this did not lead to a consistently high rate of congressional spending for the NTBP (Barreira, 2011). While funding has increased in recent years, it is far less than what is provided for the national AIDS program (Barreira, 2011; Gómez, 2013; Rich and Gómez, 2012). Moreover, TB officials have not been able to convince Congress to provide more money (Barreira, 2011). Much more funding is needed in order to acquire drugs, hire more healthcare workers, and provide technical support to the states (Barreira, 2011). Additional funding is also needed to organize international conferences, to meet with international officials, and to increase awareness and prevention campaigns through various media outlets (Barreira, 2011). In a context where Global Fund support has ended, this financial assistance is much needed.

But there also seems to be a general lack of support from within Congress — and across government — for the NTBP. Despite former Presidents Cardoso's and Lula's heightened attention to the issue, and despite current President Dilma Rousseff's support for the program's initiatives, TB is still not a national priority for the MOH. TB's association with the poor and the comparatively weak international attention and resources committed to the disease, especially when compared to AIDS, appears to have decreased the attention paid by Congress to the epidemic.

The Absence of Civic Supporters

However, there is another challenge that helps to explain why the NTBP has not been able to obtain ongoing financial support from Congress. In contrast to what we saw with AIDS, in essence it was the absence of civic supporters that failed to provide the legitimacy and influence that TB officials needed to continuously expand their programs and provide more assistance to the states. As I explained in Chapter 1, the presence of civic supporters requires the emergence of NGOs and/or social health movements resembling similar civic movements from the past while proffering historically proven policy ideas of central government intervention in response to epidemics. Nevertheless, while civil society and TB officials were certainly in agreement over the need for a centralized response, the social health movement was too small and, consequently, did not help to increase TB officials' legitimacy and influence.

Indeed, there are those who claim that the forum movements in Rio and São Paulo are too new, lacking sufficient funding and organizational skills to be effective (Gómez, 2013; Santos Filho, 2006b; Santos Filho and Gomes, 2007). While several NGOs have joined the forums, there is still insufficient funding and capacity to meet on a consistent basis as well as seek out partnerships with national TB officials and propose new policies (Gómez, 2013; Santos Filho, 2006b;

Santos Filho and Gomes, 2007). The Rio and São Paulo TB Forums were too small and did little to get involved in national policymaking decisions, monitor policy implementation, and pressure politicians for program expansion (Nogueira *et al.*, 2011; Rich and Gómez, 2012; Rodrigues *et al.*, 2007; Santos Filho and Gomes, 2007). While the forum movements have been effective at publicizing their work and increasing awareness for TB, this cannot replace the need to work closely with national TB officials and to help them obtain more resources from Congress. However, similar to what we saw with the Liga contra a Tuberculose in the past, the Rio and São Paulo Forums have advocated and supported national TB officials' interest in creating a more centralized approach to TB eradication. Forum members have repeatedly asked for more financial and technical assistance to hold meetings, provide information and, above all, ensure a steady flow of medications (Gómez, 2013). Additionally, they have requested funding for more nurses and healthcare practitioners that can ensure that DOTS therapy is effected correctly (Gómez, 2013). Despite the Rio and São Paulo Forums' interest in a more centralized approach to TB eradication, which comports with NTBP officials, until the Rio and São Paulo Forums grow in size, obtain more funding, and present themselves as well organized, influential social health movements, they will not become the body of civic supporters that national TB officials need to increase their legitimacy and influence.

Yet, there are other reasons why these officials have not viewed and used the forums as effective civic supporters. First, scholars point out that TB officials have viewed their work with civil society mainly as an attempt to obtain more funding from the Global Fund and potentially other donors, rather than genuinely caring and mobilizing on civil society's behalf and/or obtaining funding at the domestic level (Rich and Gómez, 2012; Santos and Gomes, 2007). Because TB officials have received so little support from the MOH and Congress, there have been few incentives to work closely with the Rio and São Paulo Forums. Essentially TB officials have not bothered because, even if they did work closely with the Forum, they doubt that it would do much good. Second, it seems that TB officials have realized that the unorganized, poorly financed forum network is too small and insignificant to make a difference. Even if they did mobilize with them, few in society, and especially within government, know about the TB forum movements (Santos Filho, 2006b; Santos Filho and Gomes, 2007). This realization has created few incentives for TB officials to spend a lot of time and money trying to galvanize a stronger partnership with forum members.

However, another problem has challenged the emergence of a powerful, well-organized forum movement. Moreover, it is a problem that persists for TB but not as much for AIDS: that is, the ongoing challenge of social stigma. As seen in other developing nations (Farmer, 1996), because of TB's close association with the poor and lower classes, and because most of the TB infected are not influential members of society, the stigma surrounding TB has created few incentives for medical and social elites to join the forums (Porto, 2007). People appear to be ashamed to be seen with TB victims. In Rio, for example, nurses and health practitioners have been known to be embarrassed about working with the TB community (Delcalmo, 2006). Citizens have felt the same way. In this context, it is difficult for the forums to increase their memberships and attract members that have a lot of influence and resources. This was, of course, not the case when it came to AIDS, however; by the mid-1990s, influential members of civil society, such as artists, sports stars, and famous activists joined the AIDS cause in order to embolden its mobilization efforts, and hence succeeded in garnering more attention and resources.

Conclusion

Similar to what we saw with AIDS, by the late 1980s TB reemerged as a highly contested epidemic in Brazil. During the first few years of TB's spread, the president and MOH officials believed that TB's resurgence did not pose a serious national health threat, one worthy of an immediate, centralized bureaucratic and policy response. The presence of multiple diseases, the perception that TB had been eradicated, and the absence of international criticisms and pressures convinced the government that engaging in a centralized response was unnecessary. Instead, in 1990, the MOH decided to devolve all financial and policy responsibilities to the states and municipalities, in the process destroying the historically centralized, successful NTBP. What is more, this occurred despite vehement resistance from national TB officials claiming that TB was a serious issue and that the government needed to maintain and strengthen its centralized response.

Like the situation with AIDS, however, eventually the rise of international criticisms and pressures kindled the government's interest in responding to TB. Because of Presidents Cardoso's and Lula's interests in increasing Brazil's international reputation as a modern state capable of eradicating disease, they did not take these international criticisms lightly. In response, in 1994 the Cardoso administration created the Emergency Plan for TB, followed by resurrecting of the NTBP in 1998. Despite its national campaign and the technical and financial support that it provided to the states, pundits as well as the international community soon realized that the NTBP was poorly constructed and ineffective at achieving its goals.

While at first glance the Global Fund's emergence in 2005 would help national TB officials achieve their goals, this funding was instead targeted at specific groups in civil society. Global Fund support helped to finance the implementation of new prevention and awareness campaigns, access to drugs, while saving the NTBP millions of dollars. However, the Global Fund's biggest influence was in its contribution to the preexisting development of a civic response to TB, one that was sorely lacking, especially when compared to civil society's response to AIDS.

While new TB forums emerged in the cities of Rio and São Paulo as early as 2003, the forums were too small in membership size, had insufficient funding, and, consequently, could not mobilize effectively. The ongoing stigma surrounding TB also did not help in garnering voluntary and financial support. While the forums have gradually grown in size and have been helpful in raising awareness, research, and medical support for the TB afflicted, they are still too small and, when compared to the AIDS sector, less influential. As a result, national TB officials never had access to the civic supporters that they needed in order to engage in ongoing centralized bureaucratic and policy reforms.

Thus, in sum, despite the emergence of a heightened national government response to TB, kindled by the emergence of international criticisms, pressures, and the government's reputation-building interests, this response was insufficient for guaranteeing an ongoing and effective centralized response. In the absence of civic supporters, the NTBP could not come close to achieving what the national AIDS program did, especially in terms of continued federal spending, bureaucratic expansion, and the introduction of new fiscal policies and partnerships with NGOs. Until the TB forums increase in size and resources, until other segments of the population overcome the stigma attached to TB, and until the forums are able to establish a strong partnership with national TB officials, the implementation of TB policies will continue to be challenged by the presence of municipal health departments lacking adequate financial and technical support. TB cases will continue to increase, the poor will continue to suffer, and the dangers of decentralization will persist.

References

Adeodato, S. (1991). Rio está se transformando na capital da tuberculose, *Jornal do Brasil*, August 19.

Aggleton, P. (2001). HIV/AIDS in Europe: The Challenge for Health Promotion Research, *Health Education Research*, 16, 403–409.

Altman, D. (1986). *AIDS in the Mind of America*, Doubleday Press, New York.

Baldwin, P. (2007). *Disease and Democracy: The Industrialized World Faces AIDS*, University of California Press, Berkeley.

Barreira, D. (2009). Personal interview. October 20.

Barreira, D. (2011). Personal interview. June 10.

Barrozo, J. (1993). Miséria mantém o perigo da tuberculose no Brasil, *Diario Popular*, November 8.

Basilia, C. (2006a). *Construçando uma Resposta a Controle no Tuberculose*. Unpublished manuscript, Rio de Janeiro.

Basilia, C. (2006b). Personal interview. July 26 and October 17.

Basilia, C. (2009). Personal interview. November 15.

Biancarelli, A. (1996). Tuberculose mata 40 Milhões em 15 anos, *Folha de São Paulo*, August 28, p. 5.

Delcalmo, M. (2006). Personal interview. July 18.

Durovni, B. (2006). Personal interview. July 18.

Faraone, N. (2010). Personal interview. June 4.

Folha de São Paulo (1991). Tuberculose afeta mais os aidéticos e mendigos, November 29.

Folha de São Paulo (1996). Índice alto preocupa medicos Brasilieros, August 28.

Formenti, L. (2009). Fundo rejeita proposta do país aids. *Estado do Brasil*, November 2.

Franco, C. (1991). Tuberculose aumenta no Estado do Rio, *Jornal do Brasil*, November 19.

Freitas, A. (2000). Tuberculose volta a assustar a OMS, *Jornal do Brasil*, April 12, p. 12.

Fundo Global Tuberculose (2009). Metas e ações definidas para 2010, *RedeTB*, on-line website news publication, October 8.

Galesi, V. (2006). Personal interview. July 12.

Galesi, V. (2009). Personal interview. October 13.

Gazeta Mercantil (1994a). O ministério da doença, January 14.

Gazeta Mercantil (1994b). Pesquisadores irão estudar a relação entre a doenca e os cases de tuberculose, August 1.

Gerhardt, G. (2006). Personal interview. July 6.

Gómez, E. (2007). Why Brazil Responded to HIV/AIDS and not Tuberculosis: International Organizations and Domestic Institutions, *Revista: Harvard Review of Latin America*, Spring, p. 1.

Gómez, E. (2008). A Temporal Analytical Approach to Decentralization: Lesson's from Brazil's Health Sector, *Journal of Health Politics, Policy and Law*, **33**, 53–91.

Gómez, E. (2013). An Inter-dependent Analytical Approach to Explaining the Evolution of NGOs, Social Movements, and Biased Government Response to HIV/AIDS and Tuberculosis in Brazil, *Journal of Health Politics, Policy & Law*, **38**, 123–159.

Gómez, E. and Atun, R. (2012). The Effects of Global Fund Financing on Health Governance in Brazil, *Globalization & Health*, **8**, 1–14.

Huang, Y. (2006). The Politics of HIV/AIDS in China, *Asian Perspective*, **30**, 95–125.

Jornal do Brasil (1989). Falta de examen em tuberculosos pode agravar expanção da Aids, June 27.

Jornal do Brasil (1993). Lutra contra tuberculose é destaque, September 7.

Jornal do Brasil (1994). Uma luta de US$ 100 milões, March 30.

Jornal do Brasil (1994). Bolsas para estudar tuberculose, May 5.

Jornal do Brasil (1995). Rio pode 9 mil casos de tuberculose, November 4, p. 20.

Jornal do Commercio (1994). Médico teme o avanco da tuberculose, July 14.

Jornal do Commercio (1998). Tuberculose mata mais que a Aids e a malaria juntas, March 20.

Junqueira, J. (1998). Cresce número de casos de tuberculose no mundo, *O Estado de São Paulo*, March 2.

Kritski, A. (2006). Personal interview. July 17.

Leali, F. (1999). Saúde admite aumento de tuberculose, *Jornal do Brasil*, July 24, p. 5.

Lieberman, E. (2009). *Boundaries of Contagion: How Ethnic Politics have shaped Government Responses to AIDS*, Princeton University Press, Princeton.

Lux Jornal, Diario do Grande ABC, Santo Andre-SP (1994). Cresce tuberculos em aidéticos: secretaria de saúde alerta profissionais da area em forum regional, June 2.

Lux Jornal, Tribuna da Impresa, Rio de Janeiro-RJ (1994). AIDS é a maior responsável pela volta da tuberculose, June 17.

Maherdai, F. (2006). Personal interview. June 16.

Marques, C. (1992). Guilherme Álvaro registra aumento do número de casos de tuberculose, *A Tribuna*, March 24.

Nascimento, D. (2005). *As Pestes do Século XX: Tuberculose e Aids no Brasil, uma História Comparada*, FIOCRUZ, Rio de Janeiro.

Nathanson, C. (1996). Disease Prevention as Social Change: Towards a Theory of Public Health, *Population and Development Review*, **22**, 609–637.

Neto, V. and Pasternak, J. (1995). Tuberculose, da tísica a resistencia, *O Estado de São Paulo*, June 5, p. 2.

Nogueira, J., Trigueiro, D., Duarte de Sá, L., Alves da Silva, C., Carla Santa Oliveira, L., Villa, T., and Scatena, L. (2011). Family Focus on Community Orientation in Tuberculosis Control, *Revista Brasileira de Epidemiologia*, **14**, 207–216.

O Fluminense/RJ (1997). AIDS gera surto de tuberculose, April 4, p. 4.

O Globo (1991). Avanco da Aids aumentará casos de tuberculose no Rio, November 22.

O Globo (1994). Tuberculose ameaca elevar número de mortes port Aids, August 11.

O Globo. (1998). OMS: Brasil não age para erradicar a tuberculose, March 20.

O Globo. (1999). Governo lanca plano de combate á tuberculose, August 4, p. 37.

Parker, R. (2003). Building the Foundations for the Response to HIV/AIDS in Brazil: The Development of HIV/AIDS Policy, 1982–1996, *Divulgação em Saúde para Debate*, **27**, 143–183.

Patterson, A. (ed.) (2005). *The Politics of AIDS in Africa*, Ashgate Publishers, Aldershot.

Porto, A. (2007). Social representations of tuberculosis: Stigma and prejudice, *Revista Saúde Pública*, **41**, 1–7.

Price-Smith, A. (2002). *The Health of Nations: Infectious Disease, Environmental Change, and their Effects on National Security and Development*, MIT Press, Cambridge.

Price-Smith, A., Tauber, S., and Bhat, A. (2004). State Capacity and HIV Incidence Reduction in the Developing World: Preliminary Empirical Evidence, *Seton Hall Journal of Diplomacy*, Summer/Fall, 149–160.

Rodrigues, L., Barreto, M., Kramer, M., and Barata, R. (2007). Brazilian Response to Tuberculosis: Context, Challenges, and Perspectives, *Revista Saúde Pública*, **41**, 1–3.

Rosenbrock, R. and Wright, M. (eds) (2000). *Partnership and Pragmatism: Germany's Response to AIDS Prevention and Care*, Routledge Press, London.

Ruffino-Netto, A. and Figueiredo de Souza, A. (2001). Evolution of the Health Sector and Tuberculosis Control in Brazil, *Pan American Journal of Public Health*, **9**, 306–310.

Ruger, J. (2005). Democracy and Health. *Quarterly Journal of Medicine*, **98**, 229–304.

Sanchez, M. (2009). Personal interview. November 9.

Sanchez, M. (2011). Personal interview. July 2.

Santos Filho, E. (2006a). *Politítica de TB no Brasil: Uma Perspectiva da Sociedade Civil: Tempos de Mudancas para o Controle da Tuberculose no Brasil.* Research Report, Public Health Watch, the George Soros Foundation/Open Society Institute.

Santos Filho, E. (2006b). Personal interview. June 30.

Santos Filho, E. and Santos Gomes, Z. (2007). Strategies for Tuberculosis Control in Brazil: Networking and Civil Society Participation, *Revista Saúde Pública*, **41**, 1–6.

Sen, A. (1999). *Development as Freedom*, Knopf Press, New York.

Serra, J. (2000). Tuberculose: Bicho-papão, *Folha de São Paulo*, April 20, pp. 1–3.

Stop TB Partnership (2009). *Partners Forum 2009*. Available on-line: http://www.stoptb.org/events/meetings/partners_forum/2009.

Tarantino, A. (1994). A volta de tuberculose, *Jornal do Brasil*, December 12.

Tribuna de Impresa (1998). Tuberculose Foge ao Controle e já Mata Mais que a Aids e a Malaria, April 20.

Vallgarda, S. (2007). Problematizations and Path Dependency: HIV/AIDS Policies in Denmark and Sweden, *Medical History*, **51**, 99–112.

Werlang, P. (2011). Personal interview. August 1.

Winters, D. (2009). Personal interview. October 1.

Wodtke, M. (1989). Banco Mundial preve a duplicação do custom da saúde, *Jornal do Brasil*, December 17, p. 36.

Chapter 7

Reforms in the BRICS and What They Can Learn from Brazil

In the preceeding chapters, where my goal in comparing the US to Brazil has been to accentuate the uniqueness of why and how these governments responded to contested epidemics, my arguments about the conditions under which these governments responded may also help to explain the timing and depth of government responses in other emerging nations. As an example, let us consider those nations that are similar to the US and Brazil, such as India, China, Russia, and South Africa — the BRICS nations. Like the US and Brazil, these nations are geographically large federations; each has a high level of healthcare decentralization; sub-national governments are mainly responsible for funding and administering healthcare; administrative inefficiencies, and human resource scarcity, and infrastructural capacity are also ongoing challenges. The US, Brazil, India, China, Russia, and South Africa therefore share common challenges in their response to AIDS, obesity, and TB.

Like the US, however, it seems that these emerging BRICS nations may learn several institutional and policy lessons from Brazil. Towards the end of this chapter, I explain what these lessons are and if these nations have the historical and contemporary prerequisites needed to eventually respond as effectively as Brazil.

Responding to AIDS and Obesity in India and China

By the late 1980s, and similar to the US and Brazil, India and China were delayed in their government response to the AIDS and obesity, and consequently these governments also confronted a host of international criticisms and pressures because of their delayed response. Similar to Brazil, presidents and senior health officials in India and China viewed these international criticisms and pressures as an opportunity to increase their international reputation as modern states capable of eradicating disease (Chan *et al.*, 2010; Lieberman, 2009). India and China's politicians, as well as health policymakers, wanted to show the world that they not only had the medical technology and infrastructural capacity needed to effectively respond, but that they were also committed to human rights in access to medicine while providing a safe and productive environment for foreign investment. Scholars in fact note that these reputation-building incentives motivated these governments to support previously ignored health officials responding to AIDS and obesity; more specifically, these officials were given greater policymaking autonomy and funding to pursue prevention and treatment policies while providing funding and technical assistance to the states (Gómez, 2014).

In contrast to Brazil, however, India and China ultimately failed to engage in *ongoing* centralized bureaucratic and policy reforms. That is, in both nations health officials did not obtain the ongoing political and financial support needed to continuously expand their agencies, to introduce universal prevention and treatment policies, as well as give financial and technical assistance to the states (Chandrasekaran *et al.*, 2006; Gómez, 2014; Huang, 2006; Lo *et al.*, 2005; Lieberman, 2009). This was problematic considering the fact that, like the US and Brazil, several state and municipal health departments lacked the financial and administrative resources needed to effectively respond to AIDS and obesity (Chandrasekaran *et al.*, 2006; Kaufman and Saich, 2006; Lo *et al.*, 2005; Liu and Kaufman, 2006).

Nevertheless, in a context where the national government was now committed to reform, why did these health officials have such difficulty obtaining political and financial support for their centrist policy interests? It seems that this shortcoming was attributed to the absence of civic supporters and consequently, health officials' inability to use them. The absence of these supporters seems to have been the product of a long history of social health movements and civic organizations working in isolation from government officials (Andharia, 2009; Pye, 2006; Yang Da-Huang, 2004).

Indeed, in contrast to what we saw in Brazil, in India during the early 20th century, social movements never had an incentive to engage in public health awareness campaigns and pressure the state for a centralized response to disease. This was due to the fact that the colonizing British government had already constructed a Ministry of Health (MOH) that intervened at the local level to provide prevention and medical treatment for all (Mushtaq, 2009). Because of this, civil society had no need and incentive to collectively pressure the state for these services. In this context, the only social movements that were present focused instead on addressing broader poverty and social welfare needs (Andharia, 2009).

As a consequence of all this, and unlike what was seen in Brazil, there never emerged a well-organized, influential social health movement advocating ideas of a centralized bureaucratic and policy response to health epidemics, even during the 20th century. Consequently, the absence of these movements and their centrist policy ideas did not add legitimacy to NGOs when the AIDS and obesity epidemics emerged (Gómez, 2013).

At the same time, historically public health officials were never committed to engaging in strong partnerships with civil society in response to disease (Mistra, 2013). This also failed to establish a tradition and recognition by future health officials, politicians, and civil society that such a partnership was important and that it could add legitimacy and influence to federal health officials. The upshot to this was that in response to AIDS and obesity, MOH officials never proactively tried to establish strong partnerships with non-governmental organizations (NGOs) and/or social movements (Gómez, 2013; Mistra, 2013; Schaffer and Mitra, 2004; World Bank, 2007).

Thus, in contrast to Brazil, though similar to the US, India's health officials never had access to influential civic supporters. Because of this, it seems that officials seeking to obtain ongoing financial support from Parliament did not have the legitimacy and influence needed to secure funding. In this context, establishing a strong, centralized response to AIDS and obesity was impossible.

In China, on the other hand, the historic absence of a proactive social health movement was more the product of firmly ingrained cultural beliefs. As a product of Confucian moral tradition, civil society's respect for state authority and beliefs in self-sacrifice and communitarianism generated no interest in creating a social movement challenging the state's views and policies (Pye, 1996). Instead, what emerged were civic associations that benefited the community as a whole, such as benevolent associations providing health services, public works, schooling, trade guilds, and Landsmann Halls, that is, places were people from a particular province could come together and meet in order to obtain a sense of collective security (Pye, 1996). Because of these cultural beliefs, there never emerged social health movements proffering alternative centralized policy ideas, while pressuring the government for reform — as seen in Brazil. The emergence of such a movement was also hindered by years of oppressive Communist Party rule beginning in 1949, mainly by way of the Cultural Revolution, which sought to eradicate all civic associations that were present under the previous Kuomintang regime (Keping, 2009).

Further complicating matters was the absence of federal public health officials seeking to create a strong partnership with civil society in response to health epidemics. This kind of partnership never emerged in China, mainly because the state's political and policy endeavors were far removed from civil society's communal efforts (Pye, 2006). The state was respected and revered, thus granting health officials a high level of policy autonomy, a condition that continued over several decades (Huang, 2006). In this context, then, health officials did not have a need and therefore incentive to seek out strong partnerships with civil society.

The end result was that in contrast to Brazil, by the time the AIDS and obesity epidemics emerged in China, there never emerged a robust group of civic supporters as well as health officials seeking them out. Furthermore, those NGOs and civic associations that emerged in response to AIDS and obesity in both nations were poorly organized and funded, generating a lack of social as well as political trust in their endeavors (Kaufman, 2009; Mistra, 2013; Global Fund to Fight AIDS, Tuberculosis and Malaria, 2009). Consequently, federal health officials have not had incentives to seek out and work closely with NGOs (Kaufman, 2009; Kaufman, 2010; Schaffer and Mitra, 2004; World Bank, 2007). The end product has been the inability of AIDS and health officials working on obesity and its related diseases to strategically use civil society to increase their legitimacy and influence when seeking ongoing funding and political support for their centralized bureaucratic and policy endeavors.

Responding to AIDS and TB in Russia and South Africa

My approach to explaining Brazil's success also seems to provide insight into Russia and South Africa's lackluster response to their contested epidemics, namely AIDS and TB. While Russia and South Africa were just as delayed as Brazil in their initial response, after the rise of international criticisms and pressures, Russia and South Africa's presidents did not view these conditions as an opportunity to increase their government's international reputation (Sjostedt, 2008; Sridhar and Gómez, 2011). Instead, and similar to what we saw in the US, Russia and South Africa's policymakers believed that they had nothing to learn from the international community, that they should pursue policies unique to their situation, and, more importantly, should do so at their own pace and for their own reasons, such as national security concerns (Sjostedt, 2008; Sridhar and Gómez, 2011) — as discussed shortly.

Like the US, India, and China, health officials in Russia and South Africa also did not have access to civic supporters. This had long-run implications for health officials' ability to engage in ongoing bureaucratic and policy reforms.

In Russia, historically civic organizations developed in isolation of state interference. Groups arose focused on health, education, business development, and elderly care, and were in fact encouraged by Tsarist governments (Conroy, 2006; Hosking, 2001; Topolev and

Topoleva, 2001), mainly due to the central government's inability to provide assistance in distant locations (Conroy, 2006). Social health and medical movements, such as the *feldshers*, also preferred to work alone, viewing themselves as having the best technical knowledge and awareness of what civil society needed (Hosking, 2001). Consequently, and in contrast to what we saw in Brazil, the *feldshers*, as well as other medical societies forming in major cities, such as the Society for the Preservation of Public Health and the Pharmacy Society, never advocated for the central government's interference in local health issues; they never proffered new policy ideas of a centralized bureaucratic and policy response to epidemics, or even sought partnerships with federal health officials (Hosking, 2001). In fact, Hosking (2001) writes that the *feldshers* viewed any central government involvement as an impediment to their work.

Following the Bolshevik revolution of 1917, most of these civic organizations, as well as civil society's interest in mobilization, disappeared. By the 1930s, the Communist Party sought to replace all civic organizations with those that supported the Party's communist ideas (Evans, 2006). Years later, with the fall of the soviet empire and the arrival of a democratic government under Mikhail Gorbachev (1988–1991), there was renewed hope that this history of civic activism and mobilization would rejuvenate. However, it did not, and the government became increasingly centralized and apathetic towards the needs of civil society during the subsequent Boris Yeltsin and Vladimir Putin administrations (Evans, 2006). With Putin's arrival into office, a growing fear surfaced in society as to whether to approach the state for policy reform. This was mainly due to Putin's centralization of authority, his effort to only validate civic movements supporting his government, as well as criticisms of NGOs working with international organizations and especially Western governments (Topolev and Topoleva, 2001). Under these conditions, few social movements, especially those working on AIDS, TB, and other health issues, flourished. Wallender (2005) writes, moreover, that because of these conditions, AIDS activists feared to mobilize and question the government's policies.

Amidst an ongoing AIDS and TB epidemic, then, the NGO movement was weak, neglecting to propose new policy ideas and to proactively seek partnership with health officials (Wallender, 2005). Under these circumstances the best that NGOs could do was to work in local communities, providing counseling, treatment, and preventative educational services (McCullough, 2006).

Yet, the absence of a robust network of AIDS and TB NGOs also meant that there were no civic supporters that federal health officials could use for bureaucratic expansion and policy reform. There were no NGOs that proffered historically proven — as well as socially and thus politically popular — policy ideas advocating for centralized government intervention in response to health epidemics (Gómez, 2013; Wallender, 2005). What this essentially meant, then, was that any AIDS officials seeking reform could not increase their legitimacy and influence by establishing partnerships with NGOs. This limited AIDS officials' ability to obtain the financial and political support needed to consistently develop more effective federal AIDS programs while providing ongoing assistance to the states.

This possibility, moreover, has been further hampered by the Putin administration's ongoing lack of trust in NGOs, their relationship with international agencies, and bilateral organizations providing funding (Isachenkov, 2013). This resistance stems from Putin's fear that international organizations will impede Russia's sovereign ability to respond to disease, which in turn could connote a sense of state weakness and influence from countervailing foreign interests (Bidder, 2012). With respect to domestic NGOs, by 2009, Putin withdrew funding and support for AIDS NGOs, such as the GLOBUS network of NGOS focusing on AIDS (Cohen, 2010). This has further fueled hostilities and a lack of trust between AIDS activists and the state, which continues to undermine any possibility of close state–NGO relationships in response to AIDS.

The only factor that seems to have motivated the Russian government to escalate its response to AIDS has been its threat to the national security, specifically military readiness. Similar to what we saw with the US's historic response to malnutrition and syphilis, the only time Putin seemed serious about increasing the government's response to prevention and treatment came when military officials warned the government of a burgeoning rise of HIV infection rates, brought on by poorly organized HIV screening and prevention activities (Holacheck, 2006). In 2006, a report was published in the Russian media indicating that approximately 200,000 army enlistees were discharged because of their HIV status (Central Eurasia-OSC Report, 2006). In response, Putin became increasingly concerned and escalated his commitment to AIDS, viewing the epidemic as potentially undermining military fighting capabilities (Gómez, 2013). In contrast, however, TB posed no such threat and did not motivate the president to respond in a similar manner (Gómez, 2013).

Similar to Russia, South Africa's AIDS and TB officials did not have access to civic supporters, thus limiting their ability to engage in a centralized bureaucratic and policy response to these epidemics. This occurred mainly because of the historic relationship between the state and civil society. During the Dutch and British settler period, healthcare systems were segregated along racial lines, fueled by racial hostilities (Davenport and Saunders, 2000). White European settlers of the 19th century created their own Western-style healthcare system, while the black community created their own traditional healthcare system, based mainly on tribal healers and ritual (Kalipenti, 2000; Miti, 2013). Because most of the population relied on these traditional healthcare systems (Adler and Steinberg, 2010), and because of the fear and hostility that the black community had towards the white colonists and subsequent government leaders during the apartheid, the former had no incentive to proactively mobilize, create social health movements, propose centralized policy intervention, and work with governing white public health officials (Hausler, 2013). At the same time, government health officials also had no interest in working with the black community (Hausler, 2013; Miti, 2013).

Therefore by the time the AIDS and TB epidemics emerged, there was no long history of social health movements proffering centralized bureaucratic and policy ideas and working closely with government officials — as we saw in Brazil. State–civil society relationships became even worse under the apartheid policy, which led many NGOs and activists to flee the country. Consequently, with the return to democracy in 1996 under President Nelson Mandela, the health NGO community was very inexperienced, both in their ability to mobilize and partner with the state (Schneider, 2002). What this essentially meant was that those health officials seeking greater funding for AIDS and TB did not have the civic supporters that they could use to expand national administration, prevention, and treatment programs.

Similar to Russia, in a context where the South African government was apathetic towards international pressures and where the state was essentially on its own, domestic political and social conditions were the main catalysts for reform. AIDS's threat to national security quickly became an issue. By 1988, the HIV/AIDS virus was so prevalent that President Mbeki began to address the non-health threats that the epidemic posed, such as economic and political instability (Baleta, 1998). During this period reports began to emerge stating that approximately 150,000 public servants were infected with AIDS, while economists warned that AIDS could be very harmful to economic productivity and growth (Strachan, 1997). Additionally, AIDS began to emerge in the military, thus prompting concerns that South Africa would join Angola and Zimbabwe in seeing a quickly deteriorating military defense system (*Business Day*, 1997). By 1998, all of these factors convinced Mbeki that AIDS posed a series national security threat and that the government needed to heighten its response to AIDS. Mbeki would soon call forth a Nationwide Partnership against AIDS as a catalyst to future policy reforms (SAPA News Agency, 1998).

In contrast, TB did not pose as much of a national security threat. In contrast to AIDS, because of early screening and prevention efforts, there were far fewer reported TB cases in the military (Tuberculosis Strategic Plan for South Africa, Department of Health, South Africa, 2007). Part of this aggressive monitoring response was also due to the well-known fact that the AIDS virus suppressed immune systems and could easily lead to the spread of TB (Tuberculosis Strategic Plan for South Africa, Department of Health, South Africa, 2007). Furthermore, during the 1990s no evidence suggested that TB was negatively affecting economic performance. While the mining industry was certainly affected by the disease (Stuckler *et al.*, 2010), TB's general effects on the economy were not felt. In contrast to AIDS, then, these conditions created few incentives for the government to eventually strengthen its response to TB.

Russia and South Africa's lackluster response to AIDS and TB does not suggest that no reforms efforts ever emerged. Indeed, in recent years, both nations have begun to invest in addressing these and other ongoing health threats. However, while South Africa has now engaged in very aggressive HIV/AIDS and TB prevention and treatment campaigns, Russia's efforts are still troubled by a lack of enduring political commitment and state–civil society partnerships (Gómez and Harris, 2013). This is mainly the product of President Putin's ongoing lack of trust in NGOs with linkages to Western-based NGOs and funding organizations (Isachenkov, 2013). Conversely, in South Africa, in recent years the government has sought to work more closely with AIDS and TB NGOs (Hausler, 2013; Miti, 2013). After years of neglecting civil society, the government seems to have finally realized that working with NGOs is vital for ensuring that the government can effectively respond to these epidemics.

What can the BRICS Learn from Brazil?

When compared to each other, it seems that Brazil has also outpaced India, China, Russia, and South Africa in its response to contested epidemics. Given Brazil's success, what potential lessons can these countries learn from Brazil? Moreover, can these nations ever realistically adopt Brazil's centralized bureaucratic and policy response to epidemics?

The first major lesson that emerges is that India, China, Russia, and South Africa's leaders should positively respond to international criticisms and pressures and to view them as an opportunity to enhance the government's international reputation in health. As HIV/AIDS, TB, and other diseases — especially non-communicable diseases — increase in these nations, international community pressures will continue to rise; India and China seem to have positively responded to these international pressures in order to bolster their international policy reputation for HIV/AIDS, but not for obesity and other diseases. Going forward, however, these nations should strive to strategically use domestic health policy as a *means* to not only prove to the world that they are committed to better healthcare and avoiding the perils of these diseases, but so that they can also provide more effective, credible technical assistance to those developing nations suffering from similar health challenges. Brazil indeed shows that the international image of strong state capacity can emerge through "soft power," that is, leading by example and inducing others to adopt their policies (Nye, 2005). Effectively responding to contested epidemics provides an important opportunity for these other emerging powers to achieve this goal.

Second, the case of Brazil suggests that these nations should find creative ways to overcome the ongoing challenges of healthcare decentralization. In India, China, Russia, and South Africa, the responsibility for administering and financing public health policies has increased over time. And yet, ongoing financial and administrative challenges, corruption, and lack of local political accountability appear to be challenging the implementation of prevention and treatment policies (Gómez, 2011). In this context, these other emerging nations should consider incorporating Brazil's inter-governmental fiscal transfer policies, such as the conditional fiscal transfer program — i.e., Política de Incentivos program, which is based on sub-national compliance with national MOH policy mandates. At the same time, national HIV/AIDS, TB, and obesity programs should consider following Brazil's lead in contracting NGOs to closely monitor local government policy implementation commitments, success rates, and to report any discrepancies back to the central government; the latter approach, in turn, helps to further increase sub-national political accountability to the central government as well as civil society (Rich and Gómez, 2012). Considering the aforementioned challenges with state–civil society relations — especially in Russia, China, and, to a certain extent, India, accomplishing this task may prove to be arduous. Nevertheless, given the vast geographic size of these nations, any similar processes that can help the central government understand what is going on at the local level may help to improve policy-implementation processes.

And finally, these nations should strive to continuously reach out to and partner with NGOs and other social health movements for two key reasons: first, to continuously learn new policy ideas and innovative ways of working with local communities; and second, to strategically use these connections to justify domestic spending in public health. As the NGO community continues to grow in these other emerging powers, the time is ripe for Russia, China, and India to adopt Brazil's proactive stance in achieving these objectives. Health officials in these other nations must come to realize that their power in persuasion and policymaking rests not necessarily in their technical expertise and decision making, but in their networks with civil society actors, who themselves are at times more knowledgeable of health conditions and needs, and who are working closely with the international community.

Conclusion

To conclude, while political leaders in the BRICS nations, as well as the US, started on the same path of failing to immediately respond to contested epidemics, Brazil eventually emerged as the nation that was most successful in building a centralized bureaucratic and policy response. However, the speed and depth of success in Brazil, as well as these other nations' unwillingness to pursue Brazil's path, seems to suggest that Brazil is a rather unique nation, especially from a historical perspective. But what does this mean? Does this suggest that India, China, Russia, and South Africa, as well as the US, will never be able to respond as aggressively as Brazil? Is Brazil's success historically predetermined, especially in light of its unique history of state–civil society partnerships in response to disease, as well as the government's historic interest in making a name for itself in the international sphere? Perhaps this is the case. However, this should by no means discourage the US and other emerging nations to strive for Brazil's policy strategies and to look for, and indeed learn from, other nations that have joined Brazil in exhibiting a successful response to HIV/AIDS and other contested epidemics.

References

Adler, G. and Steinberg, J. (eds) (2000). *From Comrades to Citizens: The South African Civics Movement and the Transition to Democracy*, St. Martin's Press, New York.

Andharia, J. (2009). 'Reconceptualizing Community Organization in India: A Transdisciplinary Perspective', in Butterfield, A. and Korazim-Korosy, Y. (eds), *Interdisciplinary Community Development: International Perspectives*, Haworth Press, Abingdon, pp. 91–120.

Baleta, A. (1998). Mbeki: HIV/AIDs 'Most Serious Crisis Yet' Facing S. Africa, *Johannesburg Saturday Start*, September 12.

Bidder, B. (2012). Putin vs. the NGOs: Kremlin Seeks to Brand Activists 'Foreign Agents.' *Spiegel On-Line International*, July 5, page 1. Available on-line: http://www.spiegel.de/international/world/russian-draft-law-seeks-to-label-ngos-and-activists-foreign-agents-a-842836.html. Accessed March 27, 2014.

Business Day (1997). Soldiers at Greater Risk of Contracting AIDS than Others, November 20.

Central Eurasia — OSC Report (2006). Russia: Epidemiology, Public Health Update for HIV/AIDS for 17–30 October, October 31.

Chan, L., Chen, L., and Xu, J. (2010). China's Engagement with Global Health Diplomacy: Was SARS a Watershed? *PLoS Medicine*, 7, 1–6.

Chandrasekaran, G., Loo, V., Rao, S., Gayle, H., and Alexander, A. (2006). Containing HIV/AIDS in India: The Unfinished Agenda, *The Lancet*, 6, 508–521.

Conroy, M. (2006). 'Civil Society in Late Imperial Russia', in Evans, A., Henry, L., and Sundstrom, L. (eds), *Russian Civil Society: A Critical Assessment*, M.E. Sharpe Publications, London, pp. 11–27.

Davenport, R. and Saunders, C. (eds) (2000). *South Africa: A Modern History*, St. Martin's Press, New York.

Evans, A. (2006). 'Civil Society in the Soviet Union?', in Evans, A., Henry, L., and Sundstrom, L. (eds), *Russian Civil Society: A Critical Assessment*, M.E. Sharpe, London, 28–49.

Global Fund to Fight AIDS, Tuberculosis and Malaria. (2009). *India and the Global Fund*, The Global Fund to Fight AIDS, Tuberculosis and Malaria Press, Geneva.

Gómez, E. (2011). Overcoming Decentralization's Defects: Discovering Alternative Routes to Centralization in a Context of Path Dependent HIV/AIDS Policy Devolution in Brazil, *Global Health Governance*, 5, 1–35.

Gómez, E. and Harris, J. (2013). *State-Civil Society Relations and Brazil, India, China, and South Africa's Response to HIV/AIDS*. Unpublished manuscript, King's College London.

Gómez, E. (2014). Understanding Brazil, China, and India's Response to Obesity and Diabetes: Proposing an Interdisciplinary Approach to Unifying International Relations Theory, Historical Institutionalism, and Policy-making, *Global Health Governance* (in press).

Hausler, H. (2013). Personal interview. January 22.

Holacheck, J. (2006). *Russia's Shrinking Population and the Russian Military's HIV/AIDS Problem*. Occasional Paper, The Atlantic Council, Washington DC.

Hosking, G. (2001). *Russia and the Russians: A History*, Harvard University Press, Cambridge.

Huang, Y. (2006). The Politics of HIV/AIDS in China, *Asian Perspective*, 30, 95–125.

Isachenkov, V. (2013). Putin warns Foreign NGOs against 'Meddline' in Russian Affairs, *Huffington Post*, February 14, p. 1.

Kaufman, J. (2009). 'The Role of AIDS NGOs in China's AIDS Crisis', in Schwartz, J. and Sheih, S. (eds), *State and Society Responses to Social Welfare Needs in China: Serving the People*, Routledge Publication, Florence, pp. 156–174.

Kaufman, J. (2010). Turning Points in China's AIDS Response, *China: An International Journal*, 8, 63–84.

Kaufman, K., and Saich, T. (2006). 'Introduction', in Kaufman, J., Kleinman, A., Saich, T. (eds), *AIDS and Social Policy in China*, Harvard University Asia Center Press, Cambridge, pp. 3–14.

Keping, Y. (2009). *Democracy is a Good Thing: Essays on Politics, Society, and Culture in Contemporary China*, The Brookings Institution Press, Washington DC.

Lieberman, E. (2009). *Boundaries of Contagion: How Ethnic Politics have Shaped Government Responses to AIDS*, Princeton University Press, Princeton.

Lo, Y., Shetty, P., Reddy, D., and Habayeb, S. (2005). *Controlling the HIV/AIDS Epidemic in India*, NCMH Background Papers-Burden of Disease in India, World Health Organization Press, Geneva.

Liu, Y. and Kaufman, J. (2006). 'Controlling HIV/AIDS in China: Health System Challenges', in Kaufman, J., Kleinman, A., and Saich, T. (eds), *AIDS and Social Policy in China*, Harvard University Asia Center, Cambridge, pp. 75–95.

McCullough, M. (2005). *How NGOs Respond when the State does Not: Confronting the Problem of HIV/AIDS in Russia*. Paper prepared at the conference Public Health and Demography in Russia, Davis Center for Russian Affairs, Harvard University, March 2005.

Mistra, R. (2013). Personal interview. March 29.

Miti, A. (2013). Personal interview. January 13.

Mushtaq, M. (2009). Public Health in British India: A Brief Account of the History of Medical Services and Diseases Prevention in Colonial India, *Indian Journal of Community Medicine*, **34**, 6–14.

Nye, J. (2005). *Soft Power: The Means to Success in World Politics*, Public Affairs, Washington DC.

Pye, L. (1996). 'The State and the Individual: An Overview Interpretation', in Hook, B. (ed.), *The Individual and the State in China*, Oxford University Press, New York, pp. 16–42.

Rich, J. and Gómez, E. (2012). Centralizing Decentralized Governance in Brazil, *Publius: The Journal of Federalism*, **42**, pp. 636–661.

SAPA News Agency (1998). Democratic Party wants AIDS to Become a State Priority Concern, October 14, South Africa.

Schaffer, T. and Mitra, P. (2004). *India at the Crossroads: Confronting the HIV/AIDS Challenge*. A Report of the CSIS HIV/AIDS delegation to India, CSIS Publications, Washington DC.

Schneider, H. (2002). On the Fault-line: The Politics of AIDS Policy in Contemporary South Africa, *African Studies*, **61**, 145–167.

Sjostedt, R. (2008). Exploring the Construction of Threats: The Securitization of HIV/AIDS in Russia, *Security Dialogue*, **39**, 7–29.

Sridhar, D. and Gómez, E. (2010). Health Financing in Brazil, Russia, and India: What Role does the International Community Play? *Health Policy & Planning*, **25**, 1–13.

Strachan, K. (1997). Fourfold Rise in AIDS Deaths Expected, *Business Day*, April 30.

Stuckler, D., Basu, S., and McKee, M. (2010). Governance of Mining, HIV and Tuberculosis in Southern Arica, *Global Health Governance*, **4**, 1–13.

Topolev, A. and Topoleva, E. (2001). 'Nongovernmental Organizations: Building Blocks for Russia's Civil Society', in Isham, H. (ed.), *Russia's Fate through Russian Eyes*, Westview Press, Boulder, pp. 193–201.

Tuberculosis Strategic Plan for South Africa, 2007–2011, Department of Health, South Africa (2007). Department of Health, Cape Town.

Wallender, C. (2005). *The Politics of Russian AIDS Policy.* PONARS Policy Memo, No. 389, Center for Strategic and International Studies, Washington DC.

World Bank (2007). *HIV/AIDS in India.* Policy Report, The World Bank press, Washington DC.

Yang Da-hua, D. (2004). Civil Society as an Analytic Lens for Contemporary China, *China: An International Journal*, 2, 1–27.

Chapter 8

Conclusion

Despite decades of increased democratic participation, institutional consolidation, and economic growth in the US and Brazil, both governments initially contested and failed to respond to health epidemics. Regardless of how much citizens mobilized and pressured the government for an immediate response, conservative moral beliefs, stigma, and, at times, political apathy motivated presidents and legislators to resist bureaucratic recommendations for a more aggressive bureaucratic and policy response. In both countries, historically it has only been the health bureaucrats that have constantly ignored their personal moral views, repeatedly criticizing government inaction while desiring an immediate, centralized response. Nevertheless, from the days of polio, malnutrition, syphilis, and TB during the 20th century, to AIDS, obesity, and TB today, bureaucratic criticisms and pleas for reform have been ignored by most politicians. It is only when presidents and legislatures have had a change of heart and interest in reform that bureaucratic recommendations shaped policy.

Despite their initial similarities, in this book I have argued that Brazil eventually outpaced the US in its centralized bureaucratic and policy responses. This highlighted key differences in how political leaders in both nations responded to the international community as well as the type of partnerships that they developed with civil society. Brazil eventually outpaced the US because, in light of international criticisms and pressures, Brazil's presidents sought to increase their international reputation through aggressive centralized reforms. Over time, Brazil's bureaucrats also strategically used civic supporters in order not only to build administration and policy, but also to increase sub-national accountability to the central government. None of these strategies were ever pursued in the US.

Indeed, by the late 1980s, in response to increased international criticisms and pressures from the WHO, medical scientists, and the media, Brazil's presidents saw these pressures as an opportunity to increase their government's international reputation as a modern state capable of eradicating disease. In response to TB and syphilis under President Vargas (1930–1945), fast forwarding to AIDS and TB during the late 1990s under Presidents Cardoso and Lula, respectively, it seems that Brazil's presidents pursued centralized bureaucratic and policy reforms in order to help increase their international reputation in health. When lacking sufficient funding, moreover, the Brazilians worked with the World Bank and the Global Fund to Fight AIDS, Tuberculosis and Malaria in order to hire more bureaucrats, build expertise, and fund innovative prevention programs. Engaging in these international financial partnerships therefore facilitated Brazil's ability to achieve its international reputation building objectives.

In contrast, US presidents never had such interests, nor did they ever seek international financial support to strengthen the HHS's domestic response. Instead, presidents, lawmakers, and senior HHS officials only decided to engage in a centralized response after epidemics were perceived as posing threats to national security, such as military readiness or economic performance, or when political and bureaucratic leaders personally experienced and felt threatened by a disease. As we saw in Chapter 2, while historically malnutrition and syphilis threatened the US military's ability to recruit and prepare for the two world wars, in turn prompting the creation of federal agencies as well as financial and technical assistance to the states, and while President Roosevelt's personal experience with polio motivated him to aid the states in their response to polio through the creation of the National Foundation of Infantile Paralysis in 1938, decades later, it was the lack of threat that AIDS posed to national security and political leaders that failed to engender similar reform efforts. While President George W. Bush, Fist Lady Obama, and their bureaucratic leaders have had personal experiences and interests in responding to obesity, in the absence of its threat to national security, these personal concerns have only motivated them to place obesity on the national agenda, not to create and implement policy.

Another factor accounting for Brazil's success has to do with the government's historic partnership with civil society — or what I have referred to as civic supporters: that is, NGOs and social health movements representing similar movements in the past while harboring centrist policy ideas, i.e., centralized bureaucratic and policy intervention in response to epidemics, with a historically proven track record of success. Brazil's public health bureaucrats realized early on that while the presidents' international reputation-building interests were important catalysts for reform, in order to be successful, they also needed to strategically use civic supporters in order to increase their legitimacy and influence when seeking ongoing support for their initiatives. Both historically and more recently in response to AIDS and obesity, these civic supporters were absent in the US, in turn leading to a comparatively weaker government response.

Therefore, as I pointed out at the beginning of this book, it seems that the presence of long-lasting democratic institutions, representative civil society institutions, and the possession of vast resources, experience, and knowledge are not adequate grounds to predict if governments will immediately respond to contested epidemics. There is no question that the US spends more money on healthcare, and has superior technological and human-resource capabilities when compared to Brazil. Yet, this "wealth in health," if you will, is not everything. Brazil shows that the international community, a government's geopolitical aspirations, and its strategic partnership with civil society can have a profound impact on strengthening a government's response to contested epidemics. This international context has compelled Brazil's leaders to overcome their financial hurdles, find financial resources (often from the international community), and create innovative policies. When combined with a strong civil society that is eager to get involved and that has a long history of working in partnership with the government, the case of Brazil suggests that lesser developed nations can outpace even the wealthiest of nations in their response to epidemics.

Despite these differences between the US and Brazil, it is important to point out that both nations have recently shared similarities in their policy response to other types of contested epidemics. For example, government efforts to regulate the tobacco industry and to discourage smoking have been relatively successful in both countries. Perceiving smoking as a public health threat has often been contested between politicians and bureaucrats, a debate that is typically centered on the question of whether or not smoking causes negative social externalities, such as illnesses associated with the second-hand inhalation of smoke, chronic diseases such as heart disease, high blood pressure, cancer, the diffusion of smoking habits, as well as what role the state should play in preventing a habit that is shaped by an individual's personal preferences and, thus, individual responsibilities.

Nevertheless, after years of being ignored by Congress and federal courts, in 2009 the US Food and Drug Administration (FDA) finally obtained the bipartisan congressional support needed to pass legislation regulating the cigarette industry. Called the Family Smoking Prevention and Tobacco Control Act of 2009, under this law the FDA now has the authority to restrict tobacco sales, marketing, and distribution; require stronger health warning labels on packages; reduce nicotine in tobacco products; and regulate "modified risk" tobacco products, such as electronic cigarettes (Glynn, 2012). Since the passage of this law, the FDA has used its regulatory powers: in June 2013, for instance, FDA officials rejected the sale of several unnamed cigarette products for several undisclosed public health reasons, while nevertheless approving two Newport cigarette products made by the Lorillard Tobacco Company (Tavernise, 2013). These regulatory powers are significant because before the Family Smoking Prevention and Tobacco Control Act of 2009 the FDA could not regulate the production and sale of any cigarrete products (*ibid.*). The FDA has also recently worked with the National Institutes of Health (NIH) to provide $53 million in funding to create Tobacco Centers of Regulatory Science (TCORS), which will facilitate research on tobacco's harmful effects and the types of regulatory policies that can be further effective (Federal Drug Agency, 2013).

Similarly, as the second-largest producer of tobacco and cigarettes in the western hemisphere, Brazil was one of the first nations to introduce a federal tobacco control program (DaCosta and Goldfarb, 2003).

Building on several decades of social activism and federal legislation, such as the 1986 Federal Law 7,4866/86, which founded the National Day Against Tobacco (on August 29) (DaCosta and Goldfarb, 2003), by 1987 Brazil created its first National Tobacco Control Program, as well as an Advisory Board on Tobacco Use Control (DaCosta Goldfarb, 2003). By 1998, the Ministry of Health (MOH) banned smoking in all federal buildings, while in 2001, several other progressive regulation policies were created (DaCosta and Goldfarb, 2003). For example, Brazil became the first country to prohibit the terms "mild" and "light" on cigarette packages, while legally requiring large pictorial health warnings on packages (Bulletin of the World Health Organization, 2009). In 2003, Brazil also played a key leadership role in creating the Framework Convention on Tobacco Control (FCTC). Endorsed by the WHO, the FCTC is a treaty establishing policy measures for WHO member states on what they must do, at least, to prevent and reduce over 5 million deaths annually from tobacco control (Lee and Gómez, 2011).

While the US and Brazil's government continue to face strong resistance from the tobacco industry — which in the US has recently limited the FDA's ability to require the printing of pictorial warning images on cigarette packages (Tavernise, 2013) — both governments are nevertheless fully supportive of the WHO's FCTC policy recommendations while working closely with NGOs, community-based organizations (CBOs), and, in the case of Brazil, select businesses to further prevent the harmful effects of tobacco (Glynn, 2012; DaCosta and Goldfarb, 2003). Both governments are also committed to building up the administrative capacity needed to facilitate the bureaucracy's regulatory capacity and, therefore, its ability to enforce policy at the local level (DaCosta and Goldfarb, 2003; Glynn, 2012). Going forward, more research will need to go into examining the complex international and domestic politics of how and why the US and Brazil responded aggressively to tobacco and smoking, as well as the possibility of policy diffusion and learning between both nations on how to further limit these healthcare challenges. As I will mention shortly, the US government seems to be becoming more interested in learning from Brazil on how to respond more effectively to contested epidemics.

Empirical and Theoretical Lessons

The differences in government response to contested epidemics in the US and Brazil revealed several important empirical lessons. First, national security concerns and worries about a diseases' threat to the economy may not be the only reason why governments pursue a centralized response to epidemics. Instead, perhaps policymakers should also be concerned with the international community's evaluation and judgment of their response. As one of the leaders in global health funding and policy (Bliss, 2012), it makes sense that US presidents and Congress should be concerned with how the world views their response to AIDS, obesity, and other diseases. If the US government were to ignore the international community's views and concerns, this may further deepen the government's reputation for not being a cooperative partner in the eradication of disease (Kickbusch, 2002).

Second, building effective institutions also matters. Brazil learned early on that creating a centralized bureaucratic and policy response to epidemics facilitated the government's ability to respond. As we saw in Chapter 2, shortly after political independence in 1822, Brazil consolidated all public health responsibilities under the Departmento Geral de Saúde Público (DGSP); this tradition of a centralized bureaucratic and policy response to epidemics persisted and emerged once again in response to AIDS and TB. In contrast, since the turn of the 20th century, while falling under the Department of Health, Education and Welfare, later renamed the Department of Health and Human Services (HHS) in 1979, public health agencies in the US have been fragmented and competitive, lacking in policy coordination. Beginning with the CDC's (Centers for Disease Control and Prevention) creation in 1942, its fear of eventually being dismantled instigated an ongoing need to compete with the NIH in order to justify its existence and survive. This dilemma engendered a tradition whereby every time a newly contested epidemic emerged, PHS officials would compete with each other over policy responsibilities, funding, and political attention.

When it came to AIDS, this fragmented and competitive tradition persisted, in turn hampering the US government's initial response. Although this situation did not affect the government's response to obesity, in large part because obesity did not pose as grave a medical mystery and urgency, the peril of bureaucratic fragmentation and competition persists. As we saw under the George W. Bush adminis- tration and its response to AIDS, the proposal to engender a cen- tralized bureaucratic response, such as a US PEPFAR (President's Emergency Plan for AIDS Relief), was vehemently resisted by those PHS bureaucrats fearing a loss of authority and influence. Yet, as the case of Brazil suggests, such a centralized response, even within a context of healthcare decentralization (an issue that I will return to shortly), may perhaps be considered.

When compared to the US, the case of Brazil also suggests that working closely with civil society is important for creating an *ongoing* centralized bureaucratic and policy response to epidemics. That is, bureaucrats need to strengthen their partnership with NGOs and CBOs and *strategically use* these partnerships in order to increase their bureaucratic legitimacy and influence when striving to obtain support for their federal programs. As we saw in Brazil, this kind of partner- ship requires bureaucrats to consistently meet with health victims and their activists; that bureaucrats create venues whereby these interac- tions with civil society can be achieved; that bureaucrats rely on and incorporate the views of civil society when formulating policy; and finally, that these bureaucrats hire NGOs to monitor and hold local governments to account.

Findings from the US's response to AIDS also seems to suggest that presidents and policymakers may consider providing an equal amount of attention to international and domestic AIDS policy needs. Indeed, perhaps future US administrations could consider the crea- tion of a domestic PEPFAR for those communities in ongoing need of AIDS medication and prevention services. In fact, AIDS officials in cities experiencing a consistently high level of HIV and AIDS cases, such as Washington DC, have recently proposed such an endeavor, emphasizing how PEPFAR's extensive experience in overcoming the red tape in providing drug treatment and prevention services through greater inter-agency coordination, centralized decision making, and the distribution of ARV medicine could facilitate local governments' response (Hader, 2010).

While Brazil may have eventually outpaced the US in its response to contested epidemics, this by no means suggests that Brazil's health policies are perfect. While Brazil was very successful in its response to AIDS, it was not as successful in its response to TB. The challenge for Brazil has been an ongoing bias in the government's response to AIDS versus TB and other neglected diseases (Gómez, 2013b). While political and financial support for TB has certainly increased following the rise of international criticism and pressure, congressional allocations for the national TB program still pale in comparison to the national AIDS program. Some of this also has to do with the fact that, when compared to AIDS, international pressures for a response to TB emerged much later — i.e., during the late 1990s. As we saw in Chapter 6, this delayed President Cardoso's international reputation-building incentives and, consequently, his support for a centralized bureaucratic and policy response (Gómez, 2013b). Furthermore, civil society's response to TB when compared to the response to AIDS was very late and rather weak; this led to the absence of effective civic supporters for national TB bureaucrats. In the future, the Brazilian government should consider being equally as responsive to all types of health threats.

Examining the US and Brazil in light of the theoretical literature has also revealed some important lessons. In a context of global integration and international cooperation in health, my analysis suggests that nations concerned about their international reputation will ultimately succeed in continuously strengthening their bureaucratic and policy response to epidemics. The case of Brazil supports those claiming that in response to international criticisms, reputation building through a heightened domestic policy response can lead to a more successful response to not only AIDS (Huang, 2006; Lieberman, 2009; Rich and Gómez, 2012) but other health challenges, such as infant and maternal deaths (McGuire, 2010). Nations often strive to increase their international reputation because they want to show the world that they are modern states possessing the political commitment and financial and infrastructural capacity needed to successfully contain the spread of disease (McGuire, 2010). Brazil is no different.

In addition, the case of Brazil supports those theories claiming that nations concerned about their international reputation are more likely to strategically use the creation of health policy as a *means* to achieving foreign policy objectives (Chan and Xu, 2010; Feldbaum *et al.*, 2010; Feldbaum and Michaud, 2010; Fidler and Drager, 2006; Smith *et al.* 2010). This foreign policy objective not only includes international reputation building but also a nation's "soft power" in global health. According to Nye (2005), "soft power" refers to a nation's ability to use its unique political culture and policies in order to increase the international respect that other nations have for them, in turn motivating other nations to emulate and follow suit; this is different from a nation trying to lead the world in global health financial and technical assistance, which the US and other nations may at times be trying to achieve. Because of Brazil's world-renowned success in curtailing the spread of AIDS, motivating CNN to call Brazil's response the "envy of the global health world (Gupta, 2009)," other nations have sought to emulate Brazil's response while approaching Brazil's MOH for technical assistance (Gómez, 2009). However, it is also important to note that Brazil never sought to take a global leadership role on AIDS. Instead, Brazil's government was focused first and foremost on building a strong national response and waited on other countries to seek Brazil's assistance.

Findings from Brazil's response to AIDS and TB also suggest that the theoretical literature should be combined to better explain government response to epidemics. That is, scholars to date have treated the literature focusing on international pressures (Lieberman, 2009; Oluonzi and Macrae, 1995), international reputation building (Chan and Xu, 2010; Feldbaum *et al.*, 2010; Feldbaum and Michaud, 2010; Fidler and Drager, 2006; Smith *et al.* 2010), and soft power (Nye, 2005) as separate and distinct approaches to explaining government responses to health epidemics. But the case of Brazil suggests that a more compelling approach would be to *combine* these theoretical perspectives. This would entail showing how international criticisms and pressures lead to the creation of progressive domestic policies in order to increase a nation's international reputation and soft power.

Nevertheless, my comparative analysis has also revealed that international criticisms, pressures, and reputation building are insufficient in isolation in engendering an effective, ongoing, and centralized government response. For what is also needed is the bureaucracy's ability to strategically *use* civil society for its policy benefits.

In this book, my conception of state–civil society relationships has been rather different from the traditional view held in political science and public health policy. This is especially the case when we consider the purpose, roles, and influence of interest groups and social movement pressures for health policy reform (Kwon and Reich, 2005; Weyland, 1995). That is, rather than viewing NGOs and social health movements as groups that effectively pressure the state for a reform of health policy (Kwon and Reich, 2005; Weyland, 1995), the civic groups analyzed in this book — e.g., the *sanitarista* movement and AIDS NGOs — were instead viewed as entities that existed in order to *assist* the state in achieving its policy objectives. In other words, civil society is viewed as essentially working for the state; that is, providing civic supporters that serve to increase the bureaucracy's legitimacy, influence, and ability to procure financial resources.

In contrast to what the recent literature has argued (Barnett and Whiteside, 2006; Boone and Batsell, 2001; Parker, 2009; Gauri and Lieberman, 2006; Gómez, 2006; Rau, 2006; Whiteside, 1999; Lieberman, 2009), while civil society may not be successful in immediately pressuring the government for a response to epidemics, the case of Brazil's response to AIDS and TB suggests that civil society's role and influence emerges *after* the government has responded and for reasons other than the needs of society, e.g., international reputation building. Analyzing the role of civil society in this post-reform context provides a new area of research. For example, some researchers have started to consider how NGOs provide health bureaucrats with important cultural and healthcare information, and how bureaucrats seek NGOs out to obtain this information (Garcia and Parker, 2011; Gómez, 2013a; Rich and Gómez, 2012).

It is important to note, however, that nations vary in their bureaucracy's ability to strategically use civil society in this manner. In fact, such a strategy may be historically predetermined. As we saw in

Chapter 2 in Brazil, there is a long history of non-governmental entities and social health movements working in partnership with public health bureaucrats to contain the spread of disease. In Brazil, this history engendered a rich tradition of civil society providing health bureaucrats with the information and networks needed to implement bureaucrats' centralized bureaucratic and policy reforms. Decades later, when the AIDS epidemic emerged, civil society once again mobilized itself, this time taking the form of civic supporters advocating historically proven policy ideas of a centralized bureaucratic and policy response to epidemics. Partnering with these civic supporters helped Brazil's AIDS bureaucrats in their efforts to obtain ongoing financial and political support for their centralized bureaucratic and policy strategies. However, no such history existed in the US, or the other BRICS nations — as we saw in Chapter 7. Therefore, not every nation poses Brazil's unique history of state–civil society partnerships in response to epidemics. Future research will need to explore which nations share this type of history and if civil society has served the state's interests in a similar manner.

But what were these state interests? In this book, I have argued that perhaps the best response to contested epidemics is an ongoing centralized bureaucratic and policy response. As I argued in Chapter 1, this kind of response may be advantageous when decentralization policy is poorly implemented; when sub-national administrations lack the financial and administrative capacity necessary for creating and implementing policy; and when sub-national institutions are corrupt and self-interested. While centralization strategies may not work in all political contexts and can also suffer from principle-agent problems (Pritchett, 2004), when the appropriate historical and bureaucratic context is in place, as we saw in Brazil, centralization can certainly be advantageous.

Brazil's successful response entailed a combination of formal and informal centralization strategies, which entailed the concentration of financial resources at the central government level, redistribution from the center, while partnering with NGOs to increase accountability to the central government. With regards to formal centralization strategies, in response to AIDS and TB, the president and the MOH increased the national AIDS and TB programs' policymaking autonomy and financial resources, while national AIDS and TB bureaucrats also provided financial and technical assistance to the state health officials. Moreover, the MOH also created discretionary fiscal-transfer policies, such as the national AIDS program's Fundo-a-Fundo Incentivos program, which was implemented in order to incentivize municipal health departments into compliance with the national program's policy recommendations. The national AIDS program made Fundo-a-Fundo assistance conditional on municipal adherence to the national program's policy recommendations. Informally, the national AIDS program also hired and used AIDS NGOs in order to monitor municipal government compliance to the national program's recommendations, thus increasing municipal accountability to the center. Through these formal and informal centralization strategies, Brazil's national government was able to maintain its policy influence within a context of poorly planned and implemented decentralization processes.

It is important to note, however, that pursuing these centralization strategies did not mean that Brazil's government abandoned its approach to decentralization. Instead, the case of Brazil shows that centralization can *supplement* preexisting commitments to healthcare decentralization. This occurs when national bureaucrats provide additional funding and technical assistance to those local bureaucrats implementing policy. This vertical assistance for particular diseases, such as AIDS and TB, can also provide the technical training needed to strengthen municipal hospital care and treatment. In addition, amidst these disease-specific strategies, other healthcare and social welfare sectors can be decentralized and still flourish. The case of Brazil therefore suggests that a *hybrid* of centralization and decentralization processes can emerge.

Going Forward: Responding the Brazilian Way?

My argument throughout this book is that US policymakers can learn from the Brazilians, but could this really be the case? If it were, what would the US government's policies look like? Let us imagine for a moment that the tables were turned and that for the first time, US policymakers asked the Brazilians for help in transforming the US government's response to AIDS, obesity, and other contested epidemics. What kind of policies would the Brazilian government recommend?

It is likely that Brazil's first hypothetical policy recommendation would be legislation that places the healthcare needs of civil society above all else — which is, in fact, constitutionally guaranteed in Brazil as a human right. This would entail not only amending the US constitution, but also Congress working with the HHS to guarantee universal access to medicine, treatment, and prevention for AIDS, obesity, and other diseases. Next, it would seem logical that the Brazilians would suggest centralizing *all* policy responsibilities for AIDS (as well as obesity and other diseases) within the HHS — creating, if you will, a domestically focused PEPFAR — which as mentioned earlier has been suggested by US health officials (Hader, 2010), while strengthening this agency's partnership with NGOs and social health movements. Finally, it is likely that the Brazilian government would place an emphasis on prioritizing *domestic* policies over international measures.

However, would these Brazilian policy prescriptions receive vehement resistance from US citizens and from the government? Perhaps not. According to a random poll conducted in 2001 by PIPA (the Program on International Policy Attitudes) entitled Americans on Foreign Aid and World Hunger, US citizens were asked to respond to the following assertion: "Taking care of problems at home is more important than giving aid to foreign entities." In response, 65.1% "strongly agreed" and 19.3% "agreed somewhat." In sum, a total of 84.3% completely agreed with this question, while 13.9% did not (PIPA, 2001). Furthermore, in a poll conducted by the Kaiser Family Foundation in 2012, approximately 65% of those US citizens surveyed stated that because of the ongoing economic recession, increasing US bilateral and multilateral contributions for AIDS may not be the best idea (Kaiser Family Foundation, 2012).

Why has the US government not done this already? This may be because for the longest time, US policymakers and scholars have not been interested in comparing the US to Brazil. Until very recently, Brazil has always been perceived as a developing nation, riddled with economic, infrastructural, and social welfare problems. Instead, the focus has always been on comparing the US healthcare system to other similar types of industrialized nations, especially those in western Europe, such as Germany, England, and France.

I would argue, however, that it is the emerging nations that have the best potential for providing new policy insights for US policymakers. This is because Brazil, as well as India, China, and South Africa, have a keen geopolitical incentive to strategically use the creation of effective public health policies as a means to increase their government's international reputation. Brazil, for example, is constantly striving to find bureaucratic and policy innovations in response to AIDS and other diseases, viewing themselves as world pioneers in health policy innovation. Perhaps it is time that the US began to compare herself to Brazil, and to learn from its innovations rather than other advanced industrialized nations that do not possess Brazil's passion and geopolitical aspiration.

The good news is that some US government leaders are already thinking along these lines. At a meeting held at the Council on Foreign Relations on September 9, 2012, the director of the CDC, Dr. Thomas Freiden, stated that the US has a lot to learn from Brazil, and that the US needs to start working with Brazilian health officials to find solutions to ongoing domestic health problems. Freiden talked at length about Brazil's innovative response to obesity and what the US can learn from them; he commented: "Innovation is going to be really important ... Brazil is now spending $700 million dollars of its own money to help 4,000 communities throughout the country increase physical activity. That's going to teach us what works; it's going to show what works ..." (Freiden, 2012).

That said, perhaps it is time that the US focus less on global health leadership and instead start working with the Brazilians, as well as the international community, in finding creative, effective, and enduring policy solutions to AIDS, obesity, and other contested epidemics, such as tuberculosis, polio, and mental disorders, e.g., depression, anxiety, and Alzheimer's disease. The future for the US government will be to create health policies that place the needs of civil society above all else while incorporating the policy ideas of innovative emerging nations. Going forward, perhaps a new form of US "state strength" can emerge through the government's confession of its policy shortcomings and commitment to learning from others. The first step in achieving this objective will be to continue encouraging comparisons between the US, Brazil, and the other emerging BRICS nations. For, until more of these comparisons are made, US policymakers may not develop the interest, humility, and eagerness needed to learn from these nations and to develop more innovative policy responses to America's ongoing healthcare challenges.

References

Barnett, T. and Whiteside, A. (2006). *AIDS in the Twenty-First Century: Disease and Globalization*, Palgrave MacMillan Press, New York.

Boone, C. and Batsell, J. (2001). Politics and AIDS in Africa: Research Agendas in Political Science and International Relations, *Africa Today*, **48**, 3–33.

Bulletin of the World Health Organization (2009). Brazil and Tobacco Use: A Hard Nut to Crack, **87**, p. 1.

Business Day (1997). Soldiers at Greater Risk of Contracting AIDS than Others, November 20.

Chan, L. and Xu, J. (2010). China's Engagement with Global Health Diplomacy: Was SARS a Watershed? *PLoS Medicine*, **7**, 1–6.

DaCosta, L. and Goldfarb, S. (2003). 'Government Leadership in Tobacco Control: Brazil's Experience', in Beyer, J. and Brigden L (eds), *Tobacco Control Policy: Strategies, Successes, and Setbacks*, The World Bank and the International Development Research Center, Washington DC, pp. 38–67.

Feldbaum, H., Lee, K., and Michaud, J. (2010). Global Health and Foreign Policy, *Epidemiology Review*, **32**, 82–92.

Feldbaum, H. and Michaud, J. (2010). Health Diplomacy and the Enduring Relevance of Foreign Policy Interests, *PLoS Medicine*, **7**, 1–6.

Fidler, D. and Drager, N. (2006). Health and Foreign Policy, *Bulletin of the World Health Organization*, **84**, 687.

Freiden, T. (2012). The Rise of Noncommunicable Diseases in Low- and Middle-Income Countries, Official Transcript, Council on Foreign Relations, September 9. Available on-line: http://www.cfr.org/africa/rise-noncommunicable-diseases-low--middle-income-countries/p28982. Accessed March 27, 2014.

Garcia, J. and Parker, R. (2011). Resource Mobilization for Health Advocacy: Afro-Brazilian Religious Organizations and HIV Prevention and Control, *Social Science & Medicine*, **72**, 1930–1938.

Gauri, V. and Lieberman, E. (2006). Boundary Politics and Government Responses to HIV/AIDS in Brazil and South Africa, *Studies in Comparative International Development*, **41**, 47–73.

Glynn, T. (2012). The FDA and Tobacco Regulation Three Years Later. Blog article, American Cancer Society, Washington DC, October 39. Available online: http://www.cancer.org/cancer/news/expertvoices/post/2012/10/29/the-fda-and-tobacco-regulation-three-years-later.aspx. Accessed March 27, 2014.

Gómez, E. (2006). Learning from the Past: State-building and the Politics of AIDS Policy Reform in Brazil, *Whitehead Journal of Diplomacy and International Relations*, Winter/Spring, 143–164.

Gómez, E. (2009). The Politics of Brazil's Commitment to Combating HIV/AIDS in Africa: Technological Assistance, Capacity Building, and the Emergence of a New Donor Aid Paradigm, *Harvard Health Policy Review*, **10**.

Gómez, E. (2013a.) What Reverses Decentralization? Failed Policy Implementation, Civic Supporters, Policy Ideas, and Central Bureaucrats' Expertise? The Case of Brazil's AIDS Program, *Administration & Society*, **10**, 1–31.

Gómez, E. (2013b). *De-emerging Nations? Brazil, Russia, India, China, and South Africa's Struggle to Eradicate Disease*. Unpublished book manuscript, King's College London.

Gupta, S. (2009). Why the Brazilian response to fighting HIV/AIDS is the envy of the global health world, *CNN*, August 27. Available on-line: http://edition.cnn.com/video/#/video/international/2009/08/27/vital.signs.gupta.brazil.bk.a.cnn?iref=allsearch. Accessed March 27, 2014.

Hader, S. (2010). To Fight HIV in D.C., bring PEPFAR home, *Washington Post*, January 24. Available on-line: http://voices.washingtonpost.com/local-opinions/2010/01/i_saw_pepfar_at_work_in_africa.html. Accessed March 27, 2014.

Huang, Y. (2006). The Politics of HIV/AIDS in China. *Asian Perspective*, **30**, 95–125.

Kaiser Family Foundation (2012). *U.S. Global Health Policy: 2012 Survey of Americans on the U.S. Role in Global Health*, Kaiser Family Foundation Press, Washington DC.

Kickbusch, I. (2002). Influence and Opportunity: Reflections on the U.S. Role in Global Public Health, *Health Affairs*, **21**, 131–141.

Kwon, S. and Reich, M. (2005). The Changing Process and Politics of Health Policy in Korea, *Journal of Health Politics, Policy & Law*, **30**, 1003–1026.

Lee, K. and Gómez, E. (2011). Brazil's Ascendance: The Soft Power Role of Global Health Diplomacy, *European Business Review*, January/February, 61–64.

Lieberman, E. (2009). *Boundaries of Contagion: Government Response to HIV/AIDS*, Princeton University Press, Princeton.

Nye, J. (2005). *Soft Power: The Means to Success in World Politics*, Public Affairs Press, Washington DC.

Oluonzi, S. and Macrae, J. (1995). Whose Policy is it Anyway? International and National Influences on Health Policy Development in Uganda, *Health Policy and Planning*, **10**, 122–132.

Parker, R. (2009). Civil Society, Political Mobilization, and the Impact of HIV Scale-up on Health Systems in Brazil, *JAIDS — Journal of Acquired Immune Deficiency Syndrome*, **52**, 49–51.

PIPA (2001). *Americans on Foreign Aid and World Hunger: A Study of U.S. Public Assistance*, PIPA Press, Washington DC.

Rau, B. (2006). The Politics of Civil Society in Confronting HIV/AIDs, *International Affairs*, **82**, 285–295.

Rich, J. and Gómez, E. (2012). Centralizing Decentralized Governance in Brazil, *Publius: The Journal of Federalism*, **10**, 1–26.

Smith, R., Fidler, D., and Lee, K. (2010). *Global health diplomacy*, Trade, Foreign Policy, Diplomacy and Health, Draft Working Paper Series, London School of Hygiene & Tropical Medicine, London.

Tavernise, S. (2013). In First, F.D.A. Rejects Tobacco Products, *The New York Times*, June 25, p. 1.

Weyland, K. (1995). Social Movements and the State: The Politics of Health Reform in Brazil, *World Development*, **23**, 1699–1712.

Whiteside, A. (1999). *The Threat of HIV/AIDS to Democracy and Governance*, Briefing paper, USAID Press, Washington DC.

Index